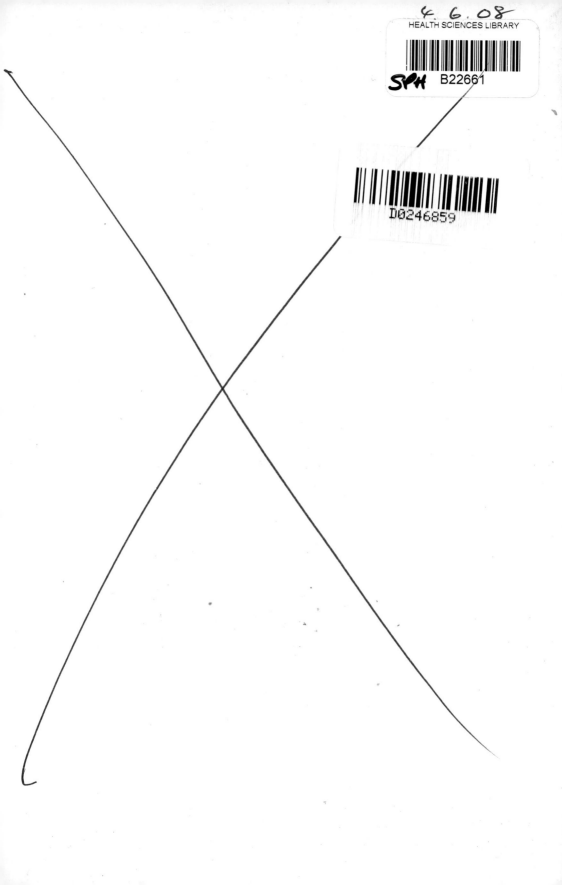

Management
for Psychiatrists

Management for Psychiatrists

Third edition

Edited by Dinesh Bhugra, Stuart Bell
and Alistair Burns

RCPsych Publications

© The Royal College of Psychiatrists 2007
First edition © The Royal College of Psychiatrists 1992
Second edition © The Royal College of Psychiatrists 1995

RCPsych Publications is an imprint of the Royal College of Psychiatrists,
17 Belgrave Square, London SW1X 8PG
http://www.rcpsych.ac.uk

British Library Cataloguing-in-Publication Data.
A catalogue record for this book is available from the British Library.

ISBN 978-1-904671-49-7

Distributed in North America by Balogh International Inc.

The views presented in this book do not necessarily reflect those of the Royal College of
Psychiatrists, and the publishers are not responsible for any error of omission or fact.
The Royal College of Psychiatrists is a registered charity (no. 228636).

Printed in Great Britain by Cromwell Press, Trowbridge.

Contents

Tables

Boxes

Figures

Contributors

Gwen Adshead, Broadmoor Hospital, Crowthorne, Berkshire

Martin Baggaley, Medical Director, South London and Maudsley NHS Foundation Trust, Maudsley Hospital, London

David S. Baldwin, Reader in Psychiatry, Clinical Neuroscience Division, Faculty of Medicine, Health and Life Sciences, University of Southampton

Simon Baugh, Medical Director, Bradford Community Healthcare Trust

Stuart Bell, Chief Executive, South London and Maudsley NHS Foundation Trust, Maudsley Hospital, London

Dinesh Bhugra, Professor of Mental Health and Cultural Diversity, Health Service and Population Research Department, Institute of Psychiatry, London

Alistair Burns, Professor of Old Age Psychiatry, University of Manchester, Manchester

Jerome Carson, Consultant Clinical Psychologist, Lambeth Directorate, South London and Maudsley NHS Foundation Trust, London

Carolyn Chorlton, Practitioner Manager, West Community Mental Health Team, Croydon Integrated Adult Mental Health Services, Croydon

Eleanor Cole, Consultant Psychiatrist and Clinical Director (Southwark), South London and Maudsley NHS Foundation Trust

Frank Holloway, Consultant Psychiatrist and Clinical Director, West Community Mental Health Team, Croydon Integrated Adult Mental Health Services, Croydon

Stephen Hunter, Medical Director and Consultant Psychiatrist, Gwent Healthcare NHS Trust

Adrian James, Associate Medical Director and Consultant Forensic Psychiatrist, Devon Partnership NHS Trust

Kalyani Katz, Consultant Psychiatrist, Central and North West London Mental Health NHS Trust, London

Manoj Kumar, Specialist Registrar, Central and North West London Mental Health NHS Trust, London

Donald Lyons, Director, Mental Welfare Commission for Scotland

Sheila Mann, Consultant Psychiatrist, Clacton and District Hospital, Clacton on Sea, Essex

Frank Margison, Medical Director, Manchester Mental Health and Social Care Trust, Manchester

Charles Marshall, Director, Healthskills Ltd, Ascott-Under-Wychwood

Stephanie Marshall, Director, Programme Development, Leadership Foundation for Higher Education, London

Roy McClelland, Professor of Mental Health, Queen's University Belfast and Consultant Psychiatrist at Belfast City Hospital Trust

Graeme McDonald, Consultant General Adult Psychiatrist, Mater Hospital, Belfast, Regional Adviser for the Royal College of Psychiatrists and Chair of the Northern Ireland Psychiatry Training Committee

Stephen Morris, National Director, Performance Support Team

Ross Overshott, Specialist Registrar in General Adult, Old Age and Liaison Psychiatry, Northwest Deanery

Sally Pidd, Consultant in General Adult Psychiatry, Lancashire Care Trust, and Associate Dean for Workforce, Royal College of Psychiatrists, London

Pramod Prabhakaran, Consultant Psychiatrist, Central and North West London Mental Health NHS Trust

Rosalind Ramsay, Consultant Adult Psychiatrist, South London and Maudsley NHS Foundation Trust

Zoë K. Reed, Executive Director, South London and Maudsley NHS Foundation Trust

Amanda Reynolds, Joint Director of Learning Disability, Norfolk Social Services and Norwich Primary Care Trust, Norwich

Diana Rose Co-director, Service User Research Enterprise (SURE), Institute of Psychiatry, King's College London

David Roy, Medical Director, South London and Maudsley NHS Foundation Trust, Maudsley Hospital, London

Eve Russell, Consultant in Old Age Psychiatry, Manchester Mental Health and Social Care Trust, Wythenshawe Hospital, Manchester

Mark Salter, Consultant in Adult General and Community Psychiatry, City and Hackney Centre for Mental Health, London

Jill Sandford, Director, Healthskills Ltd, Ascott-Under-Wychwood

Kate Silvester, NHS Osprey Programme Coach, Heart of England NHS Foundation Trust

Bryan Stoten, Director and Visiting Professor of Health Policy, Coventry University, and Fellow, Warwick Business School

Graham Thornicroft, Professor of Community Psychiatry, Section of Community Mental Health, Health Service and Population Research Department, Institute of Psychiatry, London

Koravangattu Valsraj, Specialist Registrar, South London and Maudsley NHS Foundation Trust, London

Jonathan Waite, Consultant for the Psychiatry of Old Age, Nottinghamshire Healthcare Trust, Queen's Medical Centre, Nottingham

Paul Walley, Senior Lecturer, Warwick Business School, University of Warwick

Richard Williams, Professor of Mental Health Strategy in the University of Glamorgan and Consultant Child and Adolescent Psychiatrist in the Gwent Healthcare NHS Trust

Preface to the first edition

Dinesh Bhugra and Alistair Burns

Had Rip van Winkle been a psychiatrist and woken up in the late 1980s after having been asleep for say a quarter of a century, he would have been surprised (and perhaps shocked) at the changes which had befallen his profession. The pharmacological, psychosocial and psychological advances have been well documented elsewhere. However, this is the first book to look at the management issues from a psychiatrist's perspective. In the entrepreneurial spirit of management, we have deided (colluded?) to fill this particular niche in the market, in an attempt to teach ourselves about management and, we hope, to provide an arena in which others can learn.

We have tried to achieve two aims. First, to provide a broad theoretical overview of some concepts of management, and second, to facilitate an unashamedly practical approach to the day-to-day process in which the consultant psychiatrist is involved. Whether this can be construed as management is open to debate, but by taking a deliberately broad perspective we hope we have covered most of the areas which senior registrars need to know about.

We have been tremendously fortunate in our choice of authors, Each has provided a document of quality, ranging from general concepts, through practical advice, to exposition based on personal experience. We hope these different approaches have succeeded in offering divergent views of the issues; readers can make up their own minds. Any ragged edges are our own fault.

We are grateful to all our contributors, to Dr Fiona Caldicott for writing the Foreword, to Professor Hugh Freeman, Dave Jago and Ralph Footring of Gaskell for advice, and to Dr Helena Waters, whose own management course inspired this venture. Hopefully the results will not meet the same fate as Rip van Winkle.

Preface to the second edition

Dinesh Bhugra and Alistair Burns

The second edition of this book comes out at a critical time for our speciality. Management expectations of psychiatrists are increasing and we have been gratified at how the first edition of our attempted detumescence of the process has been received. We have expanded the text into three sections – a theoretical overview, changes and conflict and the particularly popular practical issues section.

Preface to the third edition

Dinesh Bhugra, Stuart Bell and Alistair Burns

When the first edition of this book was published in 1992, two of us were still in training. Fifteen years later, it is a delight to bring out this third and completely revised edition. Since the second edition was published, there has been a seismic change in the National Health Service (NHS), with reorganisation, reforms and 'modernisation' of health delivery services as well as training. The shape of the consultant of the future is less clear now. Modernising Medical Careers (MMC) insists that there will be senior medical appointments at the end of training rather than consultnat appointments. The NHS, as a monopoly employer, is beginning to flex its muscles. The role of commissioning by primary care trusts and changes in postgraduate training, along with New Ways of Working, has inevitably meant that there will be a shift in the roles and responsibilities of the psychiatrists of the future.

Clinicians sometimes have had a confrontational relationship with managers and at other times an ambivalent one. Those clinicians who move into management are often accused of going to the other side. Yet the fundamental principles of improvement in quality of care for patients and efficient management of resources unite clinicians and managers. This book is aimed at psychiatric trainees, psychiatrists and other mental health professionals who wish to learn more about management, and at managers who wish to know more about the interrelationships between clinicians and mangers.

The 36 chapters are divided into three sections. History teaches us to learn from our mistakes; hence, we set the scene with the history of the NHS from its early days to the most recent changes. These changes have continued apace, even since this book went into production, so we apologise if the latest changes are not part of the description.

The first section also includes chapters on the politics of the NHS, medical management and the National Service Framework, with specific chapters on different constituencies within the UK and the legal aspects of psychiatry. The second section includes changes and conflicts in understanding systems, leadership, clinical governance, revalidation, confidentiality and clinical audit, along with managing change and psychiatrists' performance. The third section provides an overview of personal development and management; managing time, people and resources, informatics, quality improvement tools, managing stress and avoiding burnout. Working with the media is becoming increasingly important and requires specific skills; we hope psychiatrists will find coverage of this area helpful.

We believe that one of the major skills a consultant (or senior medical appointment) must have is the ability to manage their personal attributes: these include managing time and resources, negotiating with others, chairing and running committees and managing stress. In addition, preparing for job applications and interviews require the ability to put oneself forward in the best possible light. These are skills for lifelong learning and what we have provided here is the beginning of this process.

The authors come from a wide range of disciplines and bring cumulative wisdom to this project, for which we are grateful. They met the deadlines, often short, and put up with editorial flak. Thanks are also due to the Publications Department staff at the Royal College of Psychiatrists for their continued support and hard work. Our particularly grateful thanks go to Andrea Livingstone, who worked incredibly hard to give the book its new structure; one which, we hope, will meet the needs of the new generation of psychiatrists.

Part I
Theoretical overview

CHAPTER 1

History and structure of the National Health Service

Ross Overshott, Alistair Burns and Dinesh Bhugra

It is perhaps important for everyone working in the National Health Service (NHS) to have some idea of the origins, development and current structure of what is one of the biggest and most complicated organisations in the world. A detailed analysis of the NHS and its history is beyond the scope of this chapter; suggestions for further reading are given at the end. The purpose of the chapter is instead to outline briefly how the NHS has evolved and to put into perspective the changes it was undergoing in 2006. For more recent developments the Department of Health's website (http://www.dh.gov.uk) should be consulted.

Healthcare before the NHS

Until the middle of the 19th century, the state had virtually no control over the medical profession. Doctors had developed their own organisational structure which satisfied the need for self-regulation. Members of the Royal College of Physicians mainly worked in the London teaching hospitals and treated those who could afford their fees. Members of the Royal College of Surgeons (which had been the Company of Barbers a century before) were more experienced in the practice of medicine and treated patients both in London (in competition with the physicians) and outside. The vast majority of people were treated by members of the Society of Apothecaries, who basically prescribed medication. For a considerable period of time churches provided forms of treatment to people with mental illnesses.

The state became more involved in the health of the population and regulation of the medical profession throughout the 19th and early 20th centuries. The 1834 Poor Law was an early acknowledgement that government had some responsibility for the care of the population. Among its effects were the statutory provision of a parish medical officer to care for the poor and the establishment of parish workhouses with sick wards where able-bodied inmates could be treated when they became ill (Levitt, 1976). Free services were offered by boards of guardians to those who could pass a means test.

The Public Health Act 1848 established statutory powers that enabled a local medical officer of health (an official of the local authority) to cater for the health of the local population. Following the Poor Law reforms, the medical officers' responsibilities were extended to some Poor Law hospitals, which were considered to be providing healthcare rather than welfare. By the 1930s, their responsibilities included control of environmental hazards, infectious diseases, the school medical service and district nursing/midwifery services.

Local acts (e.g. in London and Liverpool) had proved the benefit of providing care for people suffering from infectious diseases and for those with mental illness or intellectual disability. The establishment of the General Medical Council under the Medical Act 1858 granted the profession self-regulation by establishing a basic qualification for doctors and instituting a register of qualified medical practitioners.

In the first half of the 20th century there were some important changes in the mode of delivery of healthcare and in the organisation of the medical profession (Stacey, 1988). The medical profession had gained prestige and status but lacked tools; these came about with the development of microbiology, which led to the establishment of a scientific basis for medicine.

The National Insurance Act 1911 was passed to ensure that workers were afforded some protection in the event of sickness. It involved compulsory contributions from the employee, employer and the state. The 1911 Act concerned mainly general practitioners (GPs) and the working classes; the middle and upper classes could afford their own care and the Act, which covered the cost of GP care and medication, did not include the cost of hospital care, nor did it cover workers' families. A lack of space does not allow us to look at the effects of gender and class on the establishment and delivery of public healthcare (see Navarro, 1978; Stacey, 1988).

Before 1911, only a small proportion (5 million) of working-class people could afford GP care; where it was available, it was generally through membership of friendly societies or other agencies, which set up 'sick clubs' as a form of low-cost health insurance. These offered their members and sometimes their dependants treatment through the engagement of GPs, via a committee. Around this period GPs were perhaps the least contented of the medical professions and were also the most vociferous (Stacey, 1988). They were unable to choose their patients under this system, and to be controlled by a committee of working men was 'not a pleasant matter for an educated gentleman to serve under' (*British Medical Journal*, 1875, p. 484). The 1911 Act immediately covered 15 million people and by the mid-1940s covered about 24 million (half the population).

However, the scheme established by the 1911 Act was inefficient. Local insurance committees (the forerunners of family practitioner committees) and approved societies (private insurance companies, friendly societies and trade unions, all of which tended to be confined to a particular occupation or location) formed the administrative agencies. The approved societies brought the system into disrepute. As they were not allowed to be profit making, money was purposefully wasted, for example by increasing the number of staff. They paid sickness benefit and were able to pay for specialist care only if there was a surplus at the end of a defined period, which was rare, especially in those occupations where morbidity was high and which caused the greatest drain on resources of an individual society. Those earning over the income limit were excluded. Needless to say, this limit had to be changed regularly, always against the wishes of the doctors, because of inflation.

Whereas before the 19th century treatment for most conditions was almost always offered at home, by the 20th century treatment was gradually being shifted to hospitals, in the public domain. A major consequence of the increasing influence of hospitals was a greater differentiation between general practitioners and hospital consultants under the 1911 Act (Honigsbaum, 1979). Increasing specialisation among consultants and the development of a hierarchy were two major factors that were to affect the running of the NHS subsequently. Non-clinical advances (e.g. in social services) contributed to the development of special skills and interest in specialties such as psychiatry (Stevens, 1966).

By the time the NHS was formed, in 1948, there were about 2800 hospitals in England and Wales (just over 1000 were voluntary hospitals and the rest were municipal hospitals). The voluntary hospitals ranged from the London teaching hospitals, staffed by consultant specialists, to non-teaching hospitals with little money, staffed by local doctors who combined general with hospital practice. About one-third of the voluntary hospitals were larger institutions, where the beds were controlled by consultant specialists, who were unpaid and who therefore relied on private practice to generate income. An appointment to such a hospital was regarded as a stimulus to the recruitment of such patients. This part of the hospital system was affected by the rise of specialism in the 19th century, as only very large centres were able to support all specialties.

Voluntary hospitals were run from money gleaned from endowments, donations, public appeals and some schemes whereby care from the hospital was guaranteed by means of a regular weekly payment. The municipal hospitals provided about 80% of the total number of beds. They consisted of a number of Poor Law hospitals (the former workhouse infirmaries, handed over to the local authorities when the Poor Law was reformed, and run by the local medical officers of health) and local infectious disease hospitals. Mental asylums (also under local control) accounted for half the total number of beds. Although some of the Poor Law infirmaries were of a standard equivalent to that of the voluntary hospitals, they were mainly concerned with the care of the elderly and chronically sick.

The hospital component of the health service was therefore unsatisfactory. Many of the hospitals were old and ill equipped; scant provision was made for the ordinary worker and there was relatively little available between private medicine and the Poor Law. There was inequality in the distribution of services and a financial crisis developed in the London teaching hospitals towards the end of the 1930s.

The Emergency Medical Service (EMS) was an important development in the hospital system. It was established in 1939 by the Ministry of Health to coordinate the response to the expected number of war casualties and to arrange supporting services. The EMS took over financial control of the hospitals (but not ownership), divided England and Wales into 12 regions, and categorised each hospital by its particular function. Many of the voluntary hospitals became second-line hospitals (outside the main centres of population) and specialists worked in them on a salaried basis.

It is interesting to note that by the time the NHS was formed, many hospital specialists had been paid on a sessional basis for a decade. Thus, the payment system was never a political issue in the same way that it was for GPs, who maintained their freedom of practice despite the introduction of the first scheme of National Health Insurance in 1911. It was the threat to this independence which was at the root of the GPs' suspicion of the introduction of the NHS. The EMS proved that the central administration of the hospital system could work and it was the forerunner of the NHS.

The formation of the NHS

According to Jaques (1978), a description of the general features of the NHS which need to be taken into account must take as a starting point the objective of providing the following services:

- clinics, school services, education and other services for the prevention and detection of disease
- physical treatment (medical and surgical intervention for physical and psychological illnesses and impairment)
- psychological treatment (for psychological disturbances and related physical symptoms)
- educational procedures and provision of aids to enable patients to use their abilities as fully as possible.

These features are often ignored by politicians.

The NHS provides an administrative structure by which healthcare can be properly organised and financed. The essence of the NHS is that it provides, free at the point of service, healthcare to anyone who needs it, regardless of their ability to pay. The idea of the NHS originated as far back as 1911. The originator of the Insurance Bill (the then Chancellor of the Exchequer, David Lloyd George) had the idea that the Act would eventually be extended to cover dependants, specialist care and, eventually, hospital care.

With the creation of the Ministry of Health in 1919, an attempt to extend the Act was made, embodied within the Dawson report of 1920 (named after its author, Lord Dawson, a leading physician of the day). The report recommended that preventive and curative medicine be combined, that hospital inefficiency be corrected by elected regional authorities (each of which would have a principal medical officer in administrative charge) and, in an effort to increase standards, that all general hospitals be brought into line with teaching hospitals. No mention was made of the funding of these health services, but the report specifically warned of the dangers of a salaried service, suggesting that this would 'discourage initiative, diminish the sense of responsibility and encourage mediocrity'. However, the necessary political commitment to respond positively to the Dawson proposals was absent, and it took the threat of war and the consequent creation of the EMS in 1939 to resurrect these principles.

Other reports supported the notion of change. In 1929, the British Medical Association (BMA) produced *Proposals for a General Medical Service for the Nation*, which suggested that everyone should have a GP of their choice, through whom specialist services would be available. In addition it emphasised that prevention and promotion of health were as important as the treatment of disease, and that close coordination of medical services should be promoted. The service would basically have been funded by extending the National Health Insurance Scheme.

The independent research institute Political and Economic Planning published a report in 1937 that criticised existing services for being disorganised (Political and Economic Planning Group, 1937). It also reported regional differences in infant mortality in the UK, the tendency of GPs to work where a private practice income was guaranteed rather than where there was real need, and the association between environmental conditions and ill health.

Sir William Beveridge produced his report on *Social Insurance and Allied Services* in 1942. As part of an attack on the 'five giants' impeding social progress (want, disease, ignorance, squalor and idleness), he suggested that the burden of the cost of a health service should be borne by everyone, as such a service would make the nation healthier, thereby saving on social security payments and increasing national efficiency. However, he missed the point that better health, if it leads to longer life, inevitably leads during that longer life to a greater use of services (Godber, 1975).

The wartime coalition government accepted the principle of a national health service and set about finding a formula which would be acceptable to the medical profession, politicians, the voluntary hospitals and local authorities. The Minister of Health, Ernest Brown, proposed that the service would be administered by local authorities (with voluntary hospitals retaining their independence) and that GPs would be paid a salary. The doctors effectively rejected these proposals and they were dropped when Sir Henry Willink succeeded Brown in late 1943.

In February 1944, the government published a White Paper on the NHS. The plan was to make local authorities responsible for health, directly so in the case of the municipal hospitals (as they already were) and via contractual arrangements in the case of the voluntary hospitals. Hospital doctors would be salaried and GPs would have the choice of a salaried service or capitation fees. The BMA held a postal ballot and doctors (especially GPs) came out strongly against the proposals. They were opposed to the idea of local authority control and to a scheme which would be available to all, free at the time of use, as this would restrict the scope for private practice. In contrast, among the general public there was widespread endorsement of the proposals, in particular of the fact that the services would be free at the time of use.

Before a Bill could be drafted on the basis of the White Paper, a Labour government came to power with Aneurin Bevan as the Minister of Health. Bevan took a much harder line, claiming that Willink had merely cobbled together conciliatory proposals to keep everyone happy. He objected to the political erosion of the supremacy of Parliament and made the point that one should consult, but not negotiate with, outside bodies such as the medical profession. He felt that the Minister of Health should have total control of the service. His Bill was put forward in spring 1946 and was opposed by both the Conservative opposition and the BMA. The former argued that the nationalisation of the hospitals and the loss of independence of GPs would discourage initiative, and would deprive the profession and voluntary hospitals of their freedom. However, experience with the EMS had shown that central control of hospitals could be a success. The reasons why the medical profession objected were more complex – restriction of individual freedom was one, but it is possible that they were fuelled by resentment over the Labour government's supposed attack on the middle classes (through social reform for which the middle classes thought they were paying), from which the medical profession generally drew its members. The government criticism of doctors spanned the spectrum, on the one hand, of doctors being guardians of vested interests and, on the other hand, of doctors waging a war on the government on behalf of their class.

Both Bevan and the BMA (an incredibly complex negotiating machine where its leaders had very little room to manoeuvre) stood firm. The deadlock was broken when Bevan introduced an amendment saying that he could not introduce a fully salaried service for GPs without further legislation. Leaders of the BMA (helped by the Royal Colleges) saw the chance to save face and accepted the new service. The BMA ordered a plebiscite of all its members (instead of a further meeting of the representative body, whose opposition might have become entrenched had the dispute been allowed to continue) and it was apparent that, although opposition was still strong, sufficient numbers of doctors would be employed in the new service to make it workable. Thus, on 5 July 1948, the NHS was born.

The principle of universalism which characterised welfare and health legislation in the post-war period is perhaps manifested most dramatically in the NHS (Stacey, 1988): to provide good healthcare to the whole population without a financial barrier was its original aim.

The Health Service in Scotland

The Scottish Health Service was created in May 1947, on the same tripartite principles (of hospital care, and primary and local authority health services) as that in England and Wales. The hospital and specialist services were administered by five regional hospital boards, with 65 boards of management. The community and environmental health services were provided by 55 local health authorities and family practitioner services were administered by 25 executive councils. The Secretary of State for Scotland was responsible for the whole of the NHS in Scotland (Levitt, 1976).

Under the National Health Service (Scotland) Act 1972 health boards were created for each area of Scotland to act as the single authority for administering the three branches of the former tripartite structure. Two new bodies – the Scottish Health Service Planning Council and the Common Services Agency – were created.

Developments to 1974

The NHS developed a tripartite structure as much because of vested interests as from an overall view that this structure was the most efficient. What the founders of the NHS thought they were doing and what in fact emerged are two distinct matters, for there were undoubtedly a number of unintended consequences (Stacey, 1988). Out of the negotiations leading up to the brave new world of 1948, the consultants overall, but especially those in teaching hospitals, did better than the GPs. The nurses did less well and the ancillary workers were not considered at all. The role and function of the multidisciplinary teams need to be addressed in the light of this historical development.

The hospital system was nationalised and taken away from local authorities (mainly as a result of the profession's unwillingness to work under local authority control). The Minister of Health was responsible for hospitals through hospital management committees (336 in number) and non-elected regional hospital boards (of which there were 16). Teaching hospitals retained their independent status (not wishing to 'come down' to the level of all voluntary hospitals) and were responsible through 36 boards of governors to the Minister, independent of the regional hospital boards. The Public Health Laboratory Service and the specialist hospitals were directly responsible to the Minister, although the Blood Transfusion Service remained under regional control.

General practice was unaffected by the changes and retained its independent status. The National Insurance Act 1911 was extended to cover the whole population, and general practice was controlled by 134 executive councils (the successors of the local insurance committees). The rest of the service was left to the 174 local authorities' medical officers of health, essentially because no other influential medical interest wanted them. These residual services comprised the maternity and child welfare services, health visitors, health education and prevention, the ambulance service and vaccination/immunisation services.

It is of particular importance that the readers of this book appreciate the relationship between the NHS and doctors: it has been argued that doctors are the single most important profession within the service. Changes in the shape of the NHS are impossible without a change in the relationship of power within the NHS (Heller, 1978). This is the dictum that various governments have followed to reduce the power of various factions. At the inception of the NHS, GPs retained their independent status and consultants and specialists became salaried employees of the state (although, as has been noted, the EMS had been employers since 1938). Aneurin Bevan stated that he saw the function of the Ministry of Health as providing the profession with all it needed to be used fully and without control to the benefit of patients. Consultants and specialists thus considered themselves on a par with GPs as being able to do as they wished, unworried by considerations of cost and administration. The fact that medical practitioners were on regional boards and not the hospital management committees (in charge of the day-to-day running of the hospitals) strengthened this stance.

The problem of what doctors should be paid was apparent soon after the creation of the NHS. Sir Will Spens chaired three committees dealing with the pay of GPs, consultants and specialists, and dentists. The committee on consultant's pay recommended that the salary for a consultant aged about 40 should be £2500, compared with £1300 for a GP of equivalent age (both 1939 prices). Consultants' pay before the NHS had such a wide range (from a consultant in a non-teaching voluntary hospital to one in a London teaching hospital with income from private practice) that a salary scale incorporating both ends of the spectrum was impractical. The distinction award scheme was introduced as a solution to this problem, with the top grade doubling a consultant's salary. The committee that reviewed the pay of specialists in training recommended that this should be substantially increased, to allow doctors in these grades to devote a larger part of their time to professional training without the need to do alternative work (such as teaching) to supplement their income. Much discontent still existed following the Spens committees and it took a royal commission into doctors' and dentists' pay (the Pilkington Commission) to recommend the establishment of an independent review body to advise the Prime Minister directly.

The problem of the numbers of junior doctors soon emerged. By 1950 there were 3800 registrars and senior registrars, and only double that number of consultant posts. There also existed the grade of senior hospital medical officer (devised at the inception of the NHS to employ those practitioners in hospital practice who were not of consultant calibre), many of whom were still in competition for consultant posts. The Ministry of Health attempted to force hospitals to terminate contracts of time-expired senior registrars (after three years in higher professional training), but following an outcry from the profession it was decided that their contracts could be renewed annually. The suggestion was made that consultant numbers be expanded, but this was rejected by the Ministry on the grounds of cost, and by existing consultants for fear of added competition for private patients. The result was a review by Henry Willink (the ex-Minister of Health in the wartime coalition government) of the numbers of doctors required in the UK. The recommendation was a 10% reduction in intake to the medical schools. However, the review did not take into account the numbers of doctors emigrating and the increased numbers required because of advances in medical technology; this led to a shortage of junior doctors in the 1960s, with the attendant influx of foreign graduates to fill posts in unpopular specialties, of which psychiatry was one.

The need for change

Almost as soon as the NHS was established, there was recognition that reorganisation was necessary. It was noted as early as 1952, by Dr Ffrangcon Roberts in *The Cost of Health* – see Watkin (1978) – that Sir William Beveridge was wrong in assuming that the demand for healthcare was limited. The aphorism of the NHS, 'infinite demand, finite resources', was born. A committee was set up under the chairmanship of the Cambridge economist C. W. Gillebaud with the remit of reviewing the cost of the NHS and to make recommendations for changes in administration which would make the service more efficient. The committee's conclusion was that the service was not wasteful and that a major change in organisation was unnecessary (although Sir John Maude, a former Parliamentary under-secretary in the Ministry of Health, appended a personal recommendation that the three arms of the NHS be unified). The Porritt Committee, set up by the Royal Colleges and the BMA (all the members of which were doctors), also reported (in 1962) that unification of the three arms of the service was highly desirable. Thus, there was general recognition for the need to unify the tripartite structure to ensure comprehensive planning of the service and better coordination of community, GP and hospital components.

Inequalities in the distribution of resources both geographically and within medical specialties highlighted deficiencies in the system; these caused embarrassment to successive Ministers of Health because of scandals concerning ill treatment in mental and geriatric institutions. It is not that the NHS in 1948 was perfect in any sense. Klein (1989) argues it was as much a product of messy compromises as of inspired visions, and the same remains true today.

In 1968, the government published a Green Paper on reorganisation, the basic proposals being integration of all services under 50 area boards (each to have 16 members) with responsibility for all hospital, general medical and community health services. Objections raised included the remoteness of the regional boards to local services, the problem of the continued independence of GPs and the mismatch of the 50 area boards with proposed local government reorganisation that would result in 90 local government units.

Following the merger of the Ministry of Health and National Insurance in 1968, a second Green Paper emerged, this one under Richard Crossman, the new Secretary of State of the combined departments, which recommended the following: 14 regional health councils advising the Secretary of State on planning; 90 area health authorities (the word 'authority' having replaced 'board' without explanation) to coincide with the 90 local government districts and to set up subcommittees to be responsible for services; and 200 district committees with at least half the members working in the district. The functions of the service were to be divided between health and local government, based on the skill of the provider rather than the need of the user (e.g. all social workers were to be employed by local government, all nurses by the health service).

Developments from 1974 to 1989

In 1971, the Conservative government published a further document, the thrust of which was embodied in the NHS (Reorganisation) Act 1973. The reorganisation came into being on 1 April 1974, which coincided with the reorganisation of local government. The reformed service was to have two characteristics: it was to be an integrated service and there was to be responsibility upwards to managerial authority.

The reorganisation led to the formation of regional health authorities, which for the first time had the responsibility to plan all services. The reforms led to a 30% increase in the number of administrators and the influence of managers increased, as well as to the creation of a managerial hierarchy.

The doctors insisted on retaining clinical autonomy, and this was noted:

'The distinguishing characteristic of the NHS is that, to do their work properly, consultants and general practitioners must have clinical autonomy, so that they can be fully responsible for the treatment they prescribe for the patients.' (Department of Health and Social Security, 1972)

This notion of a one-to-one doctor–patient relationship has been challenged by Stacey (1988). The clinical autonomy and security of tenure for the consultant were seen as advantageous (Beeson, 1980).

However, the final document differed from the second Green Paper in that regional health authorities were in line management with the area health authorities, and 90 family practitioner committees (replacing the executive councils) were co-terminous with the local government areas. Community health councils became essentially watchdogs of the Health Service. There were also 'district' management teams under the 1974 organisation. Some regions had 'single district areas', but more commonly each area had several such teams. It was this duplication that the 1982 reforms sought to abolish. Representatives of the professions and public were slightly different, with restriction of local authority appointees and the chairs of the regional health authority being chosen for personal qualities rather than as representatives of any particular interest. There was emphasis on professional management, with regional and area health authorities responsible for policy and teams of officers responsible for implementation. A detailed analysis of the political and practical ramifications of the relationship between central and local government and their representation on the authorities is given by Forsyth (1982).

In Scotland, the reorganisation of local government created new local authorities. The Scottish Health Service then constituted nine regional authorities divided into 56 districts and three island councils, and their boundaries were closely followed by the health board boundaries (Levitt, 1976). The 15 health boards were concerned with major policy matters and the broad allocation of resources; authority to manage the service was delegated to four senior officers of the board.

In 1982, in response to criticism of excessive administration of the NHS and the implementation of the Resource Allocation Working Party (RAWP) to ensure a more equitable distribution of resources between geographical areas and specialties, the area health authorities were abolished and replaced with 190 district health authorities.

Readers are recommended to read the account by Draper et al (1976) on the influence of the 1974 reorganisation on the NHS.

The Conservative government also introduced general management of hospitals following the Griffiths report in 1983. Sir Roy Griffiths, a supermarket executive, had been commissioned to review the management of hospitals. He concluded that the traditional NHS management by senior consultants and administrators had led to 'institutionalised stagnation'. The report's recommendations, including that hospitals should be managed by general managers, were accepted and in the middle of the 1980s they took over the role of managing hospitals. This change in emphasis brought about a large increase in general or senior managers in the NHS, from 1000 in 1986 to 26 000 in 1995, with spending on administration rising dramatically over the same period (Webster, 2002). This also resulted in a number of managers begin 'classified' into their primary professions, for example nursing, also indicating that a number of people from professions were being brought into management. There was also a new business/commercial culture in the NHS, which led to the policy in the 1980s of 'contracting out' or 'outsourcing'. The clinical work of the NHS was retained in the public sector, but, to reduce costs, support services such as laundry, cleaning and catering were contracted out to private providers. The number of non-clinical NHS employees had nearly halved by the end of 1980s. To ensure they made a profit the private companies paid the support staff less, while the quality of service reduced; in fact, the cleanliness of hospitals is still a major issue for the NHS over 20 years later.

Four themes emerge from the history of the NHS since 1983 (Klein, 2001). First, there was a sharp turn towards centralisation. This led to the second theme – that of managerialism and bureaucratic rationalisation. Third, the expansion of private medicine continued apace, along with the privatisation of ancillary services within the NHS. Fourth, there was increasing consumerism within the health sector. The increase in demand for NHS funding was accompanied by the development of healthcare as a public-policy issue. A consumer-led service was being emphasised rather than professional-led care system (Davies, 1987). Klein (2001) further argues that the 'politicisation' of the NHS between 1974 and 1989 was also related to the shifting of accountability from local to central authorities.

A crisis in the NHS developed in the second half of 1987. Since 1979, resources for the NHS had been increased by the Conservative government, from £7.7 billion in 1979/80 to £18.35 billion in 1988/89. Despite this, the Service was not doing well. Although resources were increasing, demand was outstripping this. The increasing elderly population, advances in medical technology and priority objectives (e.g. kidney transplants) meant that services had to be increased by 2% per annum just to keep up.

To reduce costs and stave off a crisis, some services provided by the NHS were effectively privatised in the late 1980s. Resources for dentistry in the NHS were reduced and as dentists were, like GPs, mostly 'independent contractors' they stopped taking on NHS patients and worked increasingly in the private sector, where they could earn more money. (By 2006 NHS dentists had become so scarce that all over the country there were large queues in the high street when spaces became available for NHS care.) In 1989, routine eye examinations became free only for children and the elderly. It was argued by the government that people could now afford to pay for tests, but the new policy led to a major reduction in examinations. Long-term care from the NHS was also eliminated, which stimulated the growth of private nursing and residential homes throughout the 1990s. These measures were implemented to reduce costs in attempt to avert the financial melt-down of the NHS. They also, however, compromised one of the founding principles of the NHS – to provide a comprehensive service.

Following the June 1987 election, when Margaret Thatcher was returned for a third term, a financial crisis began facing the health authorities. Beds began to close, charities began to shore up NHS operations, cancer patients were being denied operations and both the Institute of Health Service Management and the King's Fund announced their own independent reviews of NHS funding. Despite this, the government continued to publicise statistics about how much more was being spent on the NHS. The poor showing of the Minister, John Moore, who unfortunately became ill during this time, compounded the issue.

In early December 1987, the lack of heart operations on children in Birmingham was publicised and nurses at St Thomas' Hospital picketed the Houses of Parliament in their uniforms. Probably the most significant event, and certainly a historical one, was when the Presidents of the Royal Colleges of Surgeons, Physicians and Obstetricians and Gynaecologists issued a joint statement suggesting that the NHS was almost at breaking point (Hoffenberg *et al*, 1987). The BMA supported the Presidents and added to the media clamour for increased resources. The government responded on 16 December by announcing an extra £100 million for the NHS, but despite this the crisis continued and more nurses began to strike.

The Prime Minister reassured the public that the NHS was in safe hands and was not about to be abolished. She, however, was also still advocating tax cuts to encourage private health insurance. It was generally accepted that a government review of the NHS was inevitable. It was not until Thatcher announced it in a BBC television *Panorama* programme on 25 January 1988 that it gathered momentum (many cynics believe that she was tricked into saying this and that the Department of Health did not know of this review until she announced it).

Developments from 1989 to 1997

The results of the government's review were initially announced in the publication of the White Paper *Working for Patients* (Department of Health, 1989) on 31 January 1989. A year later the NHS and Community Care Act followed. These two policy papers instigated what was at the time the most radical reform the NHS had undergone since its inception in 1948. The policies were criticised for lacking strategic planning and many were unhappy that there had been no consultation inside the NHS. The following three measures were perhaps the principal changes made by the Act.

- *Self-governing hospitals*. Stand-alone hospital trusts were established; these were separate from the health authority and were accountable directly to central government. They were to be managed by a board of directors with a chair appointed by the Secretary of the State for Health. The hospital trusts were able to contract out services and buy and sell assets, borrow capital, employ staff on local terms and advertise their services. The government's idea was to move decision making as near to patients as possible.
- *Fund-holding GPs*. Fund-holding GPs were created. They were given their own budget, to buy hospital services directly from source. The scheme was voluntary for GPs but provided financial incentives to encourage them to sign up. Initially only larger practices (i.e. with lists of at least 11 000) could apply to be fund-holders and their budgets covered just elective surgery, out-patient and diagnostic services, prescribing and staff costs.

- *The internal market.* The 'internal market' was advocated by the US Defense Department economist Alan Enthoven, who was highly thought of by the UK government. To create an internal market, the NHS was split into 'purchasers' – health authorities and fund-holding GPs – and 'providers' – hospital and community trusts and non-fund-holding GPs. It was envisaged that providers would compete with each other (though all still within the NHS) to secure contracts with purchasers by offering higher-quality, more responsive and efficient services.

Most attention and scrutiny focused on those three reforms but there were other significant changes at this time.

- *Funding and contracts for hospital services.* A new formula on a capitation (population-weighted) basis for purchasing services for a given population replaced the RAWP. The amount to be spent was to be determined on the basis of population, with adjustments made for cross-boundary referrals and allocations to budget-holding GP practices. It was hoped this would promote resource equity between regions and allow services to be developed to meet local needs.
- *Drug budgets.* Each GP practice now has to monitor its prescriptions closely.
- *Capital charges.* The intention is to stimulate fair competition between public and private healthcare by limiting the amount of capital the government effectively provides free to the public health sector.
- *Medical audit.* This was defined in *Working for Patients* as 'systematic, critical analysis involved in clinical care' so that 'the best quality of service is being achieved within the resources available'.
- *NHS consultants.* Job descriptions were to be reviewed annually; managers were given the right to sit on appointments committees; distinction awards were to be reviewed every 5 years and were not to be awarded less than 3 years before retirement; and progression to the higher awards was not limited to those with a 'C' award.
- *Implications for family practitioner committees.* New chief executives were to be appointed and were to be responsible for organising cash-limiting budgets for GPs and monitoring the cost of GP prescribing.

The internal market did not lead to the benefits the government thought it would produce. Hospitals could not truly compete with each other as the government could not, for political reasons, allow less competitive hospital trusts to go out of business, as would happen in the real commercial world. GP fund-holding was also an unpopular policy. A two-tier system was therefore created. Fund-holders' contracts with healthcare providers gave their patients quicker access to hospital services than patients from non-fund-holding practices. There were distinct advantages for patients whose GP belonged to a fund-holding practice (the 'haves') over patients whose GP was part of a non-fund-holding practice (the 'have-nots'). The reforms of 1989 severely compromised the premise of equity that the NHS had been founded on.

The Conservatives under John Major won the 1992 general election and continued to develop the internal market in the NHS. Many still feared privatisation, as part of the 1989 reforms allowed hospital trusts to raise income from other sources, such as private beds. The collectivist model of the NHS was being threatened, although the 1992 White Paper *The Health of the Nation* (Department of Health, 1992) appeared to address the government's responsibilities for the health of the country. The document moved towards health promotion and set out 25 specific policy targets, including reducing the suicide rate by 15%, as well as reducing the proportion of the population who were obese, smokers and heavy-drinkers. The White Paper was criticised for setting targets that were easily achievable and for failing to address the effect poverty, inequality and unemployment have on health. Kearney (1992) concluded that the policy had no strategy at all and was merely 'window dressing'.

The Patient's Charter (Department of Health, 1991) reinforced the consumerist model the government had been encouraging. The document explicitly set out patients' rights, some of which reflected the original philosophy of the NHS (e.g. 'to receive health on the basis of clinical needs, regardless of ability to pay'). Other standards were promised for patients, such as waiting no more than 2 years once placed on a waiting list and to be seen within 30 minutes of a specific out-patient appointment time. A performance guide was published in 1994 (Department of Health, 1994) and hospital trusts were rated (using a five-star system) on whether they had achieved its standards. This system gave the public information on how their local NHS services were performing. Despite being 'well informed consumers', patients had no true power to choose between different NHS providers, only to opt out of the NHS and to choose private services, which they would have to pay for.

The reforms of the 1990s moved the power base of the NHS away from hospitals and towards primary care. The advent of GP fund-holders altered the relationship between hospitals and GPs. The hospitals were now in effect answerable to the GPs and therefore in essence the patients. Community service providers were also encouraged to establish themselves as separate trusts from acute hospital services, which promoted community services over hospitals.

The multitude of reforms did not lead to an improvement in services, however, although GP fund-holding was a moderate success, as a relaxation of entry requirements had allowed approximately 50% of GPs to become fund-holding by 1996. Many, however, had joined under duress, as they felt they would be left behind if they did not become fund-holders. The cost of reorganisation (e.g. the purchaser/provider split) had been covered by two short increases of funding to the NHS in 1992/93 and 1994/95. The extra money was quickly absorbed and no benefits were seen to services. The government remained prudent but its belief that the NHS would become more efficient and save money if there were strict financial pressures was misguided.

Further reorganisation was implemented and by 1996 the regional health authorities had been abolished and replaced by eight regional offices of the NHS Executive. There were 425 NHS trusts, which acted as 'providers' of services, and 8500 GP fund-holders, who were 'purchasers'. In addition to fund-holders, there were still non-fund-holding GPs, under the management of 100 health authorities. This fragmentation of the NHS into purchasers and providers made it difficult for the NHS to plan and distribute resources on the basis of the population's health needs. Many NHS trusts were failing financially and waiting lists remained static. The NHS had lurched from reform to reform, nearing a crisis many times, to the extent that come the eve of the 1997 general election the *Sun* newspaper (4 May) told its readers that they had '24 hours to save the NHS'.

Developments since 1997

The Labour Party's general election victory in 1997 brought new hope to the NHS, which in many people's eyes had been in a permanent state of crisis for over 20 years. The public were ready for change and returned Tony Blair's party with a majority of 179 following the largest two-party swing since Clement Attlee's victory in 1945. This was, however, a very different Labour Party to the one that had overseen the genesis of the NHS. Eighteen years in opposition had forced it to instigate major policy reform. Traditional party beliefs in nationalisation, central planning and state paternalism, which had underlain the creation of the NHS, were abandoned. The new government adopted what was to be known as the 'third way', mixing notions of equality and social justice with privatisation and free-market competition (Blaine, 1998). The 'third way' of running the NHS was based on partnership and driven by performance, and has led to the period of biggest reform in its history.

The newly elected government was committed to keeping to the overall expenditure plans of the previous Conservative government for the first 2 years of its term. An extra £1.2 billion was, however, invested immediately into the NHS, and was just the beginning of increased resources for the service. Following the Wanless report (Wanless, 2002), which recognised that the NHS was and had for many years been under-funded, UK taxes were increased to finance extra NHS expenditure, which for the next 5 years averaged an increase of 7.4% a year in real terms. This was to raise total health spending in the UK from 6.8% of gross domestic product (GDP) in 1997 to an estimated 9.4% in 2007/08, which would make the UK one of the higher spenders on health in Europe (Stevens, 2004).

Extra investment in the NHS coincided with a programme of major reforms, which focused on reorganising services and raising standards of health and care. In 1997 the UK's first Minister for Public Health was appointed. Subsequently, the policy document *Our Healthier Nation*

(Department of Health, 1998*a*) was published to replace *The Health of the Nation*. The new policy set a national target of saving 300000 lives over the next decade, specifically focusing on cancers, coronary heart disease, stroke and mental illness. *Our Healthier Nation* shifted the focus away from the policies of the 1990s, which implied that individuals were responsible for improving their own health, and recognised that there needed to be a framework to empower individuals, as well as strategies to reduce inequality and poverty.

The first significant health reforms by the new Labour government were set out in the White Paper *The New NHS. Modern, Dependable* (Department of Health, 1997). Although the reforms were extensive, they were by no means radical. The paper proposed the dismantling of the internal market, but many components of it were maintained. The purchase/provider split remained, but the emphasis was on cooperative relationships rather than competition. GP fund-holding was abolished and instead all general practices were obliged to join a primary care group (PCG). Primary care groups covered populations that ranged in size from 30000 to 250000 and functioned both as providers of primary care and as purchasers of secondary care. They were led by GPs, although their boards also contained representation from community groups and the health authority. The PCGs were allowed to retain any surplus from their budget, which could be spent on services or facilities of benefit to patients. Although competition was disapproved of by the Labour government, purchasers (i.e. the PCGs) were still able to switch to other providers if they were dissatisfied with the services they received.

The 1997 White Paper also began to address quality and standards in the NHS and was expanded upon by *A First Class Service: Quality in the New NHS* (Department of Health, 1998*b*) a year later. Clinical governance, which was at the time seen as a radical idea, was introduced to the NHS and a statutory responsibility for the quality of care was placed upon trust and health authority chief executives. Hospital trusts and PCGs developed systems and committees to meet the clinical governance requirements of quality assurance, audit and risk management. There has been criticism that the implementation of clinical governance in the NHS was impeded by lack of time and resources, that is, that there was too much change, implemented too quickly and with a lack of clear guidance (Roland *et al*, 2001).

The government also set up two new national bodies: the National Institute for Clinical Excellence (NICE), which was renamed in 2004 the National Institute for Health and Clinical Excellence (while retaining the acronym unaltered), and the Council for Health Improvement, which evolved into the Commission for Health Improvement (CHI), in 2000. In 2002 CHI was replaced by the Commission for Health Audit and Inspection (CHAI), which combined its work with that previously done by the Audit Commission. The CHAI also had responsibility for regulation in private healthcare (e.g. private nursing homes and hospitals). The work of the CHAI was in turn taken over by the Healthcare Commission in 2004. In simple terms NICE was expected to set standards while the Council for Health Improvement enforced them. NICE's aim to address the lack of national standards and resultant wide variations in quality of healthcare was at first very popular. There had been growing public concern over 'postcode prescribing', where the availability of effective treatments depended on where in the country the patient lived. NICE's assessment of the effectiveness of drugs and other medical technologies led to it recommending their use in virtually all cases. A large part of NICE's remit was to attempt to limit the growth of the NHS drug bill, but even when its experts asserted that the anti-viral drug zanamivir had little therapeutic benefit, they back-tracked on their original judgement and still recommended its use. The work of NICE remains controversial. In 2005, it was criticised for the speed of its evaluation of the cancer drug trastuzumab (Herceptin) and its withdrawing of support for anti-dementia drugs on cost-effectiveness grounds rather than purely on the grounds of their clinical effectiveness.

National Service Frameworks (NSFs) set out new standards for service delivery, emphasising effectiveness and outcomes. The first wave of NSFs included protocols for the management of cancer, coronary heart disease and mental health. The Council for Health Improvement instigated a rolling programme of reviews of every NHS trust (acute and primary care) every 3–4 years. Its objective was to review the clinical governance of trusts as well as their implementation of the NSFs and other guidance from NICE. CHI inspections proved truly effective only when discovering gross incompetence and negligence, as they had few solutions to offer still under-resourced trusts which were not meeting the performance standards (Day & Klein, 2002).

Other innovations to modernise the NHS and change the ways it had previously worked included NHS Direct and the National Programme for Information Technology (NPfIT). NHS Direct is a nurse-led 24-hour telephone advice service. Five years after its inception in 1998 it was handling over half a million calls a day; it expanded into an equally busy online service in 2001. The NPfIT is an ambitious project which originally aimed for NHS trusts to have electronic patient records in place by 2005 (NHS Executive, 1998). It has, however, been riddled with logistical and technical difficulties, and now aims for electronic patient records to be implemented in all acute trusts by the end of 2007 (Hendy *et al*, 2005).

The NHS Plan

The New NHS. Modern, Dependable (1997) was only the beginning of the reforms the Labour government intended for the NHS. In July 2000, its full programme to modernise the NHS was announced in *The NHS Plan* (Department of Health, 2000a), which described the government's vision for the NHS for the next 10 years. The Plan was enterprising, impressive in scope and in places daring. It concentrated on the areas of capacity, standards, delivery and partnership, but the central aim was to create a patient-led health service. It proposed an NHS that responded to the needs and preferences of patients, rather than their choice being prohibited by 'the system' or health professionals. The implementation of the NHS Plan coincided with the increase in spending on the NHS by 6.3% in real terms. Significant improvements were, however, expected for this investment:

- *More health professionals.* Over the 5-year period the extra money was expected to provide 7500 more hospital consultants (a rise of 30%), 1000 more special registrars, 2000 extra GPs and 450 more trainees. There would also be 1000 more medical school places each year, on top of the 1000 places that had been announced before the NHS Plan.
- *More hospitals and beds.* Provision was made in the Plan for 100 new hospitals over a 10-year period and 7000 more hospital and inter-mediate care beds.
- *National standards for waiting times.* By 2005, the maximum waiting time for out-patients was expected to be 3 months and 6 months for in-patients. No one should be waiting more than 4 hours in accident and emergency departments by 2004. It was also promised that all patients would be able to see a GP within 48 hours by 2004. Waiting lists for hospital appointments and admissions would be abolished by the end of 2005 and replaced with a booking system designed to give patients a choice of a convenient time.
- *Performance monitoring.* The performance of hospital trusts and primary care groups would be rated using a traffic light system by the CHI. 'Green light' organisations, the 'best performers', would receive funds from the National Performance Fund and be given more autonomy. A 'red light' rating would lead to intervention from government agencies and if necessary the installation of new management. (The traffic light system was later replaced by the equally loathed star rating system, where trusts were evaluated against performance standards such as finances and waiting lists and awarded up to three stars.)
- *Development of partnerships.* All hospitals would have a new patient and advocacy service. There would also be increased involvement and scrutiny of the NHS by local authorities.
- *Expansion of nursing roles.* To make up the shortfall of doctors, the NHS Plan also proposed training for around 20000 nurses, who would be able to prescribe a limited range of medicines.

The NHS Plan also promised to deliver an expanded NHS Direct and further national standards for more clinical specialties.

To implement the NHS Plan, the government set up the National Mod-ernisation Agency and local modernisation boards for each regional office of the NHS. The *Implementation Programme for the NHS Plan* (Department of Health, 2000b) was published at the end of 2000 and included provisional milestones and key targets for the early years of the Plan. More targets followed and many working in the NHS felt overwhelmed by the pace of change.

The reorganisation of the NHS

The NHS Plan promised greater power and authority for patients and the public. *Shifting the Balance of Power Within the NHS* (Department of Health, 2001) attempted to give that greater authority to patients as well as to decentralise decision-making. The NHS Executive was dismantled, and all English and Welsh health authorities were abolished. They were replaced with 28 new strategic health authorities, which have a strategic role in improving local health services and also in monitoring local health trusts' performance.

The PCGs evolved into new primary care trusts (PCTs), which inherited the health authorities' powers, responsibilities and resources. PCTs have become the new powerhouses of the NHS. They are responsible for health improvement, and developing and delivering primary care, but also for commissioning hospital services. PCTs hold approximately 75% of all NHS resources. While there were nearly 100 health authorities, there are now over 400 PCTs, each covering an average population of 175 000.

One of the most controversial reforms was the proposal to establish foundation trusts. Initially only top-performing trusts could apply for foundation trust status, but it is now envisaged that all NHS trusts and PCTs will eventually be eligible. Becoming a foundation trust offers more financial freedom, with organisations being allowed both to retain operating surpluses and to access a wider range of options for capital funding to invest in new services. They are also able to recruit and employ their own staff. Although they must still deliver on national targets and standards, they are not under the direction of the Department of Health and the regional strategic health authorities. There has been much resistance to foundation trusts, as many feel they indicate the break-up of the NHS, with individual hospitals having almost complete independence and determining their own priorities. Even their detractors in some hospital trusts and PCTs have realised that they are a reality, and feel obliged to prepare to apply for foundation trust status, as otherwise they, and their patients, will be left behind and disadvantaged. This is similar to the situation that GPs found themselves in over 10 years previously with regard to fund-holding.

The NHS and the private sector

For the NHS to reach the targets of the NHS Plan, it needed to increase its capacity, but extra resources to build new hospitals were unavailable. Previous governments had utilised the Private Finance Initiative (PFI), where private capital was used to build hospitals. Hospital trusts would then lease the buildings from the private companies, under contracts lasting 25 years or more. The NHS gained new buildings without raising taxes, as the public's payment was deferred, although in the long term it would be more expensive than if the buildings had been built using public money. The 2002 White Paper *Delivering the NHS Plan* announced that 55 major hospital schemes would be carried out, mostly through the PFI system (Department of Health, 2002). The PFI schemes have been renamed 'public–private partnerships' (PPPs). Some NHS services, such as psychotherapy, are contracted out to private companies. This has again been done in the hope of increasing capacity and meeting targets. Most contracts involve elective surgical procedures or diagnostic tests. The primary concern of private healthcare providers is profit and so they are prone to choose activities that will yield a profit and to leave less financially attractive services to the NHS. Because there were concerns about the quality of work provided by the private companies, contracts now specify expected performance levels. There have also been concerns that the NHS is slowly being privatised through PPPs, although at the time of writing the government is committed to a maximum of 15% of the NHS's output being provided by the private sector. For an in-depth discussion of the relationship between the NHS and the private sector, readers are recommended *NHS plc* (Pollock, 2005).

The results of the recent reforms, and the future

There has been massive investment in the NHS in the period 1997–2006: NHS spending increased from £46 billion a year to £94 billion a year. This investment has led to some modest improvements; for example, nearly 200 000 extra front-line staff have joined the NHS. Over half of the extra money has been spent on pay and pensions for staff, most significantly, in increased National Insurance contributions. General practitioners and hospital consultants received new contracts, which, while increasing the scrutiny and accountability of their work, considerably increased their pay. The average GP now earns more than £100 000 a year, making UK doctors some of the highest paid in the world outside the USA. Extra funding is due to cease in 2008.

There have been some successes. The number of patients on waiting lists, a favourite marker of success for politicians, is at an all-time low, but average out-patient waiting time has been reduced only to 6.6 weeks, compared with 7.7 weeks in 1997. In-patient waiting lists have fallen more substantially but on the whole it must be concluded that too much has been spent on delivering too little. NHS productivity has not increased enough and the Service has ended up costing more and delivering less value for money.

AT the time of writing (summer 2006) the NHS in England has a net deficit of £512 million, equivalent to 0.8% of its turnover. Services in some areas are being cut, leading to staff redundancies as trusts try to balance their books. This is likely to continue as the current level of NHS spending cannot continue. From 2008, annual increases for the NHS are expected to decrease from the current 7% to 3–4%. Further reform in 2006 included plans set out in a new White Paper to expand care outside of the hospital, with 5% of resources to be shifted from hospitals to GPs over the next 10 years. The new emphasis is on community provision of healthcare. Services previously provided by hospitals will be offered by GPs or by privately run, but NHS-funded, clinics. This will place more financial pressure on hospitals, as they will competing with each other for work: since 2005 patients have been able to choose from at least four hospitals, including one in the private sector. Under the new payment by results scheme hospitals will be paid only for the work they do, rather than being given a budget at the start of the year. Each procedure, whether it be a surgical operation or an out-patient follow-up appointment, has an attached national tariff/price and the hospital receives this payment only if it completes the activity. This system will increase the competition between hospitals, and a hospital that fails to attract enough work will face considerable financial adversity, as many already have financial deficits and are tied into long, expensive PFI contracts.

Financial difficulties will inevitably lead to further reorganisation of the NHS, but it is difficult to assess how much appetite the already reform-weary NHS staff have for further change.

Changes in the NHS management structure since 1974 are summarised in Table 1.1.

Further sources and directions of change

The Postgraduate Medical Education and Training Board (PMETB) and Modernising Medical Careers (MMC) are two key factors which will change the face of training and assessment in psychiatry. The third prong of this change is the European Working Time Directive (EWTD).

Modernising Medical Careers introduces a 'foundation year 2', with the aim of exposing trainees to three further specialties before they have to make their selection. This is a generic foundation programme for the first two postgraduate years (F1 and F2), to be followed by a Unified Training Grade (UTG) with no midpoint reselection.

The EWTD restricts the working hours of trainee doctors to a maximum of 58 hours per week, and the trainee cannot work continuously for more than 13 hours without a minimum 11 hours off; also, trainees are considered to be working if they are required to be in the hospital, whether awake or asleep. As of 30 September 2005, the PMETB is the single competent authority for postgraduate medical education, training and assessment throughout the UK. The PMETB will be responsible for all postgraduate medical education and assessment of doctors completing final postgraduate training and will be in charge of establishing, maintaining and monitoring standards relating to medical training in the NHS and elsewhere. It will issue certificates of Completion of Training and statements of eligibility for specialist registration. It has three main committees – Quality Assurance, Training and Assessment. The PMETB has taken over the approved visits

Table 1.1 Some important changes in NHS management structures since 1974

Year	Initiative
1975	*Better Services for the Mentally Ill* published, a White Paper based on a report from the Audit Commission
1982	The Korner report, from the Department of Health and Social Security's Steering Group on Health Services Information, concerning the collection and use of information on hospital clinical activity
	Abolition of NHS area health boards
1983	Management budgeting experiment started
1984	Griffiths report on Health Service management
1986	Introduction of the 'resource management initiative'
1987	*Achieving a Balance* published, which recommends staffing levels for doctors
1988	NHS review announced
1989	*Working for Patients* and *Caring for People* published – White Papers leading to the 1990 Act
1990	The NHS and Community Care Act (reforms effective 1 April 1991) and introduction of the purchaser/provider split
1991	Postgraduate and continuing medical education introduced
	First wave of trust hospitals
1992	Second wave of trust hospitals
1993	Managing the new NHS – new proposals
1994	Fourth and last wave of trust hospitals
1997	*The NHS. Modern, Dependable* published. GP fund-holders abolished. Moves away from competition. PCGs established
1998	*A First Class Service* published and clinical governance introduced
2000	The NHS Plan: increased resources, performance monitoring (traffic light system)
2001	Shifting the Balance of Power launched. PCTs set up. NHS executive replaced by strategic health authorities
2002	Wanless report highlights under-funding of the NHS
2003	Health and Social Care Act presents concept of foundation hospitals and trusts

from the medical Royal Colleges and the assessments and training have to comply with PMETB standards and principles. The assessments will be largely workplace based and trainees will become increasingly responsible for their own learning and assessment; the assessments will focus on what doctors do rather than simply knowledge. These changes will have major effects on service delivery and training. Curricula for psychiatrists have been approved and the assessment matrix has been provisionally approved.

Conclusion

It is hoped that this brief *précis* of the history of the NHS will act as an introduction to the doctor interested in management and the complex organisational structure in which we work. Two things can be learned immediately from taking this historical overview: first, that history repeats itself and it is remarkable how current plans for the NHS are similar to old ideas; second, as an administrative machine the NHS is continually evolving, and that should be borne in mind by all of us who intend to plight their troth to it for the vast majority of our professional careers.

References and further reading

Allsop, J. (1986) *Health Policy in the National Health Service*. Longman.

Beeson, P. B. (1980) Some good features of the British National Health Service. In *Readings in Medical Sociology* (ed. D. Mechanic), pp. 328–334. Free Press.

Blaine A. R. P. (1998) *The Third Way, New Politics for a New Century*. Fabian Society.

British Medical Association (1989) *Special Report on the Government's White Paper, 'Working for Patients'*. British Medical Association.

British Medical Journal (1875) Provident institutions and hospitals. II Outpatients reforms. *British Medical Journal*, 483–484.

Davies, C. (1987) Things to come: the NHS in the next decade. *Sociology of Health and Illness*, **9**, 302–317.

Day, P. & Klein, R. (2002) CHI. Who nose best? Commission for Health Improvement. *Health Service Journal*, **112**, 26–29.

Department of Health (1989) *Working for Patients*. TSO (The Stationery Office).

Department of Health (1990) *The Community Care Act*. TSO (The Stationery Office).

Department of Health (1991) *The Patient's Charter*. TSO (The Stationery Office).

Department of Health (1992) *The Health of the Nation*. TSO (The Stationery Office).

Department of Health (1994) *Hospital and Ambulance Services: Comparative Performance Grade 1993–1994*. TSO (The Stationery Office).

Department of Health (1997) *The New NHS. Modern, Dependable*. TSO (The Stationery Office).

Department of Health (1998a) *Our Healthier Nation*. TSO (The Stationery Office).

Department of Health (1998b) *A First Class Service. Quality in the New NHS*. TSO (The Stationery Office).

Department of Health (2000a) *The NHS Plan: A Plan for Investment, a Plan for Reform*. TSO (The Stationery Office).

Department of Health (2000b) *Implementation Programme or the NHS Plan*. TSO (The Stationery Office).

Department of Health (2001) *Shifting the Balance of Power Within the NHS*. TSO (The Stationery Office).

Department of Health (2002) *Delivering the NHS Plan: Next Steps on Investment, Next Steps on Reform*. TSO (The Stationery Office).

Department of Health and Social Security (1972) *Management Arrangements for the Reorganised Health Service*. TSO (The Stationery Office).

Draper, P., Grenholm, G. & Best, G. (1976) The organization of health care: a critical view of the 1974 reorganization of the National Health Service. In *An Introduction to Medical Sociology* (ed. D. Tuckett). London: Tavistock.

Forsyth, G. (1982) Evolution of (the National Health Service). In *Management for Clinicians* (eds D. Allen & D. Grimes), pp. 18–35. Pitman.

Godber, G. (1975) *The Health Service: Past, Present and Future*. Athlone Press.

Godber, G. (1988) Forty years of the NHS. Origins and early development. *BMJ*, **297**, 37–43. (Subsequent articles in the same issue, pp. 44–58, are also of interest.)

Heller, T. (1978) *Restructuring the Health Service*. Croom Helm.

Hendy, J., Reeves, B. C., Fulop, N., *et al* (2005) Challenges to implementing the National Programme for Information Technology (NPfIT): a qualitative study. *BMJ*, **331**, 331–336.

Hoffenberg, R., Todd, I. P. & Pinker, G. (1987) Crisis in the National Health Service. *BMJ*, **295**, 1505.

Honigsbaum, F. (1979) *The Division in British Medicine: A History of the Separation of General Practice from Health Care 1911–1968*. Routledge & Kegan Paul.

Honigsbaum, F. (1989) *Health, Happiness and Security – The Creation of the National Health Service*. Routledge.

Jaques, E. (1978) *Health Services*. Heinemann.

Kearney, K. (1992) Strategy for improvement or window dressing? *Guardian*, 9 July.

Klein, R. (1989) *The Politics of the National Health Service* (2nd edn). Longman.

Klein, R. (2001) *The New Politics of the National Health Service*. Pearson Education.

Levitt, R. (1976) *The Reorganised National Health Service*. Croom Helm.

Navarro, V. (1978) *Class Struggle, the State and Medicine: An Historical and Contemporary Analysis of the Medical Sector in Great Britain*. Martin Robertson.

NHS Executive (1998) *Information for Health. An Information Strategy for the Modern NHS 1998–2005*. NHS Executive.

Political and Economic Planning Group (1937) *The British Social Services. The British Health Services*. Political and Economic Planning.

Pollock, A. (2005) *NHS plc*. Verso.

Roland, M., Campell, S. & Wilkins, D. (2001) Clinical governance: a convincing strategy for quality improvement? *Journal of Management in Medicine*, **15**, 188–201.

Stacey, M. (1988) *The Sociology of Health and Healing*. Unwin Hyman.

Stevens, R. (1966) *Medical Practice in Modern England: The Impact of Specialization and State Medicine*. York University Press.

Stevens, S. (2004) Reform strategies for the English NHS. *Health Affairs*, **23**, 37–44.

Timmins, N. (1988) *Cash Crisis and Cure – The Independent Guide to the NHS Debate*. Newspaper Publishing PLC.

Wanless, D. (2002) *Securing Our Future Health: Taking a Long-Term View*. HM Treasury.

Watkin, B. (1978) *The National Health Service: The First Phase 1948–1974 and After*. George Allen and Unwin.

Webster, C. (2002) *The National Health Service: A Political History* (2nd edn). Oxford University Press.

CHAPTER 2

The politics, funding and resources of the National Health Service in England

Stephen Morris

There is probably never a sensible time to write very coherently on the topic of resources in the National Health Service (NHS). The time of writing (early 2006) seems as bad as any, with the current political debate on what is referred to as 'system reform' far from complete and its implications for how the NHS is financed possibly profound, or then again possibly not. Part of the problem is that reforming the financing of the NHS is a long-term project, whereas politics is not. Equally difficult for politicians is a requirement to have absolute wisdom about the effect of government policies, which might better be piloted on a smaller scale with some honesty about what works and, more importantly, what does not. As a result, the 50 or so years of the NHS have seen many partially completed attempts to reform its finances, but none has overcome the perception of many who deliver services that, at best, resource allocation is unfair and illogical.

It is clear that the level of spending on the NHS has consistently increased ahead of inflation, and since 1996/97 has done so at a breathtaking rate, so that the actual spend has increased from £33 billion to a projected £92.6 billion in 2007/08 (see Fig. 2.1) – an extraordinary decade by any standards,

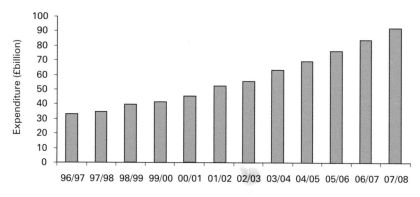

Fig. 2.1 NHS expenditure, 1996/97 to 2007/08.

especially as the first 2 years saw a very low rate of growth by historic standards. This is an effective real-terms increase of 6.5% per annum, with a cumulative real-terms increase over 11 years of 100.4%.

Two questions spring to mind:

1   For HM Treasury (and the electorate), what have we got for our money?
2   For healthcare professionals and all those working directly with patients, where did all the money go?

Right now, mental health services are complaining loudly about 'cuts' and yet more cash is being spent on mental health services than in the past. It appears as if, whatever is put in at one end, there is never enough to meet the needs of service users at the other.

Because of the domination of a performance management regime which focuses on an increasingly small number of national targets, we can provide better answers than in the past to the first question. Targets are themselves a reflection of the key government priority to know what it is getting for the cash being injected. Targets have caused quite a stir. Most accept that they work (look at the numbers), but it is a problem if what is important to you and your service is not included. Mental health services may well have cause for complaint in the absence of such clear performance indicators as waiting times for elective surgery.

Since 1997, performance indicators associated with targets have been impressive, as witness the interest internationally, not least from overseas politicians. Waiting times for elective surgery and in accident and emergency departments – the cause of the public's greatest expressed level of concern – have been reduced to a point where, although remaining a real problem for a minority of patients, they are likely by 2008 to feature as much in political debates on the health service as unemployment does in debates on the economy. That is a huge political achievement – taking this issue off the front pages and the news headlines. In mental health, the same appears to be true for the media treatment of homicides committed by people with a mental illness. This does not mean that the discrimination and prejudice held by many that stigmatise all people labelled as 'mentally ill' as violent has gone away, but the associated political impact of media coverage has diminished. Is this because the targeting of additional resources into early-onset and home treatment teams and the like has worked? It seems unlikely that anyone would wish to make such a simple connection. That illustrates the great difficulty for the NHS, and its decision-makers and leaders, in making sense of how politics, finance and resources can be made to work better.

Before considering in greater detail the financial policy environment that has emerged since 1997, what are the priorities for spending in the NHS? It is not always clear that services are free at the point of delivery, and mental health services are strongly affected by other costs and charges in the experience of mental health service users: benefits and social care costs which are means tested, as well as the need to budget for everyday living costs, often with very small amounts of available cash. Should the NHS spend more on prevention or more on treatment? Should the agenda be driven by those who make the most noise (who generally seem to call for attention to be paid to issues such as waiting times, acute episodes of mental illness, heroic surgery and pioneering drug therapies for terminal cancer) or by properly researched and tested interventions which deliver real population health improvements? There is a reasonably sound evidence base for both war and improving the performance of the local football team being effective measures for suicide prevention. Perhaps that is why these decisions are best left to the politicians.

The NHS since 1997

The election of the Labour government in 1997 provides a useful starting point for assessing the development of recent health policy as it relates to finance and resources. The Labour Party returned to power just in time to celebrate the 50th birthday of what some might see as both its problem child and its greatest achievement – the NHS. The issues facing the NHS and the government may not have especially changed in 1997, but the expectations of the electorate, NHS staff and of the Labour Party were extremely high. The obstacles to fulfilling these hopes were equally daunting.

To understand this better, the period since 1997 can be understood in three distinct phases. The initial phase culminated in the Wanless report, commissioned by the Treasury (Wanless, 2002). During this first period in office, the government came under increasing pressure to increase resources for the NHS and 2000 saw the publication of *The NHS Plan: A Plan for Investment, A Plan for Reform* (Department of Health, 2000). Over-lapping with the conduct of the Wanless report, this heralded the next phase of development, with a strong theme of modernisation and reform, backed by investment and tough performance management of the NHS against very challenging and specific targets. The final stage, which is currently in play, marks a planned move to a 'self-sustaining' system which rewards performance, is independently regulated and promotes choice and contestability. Its initiation can be associated with the publication of the *NHS Improvement Plan* in June 2004 (Department of Health, 2004).

The Wanless report

The Wanless report provided the government with a quasi-independent assessment (it was, after all, commissioned by the Treasury) that a health service, centrally funded through taxation, which provides services free at the point of delivery, is indeed the best system for the UK. It specifically rejected an insurance-based system and any of the alternatives used in other parts of the developed world. It also painted a picture which fitted well with the government's views of individual rights balanced by responsibilities. In the Wanless 'fully engaged' scenario, individuals would be enabled to take responsibility for lifestyle choices that has an impact on their health, and would be encouraged and given the opportunity actively to manage their own healthcare. This had the double advantage of supporting the government's goal of improving the nation's health while at the same time reducing incidents of avoidable illness, so that the NHS could concentrate its resources on tackling disease and improving the health of the population. It linked with the broader cross-government goal of closing the gap in the health and other outcomes between the poorest and the richest in society.

During the first 2 years of the new government, however, spending in the NHS increased by a very low level compared with historic trends. The new Labour government of 1997, determined to silence criticisms of a prior reputation for poor economic management, stuck rigidly to pre-existing budgets and gained its reputation for economic prudence. The effect on the NHS was enormous disappointment, finally voiced publicly by the Labour peer and medical academic Lord Winston: without cash the rhetoric was irrelevant. The debate about resources shifted to European comparisons and a national commitment by the Prime Minister to matching the European average spend per head. The published expenditure plan indicates that by 2007/08 the total spend on healthcare will amount to 9.2% of gross domestic product, well above the European average of 8.8%.

Increased resources – the NHS Plan

Political recognition that substantially increased funding for the NHS had to be found was matched by an absolute requirement that the money deliver results, as this would convince the public that the NHS was indeed improving. At the same time as senior NHS doctors were speaking out about the lack of anything meaningful in funding terms, the media were keeping up a relentless spotlight on the failure of the NHS to deliver an acceptable service. This spotlight focused very directly on waiting: in accident and emergency departments, for elective surgery and in primary care. Waiting times would become the political imperative of the first phase of the NHS Plan.

The NHS Plan was published in 2000. It set out ambitious targets across the health service; these reflected the public service agreement negotiated by the Department of Health with the Cabinet Office. The formerly separate roles of chief executive of the NHS and permanent secretary at the Department of Health were merged, and the new single leader was charged with delivering both the Department's public service agreement with the Cabinet Office and the NHS Plan. Following the government's return to office in 2001, the NHS Plan was supported by a major reorganisation. The regional offices and health authorities were abolished and replaced by 28 strategic health authorities (SHAs) and 302 primary care trusts (PCTs). The SHAs were given three roles: performance management, increasing capacity and supporting strategic development. The PCTs received the majority of the funding and were charged with 'commissioning' services that were sensitive to local needs and that delivered the centrally determined targets of the NHS Plan.

Perhaps most profoundly, the government directly tackled the NHS's funding gap and increased National Insurance – a straightforward price increase for the NHS's services. This meant the money was linked directly to the targets.

There were real changes in this period. Waiting times were tackled and reduced. Funding increased well beyond what even Lord Winston probably could have hoped for. The media criticism of the NHS, with its previous winter chorus of discontent over accident and emergency departments, was, if not silenced, certainly muted. New issues have since emerged – like dentistry and hospital 'superbug' infections – but there has been little interest in waiting times.

In the 5 years after the Labour Party's 2001 general election victory, the NHS grew. For instance, between 1996/97 and 2003/04 there was an increase of 75 000 in the number of qualified nurses and an extra 10 000 hospital consultants. In primary care over 5000 more general practitioners (GPs) and nearly 4000 more practice nurses were appointed. New hospitals and community and general practices were built. The number of finished consultant episodes in hospitals for the same period increased from 11.1 million to 13.3 million. However, during this period the NHS did not look hard enough at its resource base. Recent improvements could be reversed if costs cannot be contained within projected resources. This may become even more problematic when the very high rate of growth in resources in recent years returns to a more normal level in 2008–2009.

There are two structural reasons why spending has grown as quickly as it has. Both are to do with addressing previous shortfalls. The first issue is staff. In renegotiating its contracts with all its staff, the NHS has sought much greater flexibility, but the significant extra staff salary cost has yet to be translated into improved productivity. The second issue is the NHS's buildings. Much of the NHS's estate was in very poor shape, reflecting the low priority often given to maintenance and the shortage of capital expenditure. Modernisation requires this to be addressed. The procurement of new building through the Private Finance Initiative means that the cost of that capital investment counts against the revenue budget in much the same way as a mortgage. It also means that the maintenance and replacement costs of the investment are built into the contract, so slashing the maintenance budget to balance the annual budget and defer the cost until the building falls down – a traditional NHS approach to making ends meet – is not now possible.

A separate, but essential, area of costly investment where there was a history of low comparative spend on uncoordinated systems was information technology (IT). This has now been reversed, with substantial investment through the Connecting for Health programme (see below).

Sustainable system reform

The developments over the period 2001–06 were hard won politically, financially and clinically. Arguments over the impact of targets were fierce – it was claimed they had the potential to distort clinical priorities, to concentrate new funding in acute hospitals and to work against the goal of increased community care and better care for the majority of patients, specifically those with long-term conditions. Equally, the progress not just in terms of waiting times but also in terms of reduced morbidity for cancer, coronary heart disease and suicides is compelling. Narrowing the gap on health inequalities was not achieved, which does challenge policy-makers on how to implement effective delivery in a way which matches the other targets. Politically, the middle classes have not walked away from the NHS. Private health provision is having to find different ways of competing for business. The accident and emergency service is a victim of its own success and is now a very popular route into healthcare. Far fewer patients experience waiting for elective surgery as a major problem, although the goal of eliminating this as a problem altogether has not been achieved, largely as a result of the waiting times for diagnostic tests.

The buts are twofold. First, the increases in costs have outpaced the increased funding. When funding growth returns to more normal levels, the NHS will need to find other ways of solving problems than simply spending its way out of trouble. This means looking at length of stay, effectiveness of community interventions, case management of long-term conditions and better and closer working between primary and secondary care. In fact, this is what mental health services having been doing to good effect for some time, but it does not happen overnight and is never easy. Second, the rigour of performance management – the holding to account of hospital trust and PCT chief executives for the delivery of a small number of targets – does not appear desirable as a long-term solution to assuring a smoothly running health delivery system. It has achieved focus on the delivery of a small number of goals, but is this really the most sensible approach to making success routine?

Hence, policy has shifted to addressing a separate question. How do you design a system which both rewards productivity (the first 'but', of controlling expenditure) and delivers a consistently good service (the second 'but', of replacing hands-on central command and control). In essence, how do you make the system self-sustaining?

The foundations of system reform were laid before the 2005 general election, with the much contested creation of NHS foundation trusts through the Health and Social Care (Community Health and Standards) Act 2003. NHS foundation trusts are described as 'public interest companies';

the intention is that, by making hospitals accountable to the membership of the local NHS foundation trust that elects the governing body, they would be more locally accountable. Equally important, they are no longer accountable to the Department of Health but are independent and regulated by an independent body, Monitor, which as the licensing body has sole discretion in the suspension of their authorisation. As independent organisations, they have some (limited) ability to raise capital commercially. However, the first NHS foundation trusts have expressed some disappointment that this is not all it was promised to be. Of the 170 acute trusts in England, 32 have achieved NHS foundation trust status to date. Until recently the first hurdle to authorisation by Monitor was 'three star' status. This has subsequently been relaxed, but not Monitor's rigorous approval process (see www. monitor-nhsft.gov.uk). NHS foundation trusts are still obliged to deliver NHS Plan targets, for example the 18-week limit on the interval between referral and treatment set for 2008, and these continue to be assessed through annual ratings. Even the reduction in bureaucracy through fewer data demands from the Department of Health and SHAs has been less than hoped by early exponents of NHS foundation trusts.

Initially, NHS foundation trust status was reserved for acute hospital trusts. Now NHS mental health trusts are achieving NHS foundation trust status. However, this route is not open to PCTs, which have been vociferous in their criticism of acute-based targets skewing the allocation of new resources to acute trusts. This is despite the supposed role of the PCTs as 'commissioners' of services, that is, determining not just the level of planned service but also how services should be developed to maximise their effectiveness – this, rather confusingly, is often referred to as market or system management.

How do we manage demand through better routes into services and more efficient use of resources for patients? For example, long-term conditions such as chronic obstructive pulmonary disease should not be treated in crisis through accident and emergency departments and in-patient admission. In many ways, the rate at which funding has increased and the insistent performance management of targets has meant that issues of effectiveness – and the appropriateness of treatment, including patient preference – have figured less. Such, at least, is very much the view from PCTs.

In order to address this, system reform has led to changing roles for SHAs and PCTs. The number of PCTs has been reduced from 302 to 150, and the number of SHAs from 28 to 10. The role of the larger PCT is to commission in more than name and the role of the SHA in overseeing the system is to ensure that commissioning is effective. Thinking forward, in a world where the majority of secondary and tertiary care providers in England are NHS foundation trusts, there will be no ability, except through PCTs and commissioning, to performance manage traditional areas such as waiting lists. If patients are waiting more than 18 weeks from referral to treatment in 2008, this will be the PCT's problem, not the hospital's.

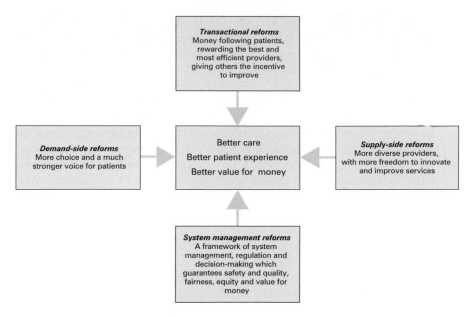

Fig. 2.2 The components of system reform (Department of Health, with permission).

The more forceful commissioning role planned for PCTs and the establishment of a much larger proportion of secondary providers with NHS foundation trust status is only part of the system reform story (see Fig. 2.2). There are four other key elements:

- *Payment by results*. This is currently restricted to 'spells' of care with acute providers but it is intended to be extended to mental health. It is the mechanism by which hospitals are rewarded for the work they actually undertake. For this to be open and transparent, payment is on the basis of a fixed tariff, so that more efficient hospitals are rewarded.
- *Patient choice*. Choice is planned to be offered by GPs to all patients, who will be able to choose from initially four and by 2008 all available providers for referral.
- *Contestability*. Contestability assures that the NHS is no longer regarded as the automatic provider, but rather as the guarantor that the provider, which may be from the independent (including profit-making) sector, matches NHS standards. From 2006, GPs will be compelled to offer at least one provider from the independent sector as one of the four providers for referral.
- *Independent regulation*. Independent regulation, currently vested in the Healthcare Commission and Monitor (for NHS foundation trusts), provides assurance, independent of the NHS and the Department of Health, that NHS organisations and services in the independent sector are providing high-quality care and value for money.

System reform remains at a very early stage. Critical to determining whether or not it is successful in creating a self-sustaining system capable of year-on-year improvement without central command and control is information. Without information, patients cannot exercise choice, GPs will not know what is available, regulators cannot assess quality and value for money, commissioners cannot monitor their contracts, and payment by results will not be possible. The NHS starts, as with its estate, from a very low level of historic investment in IT and information systems – itself an area notorious for non-delivery. Perhaps this is the most critical element, wrapped up in the project referred to as 'Connecting for Health', which faces a huge challenge in delivering one of the biggest IT programmes ever attempted across the world.

Why is system reform important to the politics, funding and resources of the NHS? Because this is where all three come together. In terms of politics, 'choice' will replace, or at least be an equal player with, 'voice' when it comes to determining the future of local services. 'Use it or lose it' will be the response when much-loved services face closure. PCTs will no doubt continue to argue over formulas for allocating resources by population and point to inequity on the basis of health need – resulting from age, ethnicity and other demographics – but, in the short term at least, the availability of resources to clinicians will be at the mercy of organisations which are most effective in matching their costs against the pricing regime of payment by results, most effective in winning commissioning from PCTs and best able to attract the right number of referrals and patients through other routes, such as accident and emergency departments.

Finally, system reform envisages a system in which an individual organisation can fail. This does not mean that essential services such as accident and emergency departments will close. It does mean that there will be a process equivalent to insolvency for a failed health organisation, with, for example, its contracts and assets taken over by a more successful health provider, be it from the public or independent sector.

Managing resources in the current environment

To conclude this chapter, it is important to emphasise that the requirements to manage effectively as a doctor – whether as a consultant, clinical director, medical director or chief executive – remains perhaps little altered. Furthermore, as set out at the start of this chapter, practically no government policy survives sufficiently long to see to an absolute conclusion in terms of planned benefits. This will be as true for system reform as it has been for the internal market. In politics it is, as ever, events, especially unforeseen events, which count and all we can be certain of is that we do not know what these are likely to be. Whoever predicted in 1995 that the NHS would receive the biggest cash injection in its history, with a tripling of its funding over the next 13 years, would surely have been referred, choice or no, to a local mental health service. The rest is speculation and belongs more to the lounge bar than the board room.

Finally, by way of a straightforward practical guide, set out below are the key elements of successful financial management for clinicians in the NHS:

- *Don't overspend.* It can look very tempting; after all, why should you care and surely users' needs are the ultimate law? Two cautions. First, if you overspend, then you will always be concerned about recovering the position and the pressure will throw current and longer-term plans into disarray. Second, in the end it is staff, mainly nurses, who pay for overspends, through reduced headcount, because that is where the money is tied up.

- *Don't argue on the basis of equity.* Given the complexity of healthcare funding and the relative shortness of life, let alone careers, developing epidemiologically brilliant demonstrations of funding shortfalls on the basis of comparative and absolute population information is largely a displacement activity for frustrated clinicians. Managers will often seek to distract you with this idea, as it at least gives them the comfort that they are coming up with something to do.

- *Do act opportunistically.* This is not the same as acting unethically but is about not looking gift horses in the mouth. Funding often arrives on the back of some half-baked initiative or under-spending. Have ready-made projects and ideas which show that money spent with you really is value for money.

- *Do work with partners.* Social services, other mental health services and the local acute trust are all sources of extra resources if you can find ways of allying your goals with theirs. Resources are about much more than just money. Endorsement by a clinician, buildings, expertise, kind words are all tradable commodities – use them.

- *Do reward productive behaviour.* Groups of human beings are good at thinking up better ways of doing things. The resource you already control is often the easiest, and least noticed, source for funding new initiatives and getting improvement.

- *Do hire a first-rate manager/management team.* Someone numerate, determined, good at negotiating and focused on the needs of your service is critical to achieving a healthy and wealthy service. But do not forget that it is clinical decisions which determine the vast bulk of how resources get used. Clinicians may not like it, but they are the ones who determine success or failure for their services. You are a critical part of management.

And if there is time after getting that sorted out, worry about the politics of resource allocation.

References

Department of Health (2000) *The NHS Plan: A Plan for Investment, a Plan for Reform.* TSO (The Stationery Office).

Department of Health (2004) *The NHS Improvement Plan: Putting People at the Heart of Public Services.* TSO (The Stationery Office).

Wanless, D. (2002) *Securing Our Future Health: Taking a Long-Term View.* HM Treasury.

CHAPTER 3

Medical management

Martin Baggaley

Psychiatrists are key members of staff in mental health trusts (or social care or mental health foundation trusts) and the relationship between them and the trust management is crucial to the day-to-day running and development of the organisation. Ideally, psychiatrists should work together with the management team in a collaborative way, in pursuit of a common goal. Unfortunately, in some cases this happy circumstance does not occur and there can be mistrust and antagonism between the two groups. Most mental health organisations have psychiatrists in a management position, either as a medical director or as a clinical director (these two roles are looked at in turn below, before some more general points are made). Such psychiatrists usually continue to have some clinical responsibility. Indeed, one of the challenges of such positions is to retain credibility with both clinical and management colleagues, and without continuing clinical work it is difficult to have either credibility or up-to-date knowledge of issues 'on the ground'. However, there are often competing demands between the management role and the clinical role.

Effective medical managers can have an important role in developing a collaborative way of working and in encouraging psychiatrists to have some corporate responsibility, as well as in maintaining professional standards. The role of a medical manager is usually very challenging and can be stressful but at the same time can be exciting and enjoyable. It is important that a medical manager does not become too closely identified with one or other constituency. In other words, he or she must not become too much of a manager or too much one of the consultant body. The difficulty of the job will depend on the context of the service at the time. It is easier to do the job when services are stable or developing, but less easy when money is short and services are contracting.

Medical director

The medical director has the responsibility to ensure that appropriate systems and mechanisms are in place to safeguard the quality of the clinical

---

Box 3.1 The responsibilities of the medical director

Corporate responsibilities

- Quality of the service
- Service policy development
- Response to a major clinical problem
- Clinical risk management
- Medical workforce planning

Specific trust responsibilities

- Leadership role for psychiatrists
- Clinical governance
- Appraisal of psychiatrists
- Performance management of psychiatrists
- Managing psychiatrists
- Managing the clinical service

External liaison

- Media
- Clinical networks
- Local community
- Service user and carer groups
- Deanery and Royal College

---

service. These responsibilities can be divided into corporate responsibilities, specific trust responsibilities and responsibilities external to the trust, as set out in Box 3.1.

As can be seen from Box 3.1, the remit of the medical director is wide and demanding. It requires a broad range of skills and competencies. In many trusts some of the responsibilities are delegated to other managers, either medical or non-medical. For example, one or more associate medical directors may take responsibility for specific areas, such as clinical governance. There may well be one or more clinical directors who can be delegated tasks (on clinical directors, see below). They, together with associate medical directors, can form a supportive group of medical managers within the trust, as well providing some cross-cover for sickness and leave absence.

The medical director usually sits on the trust board as a director and becomes a key member of the executive. The relationships with the chief executive and chair of the trust in particular are crucial to being a successful medical director. Indeed, it is virtually impossible to be medical director without the support and backing of the chief executive.

Corporate responsibilities

Quality of the service

The medical director has a key role in ensuring that a high-quality service is delivered. This is done by ensuring that:

- the best doctors are recruited and retained
- their morale is high
- they are well trained and have appropriate skills, through excellent and well-funded programmes of continuing professional development (CPD)
- they work well with colleagues of different disciplines in multi-disciplinary teams
- they operate the latest evidence-based practice
- they work to the highest ethical standards
- they understand, help develop and work towards the objectives and policies of the trust.

In a large trust it can be difficult to know how one individual can implement such a list of worthy objectives. However, the behaviour of consultant colleagues is often strongly influenced by the culture of the organisation, which in turn is influenced by the behaviour of those at the top. The medical director, together with other members of the trust executive, therefore has a key role in modelling appropriate behaviour. If the medical director lacks vision and strategic direction, for example, it would not be surprising to find similar deficiency in the consultant workforce as a whole.

Clinical risk management

Risk is an integral part of psychiatric practice and the medical director has a role in ensuring that all clinicians, including psychiatrists, are appropriately trained in clinical risk management and that their practice incorporates good risk management principles. Success in this area can reduce the number of serious clinical incidents which medical directors may be asked to investigate. Part of the process of risk management is ensuring the organisation has robust systems to examine what has gone wrong after a serious untoward incident and why, and to try to prevent it happening again.

Workforce planning

The medical director has a responsibility for ensuring that the trust has the appropriate numbers of medical staff with the necessary skills. The Department of Health's policy is for strategic health authorities to work with the workforce development confederations on what are known as 'local delivery plans' to determine the requirements of trusts for various members of staff, psychiatrists included. Unfortunately, many of the factors that determine the number of good doctors applying for training in psychiatry are beyond the control of medical directors. Furthermore, it is often not possible to expand the numbers of training posts even if there are suitable potential recruits. It is unclear what effect the forthcoming changes to medical training (Modernising Medical Careers, changes to the Royal College of Psychiatrists' Membership examinations and increased emphasis on work placement assessment) will have on recruitment into psychiatry. However, it is likely that for the foreseeable future there will be a shortage of good candidates for consultant posts. Medical directors (and clinical directors) have a key role in recruiting and retaining high-quality doctors. This can be achieved through ensuring that the morale of the consultant workforce is good, making the individual jobs manageable and giving consultants a feeling of being valued by the organisation. In addition, attention should be paid to the experience of doctors coming through the organisation in training posts, as these doctors often prove to be high-quality candidates.

One of the skills is to realise that not all doctors should be managed the same way, although they should be treated equally. In other words, understand their different motivations and worries, and try to find ways to keep people motivated, interested and pushing in the same direction.

Specific trust responsibilities

Appraisal

All psychiatrists require an annual appraisal and it is the responsibility of the medical director (and individual consultants) to ensure that this occurs. It is usually impractical for the medical director to perform all appraisals in the trust; certainly some appraisals may be delegated to clinical directors or other lead consultants.

An appraisal serves a number of purposes: it helps to prepare staff members for revalidation; it is an opportunity to review the job; and it allows for a discussion of career development. The nature and tone of such activities often depends on the state of the relationship between the trust management and the consultant body and individual consultants. In an ideal world, an appraisal should be a positive, enjoyable experience. Increasingly, there is a requirement for a large number of forms to be completed, the exact format of which varies from trust to trust. Provided the documentation is saved electronically, doctors usually find that the process becomes less painful from year to year.

All doctors are now required to have prepared a portfolio for revalidation, for which the appraisal forms a key component. The appraisal documents can form part of this portfolio. It is useful to have the information presented so that it would make sense to someone external to the organisation.

One of the key guiding principles of appraisal is that there should be no surprises. That is, if there are major performance issues which need to be discussed, these should be known about before the actual appraisal meeting. Many consultants genuinely believe that their job is the busiest, least supported and most stressful job in the trust. All consultants cannot be correct about this! It is important, therefore, that as much objective information as possible is available to inform the discussion.

Appraisal is closely linked to job planning and in some organisations the two activities occur simultaneously. This may be impractical however, as the two meetings together would last several hours.

Performance management of psychiatrists

One of the most challenging roles of a medical director is to deal with situations where a psychiatrist is not performing appropriately. There may be one particular incident, such as a serious complaint from a service user or colleague. Alternatively, there may a long history of minor complaints. Many difficulties relate to problems of personality and being unable to work easily in a multidisciplinary team. Others may relate to illness or even to criminal behaviour. In these circumstances it is important to work closely with the trust's human resources/medical staffing director and to follow the appropriate trust policy, which should be compatible with appropriate national policy.

The first step is to investigate the facts fully and this is best done by an independent team before any decision is reached regarding the next step. It is important to follow the process through to its conclusion, which may include a disciplinary hearing and dismissal, although the latter outcome is rare. It is important to keep careful notes at every step. For further information see Department of Health (2003).

Managing psychiatrists

The majority of consultants in England have moved on to the new consultant contract. This is based on a 10-session contract, of which 7.5 sessions are typically involved in patient contact and 2.5 in supporting activities. Each session is 4 hours long. Consultants with extra responsibilities, such as clinical tutors, may have some of their supporting activities dedicated to this purpose. Consultants may negotiate extra sessions if they can show they are working the required number of hours, but these are not pensionable and need to be reviewed each year. There will be pressure to bring most consultants down to ten sessions in due course and consultants are not supposed to be appointed with more than ten sessions. The new contract places specific expectations on consultants and in theory at least allows the trust more control over how consultants spend their time. It was anticipated by the Department of Health that the new consultant contract would increase productivity in return for increased pay. However, to date there is little evidence that this has proved to be the case.

The job planning process is a way in which the needs of the service can be met more effectively by the consultant workforce, such that the day-to-day working practice of the consultant can be changed to meet the needs of the clinical team. This process should be managed by negotiation and mutual agreement. To some extent, as there is a shortage of consultant psychiatrists, it is important to ensure that similar policies exist across neighbouring trusts, to prevent consultants being encouraged to move to whichever trust pays more sessions.

Managing clinical services

The management of clinical services is typically delegated to clinical directors (see below); usually it is a matter of managing psychiatrists within clinical services rather than of managing complete operational services.

External liaison

This should be one of the more enjoyable roles of the medical director, although appearing as a spokesperson following a homicide by a service user under the care of the trust would not be.

It is important to build up relationships with other medical directors and board members in neighbouring trusts (both mental health and acute). At times of crisis, it is much easier if the medical director has a good personal relationship with someone senior who is able to give advice and support. In some parts of the country, for example London, there is a formal meeting of mental health medical directors.

Key relationships with external groups and organisations include those with the Royal College, the Department of Health, the local strategic health authority and the deanery.

The medical director also has a responsibility for developing good relationships with local stakeholders, such as service user and carer groups.

Clinical director

Organisations vary in terms of their structure and therefore the exact role of the clinical director will differ. Some services are arranged along directorate lines (i.e. adult services, old age services, etc.), others along geographical areas (i.e. a borough or primary care trust). Whatever the local circumstances, clinical directors will usually: be involved in directorate management; be responsible for a range of members of staff; have some (often delegated) responsibility for clinical governance; and carry some corporate responsibility.

Directorate management

Clinical directors have operational responsibility for the doctors in the directorate. They may become involved in the organising of rotas and ensuring complaints are dealt with. They may be required to resolve issues such as who is responsible for which patient in case of disputes.

Clinical directors usually have responsibility for the medical budget. In practice the majority of the budget is taken up by salaries and there is therefore often little control over this. It is helpful to have a good relationship with the financial director or accountant and to understand how to read a budget report.

Locums can be very expensive, especially those from agencies. It is useful to have good networks with colleagues who run the local training schemes, as such individuals may know of doctors interested in doing a locum and they can be employed directly, which can work out considerably cheaper.

It is important to have a clear sickness policy and to consider holding 'return to work' interviews for doctors who have had time off, as this can reduce absenteeism.

Responsibility for individuals

Clinical directors manage the doctors within their area of responsibility, including carrying out appraisals. They have a role to play in recruitment and retention of consultants. They should know their colleagues well and be able to identify their strengths and weaknesses and be aware when they are particularly stressed or under pressure.

It is important to treat all colleagues equally and to be open and transparent. Although it may be tempting to respond to colleagues who complain the most, giving in and, say, allocating extra resources without clear justification will cause resentment in others.

Clinical governance

Clinical directors are likely to have responsibility for those areas of clinical governance that relate to medical staff. This role is carried out in conjunction with the trust's clinical governance structures. There is a formal part of the role in ensuring that appropriate meetings are held and minuted. It is more difficult to inspire and encourage clinical teams and psychiatrists within clinical teams to understand fully and to take up the challenge of what clinical governance means at a local level.

Corporate responsibility

Clinical directors are responsible for helping develop the directorate and taking forward the trust vision. This involves engaging colleagues in the agenda the trust is developing and the direction in which it is moving – trying to explain the 'bigger picture' to colleagues and giving an explanation and justification for changes.

Consultant psychiatrists can be surprisingly unaware of organisations and issues at the level of the primary care trust, strategic health authority or Department of Health. They may take a pride in their clinical work but be dismissive of other things. It is the job of the clinical director to inform colleagues of important developments and to suggest which policy statements can be skim read and which are important enough to give some time to read and digest.

Succession planning

There are often few psychiatrists who are either prepared, or have the skills, to take on the role of a medical manager. On some occasions it is possible to recruit medical managers externally, although it can be difficult to attract suitable candidates and there may be problems of acceptance of an external consultant by the existing consultant group. Therefore it is important to identify and develop any potentially suitable internal candidates and engage in succession planning.

Leadership

A successful medical manager must show strong leadership skills. Leadership is often most noticeable when absent in a clinical or medical director. The King's Fund, the NHS Leadership Centre and the British Association of Medical Managers (BAMM) all run courses to help clinicians develop leadership skills (see 'Relevant organisations', below). The process of mentoring by or coaching from a fellow medical director or suitably qualified person may also help a manager develop the necessary leadership skills.

'Leadership' is, though, a much misused term; Kouzes & Posner (2002) suggest that 'Leadership is the art of mobilising others to want to struggle for shared aspirations'. Others have suggested that managing consultant psychiatrists is more akin to attempting to herd a group of cats.

Creating a career pathway

One of the difficulties of becoming a medical manager is planning a satisfactory career. It has been a tradition to become a clinical or medical director for a number of years and then stand down. Some organisations have an informal system of taking turns. This can lead to very unsuitable medical managers being appointed, to the detriment of their own working life and the smooth running of the trust. It is not always easy to return to being an ordinary consultant after having been a leader and manager. It can also be awkward for the colleague who assumes the role to have to manage the ex-director. In addition, there is usually extra remuneration associated with the role, which may not be easy to lose.

Training in medical management

Psychiatrists in training, usually specialist registrars, often request experience in management, and this should be encouraged, considering the importance of succession planning. This can include attendance at various management meetings, attendance at courses (see below) and specific projects. Some psychiatrists undertake a Master of Business Administration (MBA) course in preparation for a career in medical management.

Relevant organisations and further reading

The British Association of Medical Managers (BAMM)

'BAMM exists quite simply to help clinical professionals, whatever their role or specialty, develop and use their leadership and management skills to improve care for patients.' (Dr Jenny Simpson OBE, Chief Executive, BAMM)

'BAMM provides much useful information for medical managers and has regular meetings, produces publications and provides support for medical managers, including psychiatrists.'
Website http://www.bamm.co.uk

NHS Leadership Centre

The NHS Leadership Centre has produced a Leadership Qualities Framework and runs a number of programmes aimed at developing leadership qualities among NHS staff.
Website http://www.nhsleadershipqualities.nhs.uk

King's Fund

The King's Fund is an independent charitable foundation that works for better health, especially in London. It runs a number of leadership programmes for medical and clinical directors.
Website http://www.kingsfund.org.uk

References and further reading

Department of Health (2003) *Maintaining High Performance Standards in the Modern NHS: A Framework for the Initial Handling of Concerns about Doctors and Dentists in the NHS*. (Health Service Circular HSC 2003/012). Department of Health
Kouzes, J. & Posner, B. (2002) *The Leadership Challenge*. Jossey-Bass.
Rogers, J. (2004) *Coaching Skills*. Open University Press.

CHAPTER 4

Doctors and managers

Stuart Bell

Historical background

In his book *The Rise of Professional Society*, the social historian Harold Perkin (1989) examines the change that took place in England between 1880 and the 1980s and established professions as a dominant form of social structure. In 1880, he notes, 'there were still only twenty-seven qualifying associations … (counting the four Inns of Court for Barristers and the two Royal Colleges and the Society of Apothecaries for medical doctors), but thereafter there was enormous expansion'. By 1970 another 140 had been added, plus an even larger body of non-qualifying but professionally oriented associations. Society, in short, had become professionalised, reflecting both the growing specialisation of skills following the Industrial Revolution and the growing role of government and its agencies in everyday life. As the roles and numbers of professions grew, so more and more people became correspondingly 'lay' with respect to an increasing number of areas of expertise.

The high point of this professional dominance may have been the establishment of the welfare state in the aftermath of the Second World War, when the very institutions of the state's social welfare programme itself were shaped around pre-existing or rapidly developing professional groups – the education system around teachers and lecturers, family and individual welfare around social workers, and so forth. In the National Health Service (NHS), for example, before the mid-1980s, separate, professionally determined hierarchies existed for hospital doctors, public health doctors, general practitioners (GPs), nurses, administrators, accountants and, at lower levels, the other clinical professions. No one was in charge overall and each of the different groups had substantial autonomy to run its own realm. Where decisions required agreement between the different groups they were not guaranteed to be made. Regulation and setting of standards was left to each of the different professional groups to determine for itself, and so professional bodies like the Royal Colleges exerted considerable influence over NHS policy – it was expected that they should – and when the Ministry of Health needed advice on policy it would turn first to them.

Writing in the late 1980s, Perkin sought to explain the apparent attack on the autonomy of professionals which began to emerge then. Doctors, teachers, lawyers and others were all being enjoined to become more accountable and began to lose some of their historical privileges. Rather than seeing this as a turn against the growth in professionalisation across society as a whole, he interprets it instead as part of a struggle for hegemony between the older established professions and the newer, emerging professions, such as economics, marketing and accountancy. The paradox is that as society has become more and more dominated by professions – as the model established by the church, the law and medicine has become pervasive – so the power and authority of any one individual profession has been weakened, and the rivalry between them has grown. When governments have required advice on health policy, since the 1980s they have turned successively to civil servants, NHS managers and management consultants before settling most recently on think-tanks and policy specialists, whose principal occupation is to develop policy rather than to put it into practice – professional advisors and policy-makers.

The nature of management

Is management itself a profession participating in this struggle? There have undoubtedly been attempts to cast it as such, and there are sub-components of managerial activity which have certainly become professionalised, be they the use and application of information technology, or accountancy, or the various forms of analysis and modelling – economic and otherwise. Nevertheless, management in its most general sense has proved remarkably resistant to traditional professional categorisation. It remains, in the UK at least, an unrestricted occupation – anyone can become a manager. The 'mystery' at the heart of the profession – the ability to organise and direct collective activity – is hard to pin down as a body of knowledge which can formally be imparted (it sometimes sounds rather more like trying to teach common sense). Attempts in recent times to establish it as a quasi-profession – the Management Charter Initiative in the 1990s, for example – have never really gained momentum.

Management, in short, fails to meet the essential conditions to be a profession, although it does draw on, and is heavily influenced by, bodies of knowledge and theory developed by some of the newer professions, with which it is often closely connected. However, this distinction is not clearly drawn, partly because there are some managers who would very much like their occupation to be, or to be seen to be, a profession, and partly because there are those – perhaps some management consultancies, for example – who might wish, for business reasons, to turn it into a 'mystery' which is inaccessible to those who are not initiates. This has become particularly confused in the development of management education – especially the

Master in Business Administration (MBA) (surely the litmus test of professionalism is the qualifying degree?).

Henry Mintzberg, a distinguished US professor of management, who was instrumental in the development of the MBA as a qualification, now argues that its dominance has distorted our understanding of the nature of management:

'It is time to recognize conventional MBA programs for what they are ... specialized training in the functions of business, not general educating in the practice of managing. Using the classroom to help develop people already practicing management is a fine idea, but pretending to create managers out of people who have never managed is a sham' (Mintzberg, 2004: p. 5).

Mintzberg argues that management is a blend of three distinct elements: the craft – experience; the art – insight; the science – analysis. The MBA really only equips people for the last of these, and gives a misleading quasi-professional veneer, which at best only partially equips people for managerial jobs, while at worst giving them an inflated sense of their preparedness and competence to undertake them. Instead, he argues that management is neither a science nor a profession, and therefore it cannot be taught to people without experience – 'there is no one best way to manage; it depends on the situation'.

Above all, then, management is dependent on, and must respond to, context. It is perhaps also worth making the point (as it is often missed) that as well as drawing on some of the newer professions for its techniques and models, where longer-established professions are an important part of that context – as in the health service and, indeed, in any of the sectors established by the welfare state in the 1940s – management will, sometimes indiscernibly, assimilate much of the thinking behind their traditions. In health, of course, this will not be confined to the profession of medicine – nor should it be – but it is often underestimated how much it does matter to the ability to manage health services to have a deep knowledge of the way the 'industry' works, in detail, at the clinical level.

Health service management

Good health service managers learn as they develop, just as good supermarket managers must learn how their stores work if they are to run them successfully, or good investment bankers must understand the financial markets. It must be added, of course, that all must also have the imagination to be able to see how their enterprises work from the perspective of their clients (patients or customers) as well. One of the more bizarre and interesting myths perpetrated when general management was introduced to the NHS in the mid-1980s was that bringing in managers from industry was all that was needed to sort matters out (it still resurfaces from time to time). Some who came made a success of it – they learnt quickly and well – and the bringing in of new blood was useful in making the point that the NHS should not be regarded as the exclusive preserve of those who had always inhabited it. In contrast, those who thought it possible to apply some abstract form of management without learning the context – the detail of their adopted industry – rapidly came to grief.

There are obvious attractions in an approach to management that is affected by, and therefore alert to, the values and ideas of those professions inhabiting the world with which it has most to do, and that is also realistic about the dominance that management may obtain at a particular point in time. Does this, though, mean that management itself is inherently devoid of underlying values and principles? Perhaps so, but that is a far cry from individual managers being devoid of either. Indeed, it is difficult to manage large groups of people for a sustained period if it is not possible to generate some sense of shared purpose, which must, in the end, be more than a short-term tactical or transactional community of interest; that shared purpose relies on a strong sense of shared collective value. The difference is that management does not come with a preset collection of values to be applied to whomever and whatever is managed and irrespective of the circumstances.

The values come from the individuals involved, the context of the industry and the nature of the task in hand. There is now also a well-established body of management theory which managers can use, examining how and why people and systems work together more or less successfully. It draws on a wide range of other disciplines and ways of thinking, from the hydraulic to the psychotherapeutic, but, in the end, individual managers will need to formulate their own views of how their managerial world works – how the external environment looks, what motivates the people they work with, what sets the culture, and what of that is to be built on and what must be challenged. In doing so, they will be obliged to address issues of principle and to set out their values; if they are purely synthetic and designed solely for the circumstances, that is very likely to be detected, and will not work for long.

How, then, is this phenomenon – not properly a profession, eclectic in its choice of theory, hugely sensitive to context and difficult to pin down precisely – viewed from the standpoint of a much more clear-cut profession like medicine, which apparently enshrines the scientific evidence base, the defined (if ever-expanding) body of knowledge and formally policed professional codes of conduct? A familiar response is to judge it as though it were a conventionally understood profession – 'either they don't know what they're doing, in which case they're useless, or they do know what they're doing, in which case they're not telling us about it' – and to find it lacking. This misses the essential point that we are examining a fundamentally different phenomenon. Managers often make the same mistake in reverse – exasperated by the apparent rigidity of professional groups in the face of what to them appears a decisively changed context, they can see the characteristics of a profession as a set of rather selective and perhaps even self-serving artificial constructs designed to preserve the status quo and to resist necessary change.

Where this mistrust occurs it creates problems – of divergence of priorities, poor-quality decision-making, failure to tackle issues which must be faced, putting off that which must be done sooner rather than later, with delay leading only to problems of even greater intractability. Such failure of mutual understanding is also susceptible to exploitation by others – by other professions, which can be tempted to use mutual incomprehension between doctors and managers to advance their own positions – and perhaps most of all by the external world, be it in the form of politicians, the media or the general public. Notice how frequently the tactic of fastening on the rather abstract notion of the numbers of managers in the NHS is adopted as a means of redirecting an uncomfortable debate about some aspect of healthcare. (What is the correct number? How does it compare with other healthcare systems or comparable industries? These questions are rarely part of the discussion.) A favourite alternative device is to portray the apparent intransigence of doctors as a professional group – conservative, self-interested and shroud-waving – again as a distraction from a significant issue or as a way of weakening influence.

Is this an international phenomenon? That is harder to say, as the structures of the healthcare industry vary so much from country to country. In some parts of the world there is a much older and more established tradition of the direct involvement of doctors in managerial activity – the development of specific branches of the profession for those who undertake such roles on a more or less full-time basis, for example. Curiously enough, this was a model which was common in mental health services as they developed in the 19th century in the UK – indeed, it was an important part of the origins of the Royal College of Psychiatrists – but it lapsed as the asylums closed and community services were developed. Perhaps it was a victim of the apparent triumph of the professions at the point the welfare state was established – they no longer needed to exercise a significant managerial role, because the very structures of their industry as it was established at that time allowed them to exercise control through purely professional structures.

The extent to which healthcare is provided directly by the state also makes a difference – the model of the independent practitioner being paid for specific interventions by insurers leads to a different tradition of management. Interestingly, the impulse towards a much more managed approach to care in the United States is being driven as much by concerns over the quality and reliability of care as by the need to manage resource use familiar in state-funded systems (Lawrence, 2002). In the UK, private healthcare has traditionally tended to keep the management of institutions separate from the management of clinical practice, but it has operated in a relatively unchallenged, profitable and uncompetitive market until recently.

Now there is much more of a tendency among private healthcare providers systematically to introduce managed care pathways and protocols and to exert more control over individual clinical practice to adapt to changing market conditions. As expenditure on healthcare grows, and as the boundary between state and privately funded systems becomes more permeable, this tendency is likely to continue.

Healthcare and management

The separation of the management of the institution from the management of clinical practice was for a long time a strong feature of the relationship between doctors and managers. When the last edition of this book was published (in 1995) there was a detailed discussion of clinical freedom and rationing, as the tension between the overall availability of resources and the ability of doctors to act as they thought best for their individual patients was played out. At that time, the manager's responsibility extended to ensuring that an institution balanced its books overall, but, other than in exceptional cases, it did not play a key role in the operation of clinical practice. There has been a decisive change since then, with the advent of clinical governance, which very clearly places upon an institution – an NHS board – the responsibility for the clinical quality of the services it provides; that is now just as much a part of its statutory duty as the need to manage its finances.

This has developed in parallel with the growing challenge within professions, as part of their development as professions, to the notion that, once qualified, members are sent forth to respond as they see fit to any circumstances they may encounter. The notion has taken hold of an increasingly well defined body of appropriate practice, based on a systematic and regularly reviewed appraisal of the evidence available, as the benchmark of what one would expect to see in the majority of cases, the exceptions being those where an alternative approach is explicitly justified. This has replaced the idea of individual professionals carrying around a personal body of knowledge, which they then apply as they think best in a succession of individual circumstances, over which they hold considerable discretion, the adequacy of which was a matter principally for their profession to judge.

This has come with the growth of guidelines and systematic reviews and, perhaps above all, the phenomenal growth in the sheer body of knowledge available – way beyond the capacity of any individual to assimilate in its entirety. It also reflects the growing willingness of society at large to challenge, or at the very least to expect justification for, professional practice. This growth has had an interesting effect on the relationship between doctors and managers in the realm of clinical practice. On the one hand, there is much more mutual interest in clinical practice for its own sake – how effective is it, how good is it, how unusual is it? It is no longer possible to take an interest merely in how expensive it is. While debates about rationing still occur, they now tend to contain a significant element about the effectiveness of a particular treatment, although that can get mired in the complexity of processes for determining effectiveness. On the other hand, these questions are now legitimately – even, given the statutory responsibilities, necessarily – in the managerial domain, too. While that is a far cry from the managerial determination of what constitutes good professional practice (although it is true that such questions have also been opened up much more widely in recent years, most importantly to patients themselves), it is now much more of a collective than an individual decision, and that alters the nature of the discourse.

There is also a growing international recognition that even when there are no constraints on individual doctors' activities – where they are paid for each specific thing they do – this:

'encourages doctors to do too much and rewards those who perform procedures and surgery instead of focusing on diagnosis, prevention and education. Dr William Richardson, chair of the Institute of Medicine studies on quality and safety, describes that system as "toxic to quality"' (Lawrence, 2002: p. 25).

Thankfully, given these dramatic changes, there is now much more movement between managerial and medical roles than during the first 50 years of the NHS, and distinctive medical management roles have emerged and established themselves as an essential component of a successful service (as discussed elsewhere in this volume). This has undoubtedly improved mutual understanding between doctors and managers. It is also the case that very many full-time managers in healthcare – perhaps most of all in mental health services – come from some kind of clinical background, although nurses, social workers, psychologists and occupational therapists are much better represented than doctors. In part this is because of the structure and length of medical training and the absence, still, in the UK, of a structured career path for doctors who wish to develop into a managerial role at an early stage. Perhaps national cultural assumptions about the role of management have a role to play too – French institutions, for example, exalt the technocrat, but it is part of the English tradition to look down upon 'trade'. It is still an occasional put-down to refer to a manager as an 'administrator', but one which these days reveals more about the speaker than about the subject. Such an epithet would be seen as a distinct social advantage in France.

Management in psychiatry

But is medicine all one amorphous mass in this respect? Is it not just as easy to caricature doctors as managers and at the same time to misunderstand important differences in approach and culture between the varieties of medicine? This question relates not only to the various specialties but also to the nature of medicine as it develops over time. Thomas (1984), in his delightful book *The Youngest Science*, describes the evolution of medical practice in the United States over the course of the 20th century, from his father's time before the First World War to the end of his own career in the 1980s. He trained at Harvard in the 1930s and describes the proficiency of his professor at diagnosis as follows:

'so far as I know from that three months of close contact ... he was never wrong, not once. But I can recall only three or four patients for whom the diagnosis resulted in the possibility of doing something to change the course of the illness... For the majority, the disease had to be left to run its own course for better or worse' (p. 31).

There followed a revolution in the scientific basis of intervention in medicine and he goes on to describe how this transformed the task of the doctor from that of being an accurate diagnostician and impotent but valued describer of the course of an illness to that of scientific researcher into the basis of disease and a skilled intervener in its course.

At the same time, the promise of all-conquering science sometimes raises expectations to a point where they cannot be met, and so the paradox is, despite unprecedented success, there is disappointment for patients and frustration for practitioners. The very nature of the development of medical science – in its various specialties – has a bearing on how its practitioners are constrained to interact with those around them.

Perhaps of all the medical specialties psychiatry comes closest to many of the preoccupations of management: it has to deal with high levels of uncertainty; it draws from a wide range of theoretical traditions – the biological, psychological and social; context is as important as technical diagnosis in understanding how to institute effective treatment. Are managers and psychiatrists in mental health services then closer together than at first sight might appear to be the case? This suggests great potential for even better mutual understanding and respect, but the two occupations are not the same, and there is sometimes a greater risk of misunderstanding between those who are closest together than between those where the differences are clear and distinct.

Nevertheless, the opportunity exists for collaboration and the converse is true – where relationships are chronically poor between doctors and managers, the service and the patient and the business will suffer. There may be many reasons for poor relations and a similar range of solutions – including at the extreme, getting new managers, or new doctors, or both – but the task for those who are interested in making things better, irrespective of whether they are good or bad to start off with, is to find ways of understanding what the other is trying to do, the constraints upon them, and how they are viewed by their wider professional community or the spheres which influence them.

How, then, to find out more about this – to understand what makes managers tick? Conventional medical training offers limited opportunities for this, and where they exist they are at a relatively late stage – mostly at specialist registrar level. There are short courses in management run as a part of some schemes and also by the Royal College of Psychiatrists and institutions like the King's Fund. They are worthwhile, but they are very much a snapshot. There is the British Association of Medical Managers (BAMM), which has gone some way in recent years to remedy the historic deficit in institutions supporting and promoting medical management in the UK. There are good opportunities in every trust to find out more by attending board meetings (they are usually held in public), by shadowing managers as they go about their work (and by having managers shadow clinicians as they go about theirs) and by undertaking projects (as part of a special interest) which relate to management problems. One of the most valuable experiences in my own development as a health service manager was working closely with a doctor – a medical administrator from the Australian tradition – and learning to see the functioning of the hospital from that perspective.

Conclusion

What, then, is the joint enterprise between doctors and managers when they are working together effectively? Increasingly, it is the success of the clinical business. An important recent shift in the system of care – affecting public and private operators – is the growing distinction of the role of provision from that of commissioning services. This is something we are still working through, and one that is never, in practice, as clear cut as it might seem at first glance, but the essential point is that an organisation providing services is there to fulfil a task – not simply 'to be'. That being the case, those in charge of it must concern themselves with the quality, reliability, coverage and scope, effectiveness, outcomes, productivity and profitability of the services they run. If they do not, then they will ultimately fail, to the disservice of patients, practitioners and the institution as a whole. Now more than ever, success can come only as a result of joint enterprise between doctors and managers, built on a sound, shared understanding of the world in which they work and a good knowledge of what each brings to the task.

References

Lawrence, D. (2002) *From Chaos to Care – The Promise of Team Based Medicine*. Perseus Publishing.
Mintzberg, D. (2004) *Managers not MBAs*. Prentice Hall.
Perkin, H. (1989) *The Rise of Professional Society*. Routledge.
Thomas, L. (1984) *The Youngest Science*. Oxford: Oxford University Press.

CHAPTER 5

The National Service Framework for Mental Health, the NHS Plan and *Valuing People*

Graham Thornicroft and Amanda Reynolds

This chapter looks at three key policy documents for the National Health Service (NHS): the National Service Framework for Mental Health (currently one of nine National Service Frameworks, which were introduced from 1998 in a rolling programme); the NHS Plan (published as a command paper in 2000); and *Valuing People*, the White Paper on intellectual disability (also known as learning disability in UK health services). Together these form the cornerstones of mental health policy in England.

The National Service Framework for Mental Health

The National Service Framework for Mental Health (NSFMH) (Department of Health, 1999*a*) is a strategic blueprint for services (to 2009) for adults of working age. It is both mandatory, in being a clear statement of what services must seek to achieve in relation to the given standards and performance indictors, and permissive, in that it allows considerable local flexibility to customise the services which need to be provided to fit the framework. This section of the chapter summarises the process by which the NSF was created, and its content.

Scope

The stated aims of the NSFMH are:

- to help drive up quality
- to remove the wide and unacceptable variations in provision
- to set national standards and to define service models for promoting mental health and treating mental illness
- to put in place underpinning programmes to support local delivery
- to establish milestones and a specific group of high-level performance indicators against which progress within agreed timescales will be measured.

The scope includes health promotion, primary care services, local mental health and social care services, those with mental health problems and substance misuse, and more specialised mental health services, including all forensic ones.

The NSFMH therefore encompasses a wide range of service activities, including those provided by local authorities as well as health authorities. It draws upon a review of a vast array of evidence, including some from other countries, especially in relation to the national standards set by the NSFMH. In that review, each part of the evidence base was graded according to the strength of the research in five categories:

- type I – at least one good systematic review and at least one randomised controlled trial (RCT)
- type II – at least one good RCT
- type III – at least one well-designed intervention study without randomisation
- type IV – at least one one well-designed observational study
- type V – expert opinion, including the opinions of service users and carers.

Before writing its NSFMH, the Department of Health established an External Reference Group (ERG), chaired by Graham Thornicroft, to offer advice on its content. The ERG met from July 1998 and submitted its advice to ministers at the end of January 1999. The group included over 40 members, and also co-opted a further 30 members from a wide range of stakeholders, including service users, managers, nurses, psychiatrists, national voluntary organisations, social care and primary care services, and national carers' organisations.

At an early stage, the ERG established seven critical issues facing services for adults with mental health problems, which the NSFMH had to address if it was to succeed:

1 insufficient involvement of users and carers
2 stigmatising public attitudes
3 poor agreement on service aims and boundaries
4 patchy and sometimes limited provision of services
5 lack of financial resources
6 workforce problems
7 lack of clear accountability.

Core values and principles

The ERG also established a consensus on the fundamental values that should be used to guide practical service developments, namely that services should:

- show openness and honesty
- demonstrate respect and offer courtesy

- be allocated fairly and provided equitably
- be proportional to clients' needs
- be open to learning and change.

Upon this foundation, services should also be guided by the following core fundamental principles:

- services meaningfully involve users and their carers
- they deliver high-quality treatment and care which are effective and acceptable
- they are non-discriminatory
- they are accessible (i.e. help is given when and where it is needed)
- they promote the safety of service users, their carers, staff and the wider public
- they offer choices which promote independence
- they are well coordinated between all staff and agencies
- they empower and support their staff
- they deliver continuity of care as long as needed
- they are accountable to the public, users and carers.

National standards

In the NSFMH, standards have been set in five areas:

- mental health promotion (standard 1)
- primary care and access to services (standards 2 and 3)
- effective services for people with severe mental illness (standards 4 and 5)
- caring about carers (standard 6)
- preventing suicide (standard 7).

Standard 1: Mental health promotion

Health and social services should:

- promote mental health for all, working with individuals and communities
- combat discrimination against individuals and groups with mental health problems, and promote their social inclusion.

Standard 2: Primary care and access to services

Any service users who contact their primary healthcare team with a common mental health problem should:

- have their mental health needs identified and assessed
- be offered effective treatments, including referral to specialist services for further assessment, treatment and care if they require it.

Standard 3: Primary care and access to services

Any individual with a common mental health problem should:

- be able to make contact round the clock with the local services necessary to meet their needs and receive adequate care
- be able to use NHS Direct, as it develops, for first-level advice and referral on to specialist helplines or to local services.

Standard 4: Severe mental illness

All mental health service users on the care programme approach (CPA) should:

- receive care which optimises engagement, anticipates or prevents a crisis, and reduces risk
- have a copy of a written care plan which:
  - includes the action to be taken in a crisis by the service users, their carers and their care coordinator
  - advises their general practitioner (GP) how to respond if the service user needs additional help
  - is regularly reviewed by their care coordinator
- be able to access services 24 hours a day, 365 days a year.

Standard 5: Severe mental illness

Each service user who is assessed as requiring a period of care away from home should have:

- timely access to an appropriate hospital bed or alternative bed or place, which is:
  - in the least restrictive environment consistent with the need to protect the service user and the public
  - as close to home as possible
- a copy of a written after-care plan agreed on discharge which sets out the care and rehabilitation to be provided, identifies the care coordinator and specifies the action to be taken in a crisis.

Standard 6: Caring about carers

All individuals who provide regular and substantial care for a person on the CPA should:

- have an assessment of their caring, physical and mental health needs, repeated at least annually
- have their own written care plan which is given to them and implemented in discussion with them.

Standard 7: Preventing suicide

Local health and social care communities should prevent suicides by:

- promoting mental health for all, working with individuals and communities (standard 1)
- delivering high-quality primary mental healthcare (standard 2)
- ensuring that anyone with a mental health problem can contact local services via the primary care team, a helpline or an accident and emergency department (standard 3)
- ensuring that individuals with severe mental illness have a care plan which meets their specific needs, including access to services round the clock (standard 4)
- providing safe hospital accommodation for individuals who need it (standard 5)
- enabling individuals caring for someone with severe mental illness to receive the support which they need to continue to care (standard 6).

Primary care trusts

Primary care trusts are set to take over the commissioning, and also in some cases the provision, of what are currently known as secondary, or specialist, mental health services, including general adult in-patient units, if they can satisfy the following criteria of having:

- service user and carer involvement
- advocacy arrangements
- integration of care management and the CPA
- effective partnerships with primary healthcare, social services, housing and other agencies, including, where appropriate, the independent sector
- board membership that includes competent management of specialist mental health services
- proportioned representation of mental health professionals on the executive of the primary care trust.

Implementation of the NSFMH

The importance of such ambitious and far-reaching plans can be measured by the extent to which they are implemented. Already, a concerted implementation strategy has been initiated, including:

- establishing a multi-agency National Service Framework national implementation team
- starting regional implementation teams
- bringing together local teams to produce a strategic plan on how to implement the NSFMH.

It is therefore clear that the government is serious about putting this strategy into practice. It has also set a series of more specific milestones, with clear deadlines:

- The White Paper *Saving Lives: Our Healthier Nation* (Department of Health, 1999b) sets the target of a reduction in the suicide rate by at least one-fifth by 2010.
- NHS Direct was set to be rolled out to cover 60% of the country by the end of 1999 and the whole of England by the end of 2000.
- Mixed-sex accommodation was to be removed from hospitals and no new mixed-sex wards will be approved. By the year 2002, 95% of health authorities should have removed mixed-sex accommodation.
- A reduction of two percentage points was due in the rate of psychiatric emergency readmissions by April 2002, from 14.3% to 12.3%.
- Health improvement programmes (HIMPs) should have demonstrated by April 2000 linkages between NHS organisations and partners to promote mental health in schools, workplaces and neighbourhoods for individuals at risk and for groups who are most vulnerable, and to combat discrimination and social exclusion of people with mental health problems.
- Clinical governance reports should have been introduced before the end of 2000.
- By the end of 2001, protocols were to be agreed and implemented between primary care and specialist services for the management of depression and postnatal depression, anxiety disorders, schizophrenia and drug and alcohol dependence, as well as for those requiring psychological therapies.

In addition to this, further work has been commissioned for the Department of Health, including workforce planning, education and training, research and development, clinical decision support systems, and the introduction of a national minimum psychiatric data-set from 2003.

Workforce planning

Since little of the NSFMH can be practised without sufficient capacity of a competent workforce, a Workforce Action Team was set up:

- to review the current staffing position for psychiatric sub-specialties, mental health nursing, child psychology, professions allied to medicine (therapies), social work, link-workers and advocates, and care and support staff
- to establish the staffing profile in relation to the level of services needed by the population, service users and carers
- to commission work on skill mix to inform future workforce planning (this was to include an advisory group on the delivery of psychological therapies through the range of health and social care staff)
- to establish future workforce requirements for 2002 and 2005, and the planning assumptions to meet them

- to verify the availability of suitably qualified staff and the timescales required to provide the necessary training
- Need to mention "capable practitioner" published by Workforce Action Team, spring 2001. Also skills audit? Autumn 2001. Both are being taken forward as part of NSF

Does the Framework work?

This government document is unlike many others in recent years, in that it is clearly built upon an evidence base, it has a very wide remit – covering all services relevant to adults of working age who have mental health problems – and it has specific performance indicators, with clear timescales, by which its implementation can be monitored. It contains some elements which build upon current good practice, such as the recognition and treatment of common mental disorders in primary care, but it also includes new standards that are designed to effect a step-change in clinical practice, such as the requirement to assess the needs of carers formally, and the option for primary care trusts to provide specialist mental health treatment and care. It is in this mix of extending the best of current practice and through adding new demands of mental health services that the NSFMH is a challenge to practitioners to provide better in the future than in the past for both patients and families.

The NHS Plan

The NHS Plan was presented to Parliament in July 2000. It reinforces and reintroduces the key principles of the NHS, in stating that the NHS will:

- provide a universal service for all, based on clinical need, not ability to pay
- provide a comprehensive range of services
- shape its services around the needs and preferences of individual patients, their families and their carers
- respond to the different needs of different populations
- work continuously to improve services and to minimise errors
- support and value its staff
- devote public funds for healthcare solely to NHS patients
- work together with others to ensure a seamless service for patients
- help keep people healthy and work to reduce health inequalities
- respect the confidentiality of individual patients and provide open access to information about services, treatment and performance.

The reforms set out in the NHS Plan are intended to be challenging for every part of the NHS. The executive summary states:

'This is a Plan for investment in the NHS with sustained increases in funding. This is a Plan for reform with far reaching changes across the NHS. The purpose and vision of this NHS Plan is to give the people of Britain a health service fit for the 21st century: a health service designed around the patient'.

The NHS Plan promises reforms around every area of the NHS, in what is provided and the style of care delivery (Chapter 9 considers its effect on community care). It seeks to increase the involvement of patients in how the NHS is run.

At a national level, the NHS Plan provides for:

- a monitoring role for the National Institute for Health and Clinical Excellence (NICE)
- best practice and change to be overseen by the newly created Modernisation Agency
- quicker government intervention over failing hospitals
- the establishment of a National Performance Fund to support hospitals that are improving
- care trusts to pool health and social services staff and resources for vulnerable client groups (i.e. elderly people and those with mental health problems)
- new NHS contacts for GPs and hospital doctors
- patient power through the establishment of PALS (patient advice and liaison services) in every hospital to provide better information, access to their own clinical information, patient surveys and regular forums.

Targets for mental health services

The NHS Plan contains key targets and milestones for the health and social care sectors. There are in fact 640 targets, covering all areas of healthcare. The 10-year plan for mental health services set out in the NSFMH is reinforced in the NHS Plan, but it also goes further, by introducing new structures for mental health services:

- To ensure that mental health and social care provision can be properly integrated locally, statutory powers will be taken to permit the establishment of combined mental health and social care trusts.
- The Mental Health Act 1993 is being reformed to create a new legislative framework reflecting modern patterns of care and treatment for severe mental illness. The focus will be on managing risk and providing better health outcomes for patients.
- The government is also considering proposals for those people with severe personality disorder who present a high risk to the public. By 2004, an additional 140 new secure places and 75 specialist rehabilitation hostel places had been provided for people with severe personality disorder; in total these employ almost 400 extra staff.

Valuing People: a strategy for services for people with intellectual disability

Since the launch of the NSFMH in 1999, local health and social care services have been busy planning the changes required to implement the new models of care. Meanwhile, a revolution has been going on in intellectual disability services also. When the White Paper *Valuing People: A New Strategy for Learning Disability for the 21st Century* was published in March 2001, it was the first strategy for intellectual disability services in 30 years (Department of Health, 2001). The strategy promises to revolutionise these services and how they might relate to mental health services, and therefore the White Paper needs to be considered alongside the implementation of the NSFMH.

The key themes and provisions of the White Paper included the following:

- Partnership boards in each area are to oversee the implementation of the strategy, and should include all key agencies.
- The important role of housing, education and employment is to be emphasised.
- All people with intellectual disabilities should be supported to access primary care and mainstream health services.
- A small number of people with intellectual disabilities will require access to specialist health services.
- Community intellectual disability teams are to refocus, to become health facilitators.
- A 5-year programme to modernise council day services was set up.
- The first national performance targets for intellectual disability services were set out.
- Advocacy services were introduced as a right and were to be developed in each local system.
- People with intellectual disabilities and their carers were to be involved in decision-making.
- An intellectual disability awards framework was to provide a new qualification route for care workers.

Implications for mental health services

The White Paper reminds us that most psychiatric disorders are more common among people with intellectual disabilities than in the general population. It goes on to require the NSFMH to incorporate adults with a intellectual disability who also have a mental illness. It assumes that those with an intellectual disability should also be cared for within the framework of the CPA/care management. It also sets some specific objectives:

65

- Clear local protocols are to be put in place for collaboration between specialist intellectual disability services and specialist mental health services.
- Specialist staff from the learning disability service will if necessary provide support to crisis resolution/home treatment services or other alternatives to in-patient admission wherever possible.
- Each local service should have access to an acute assessment and treatment resource for the small number of individuals with significant intellectual disabilities and mental health problems who cannot appropriately be admitted to general psychiatric services even with specialist support.
- Specialist local services are to be developed for people with an intellectual disability and challenging behaviour.
- Intellectual disability community services are to refocus, to become health facilitators to primary care. The role will include health promotion, health facilitation, teaching and service development

The strategy for intellectual disabilities is clear: for the majority of people, their needs are social and we must move away from the tendency to medicalise those with an intellectual disability. A small number of individuals have both mental illness and an intellectual disability, and there is now a need for services (intellectual disability, mental health and more generally primary care) to collaborate at many levels to improve access.

At present, people with an intellectual disability and mental health problems fall in between services and their needs are not met. The situation is even worse for those who have a borderline cognitive impairment and who are caught in the grey area of intellectual disability and mental health services. In some areas local community mental health teams report that about 15% of their population has a degree of intellectual disability or borderline cognitive impairment and would benefit from input from intellectual disabilities services. Several of these people may also have autistic spectrum disorders, including Asperger syndrome. They would have been admitted to one of the long-term institutions in the past, but now with community care their needs should be met by community resources. In some areas, and particularly London, several hundred people with intellectual disabilities have been placed far away from their families and their local neighbourhoods because of lack of local services.

For the future, a range of exciting areas of collaboration exist, for example to address the needs of mental health user groups of people with both intellectual disabilities and mental health problems, and responding to the challenges of providing services to Black and ethnic minority groups.

References

Department of Health (1999a) *The National Service Framework for Mental Health. Modern Standards and Service Models*. Department of Health.

Department of Health (1999*b*) *Saving Lives: Our Healthier Nation.* TSO (The Stationery Office).

Department of Health (2000) *The NHS Plan. A Plan for Investment. A Plan for Reform.* TSO (The Stationery Office).

Department of Health (2001) *Valuing People. A New Strategy for Learning Disability for the 21st Century.* TSO (The Stationery Office).

CHAPTER 6

Resources

Stuart Bell

The overwhelming majority of UK health service resources are raised from general taxation and National Insurance contributions, and that fact has a direct bearing on their size, their allocation, their use and how they are accounted for. Monies for the National Health Service (NHS) are voted by Parliament as part of the wider mechanisms for the allocation of public funds. Those used to operate on an annual cycle, determined in part by the projected availability of tax revenues, which were shaped in turn by the performance of the wider economy. There was often a complex and hurried wrangle of bidding and negotiation between the main spending departments of state and the Treasury. That sometimes led to difficulty in longer-term planning, often with stop–start discontinuities in funding, and so, more recently, a system of comprehensive spending reviews (CSRs) has taken a periodic 3-year forward look across all public services. The CSRs set overall resource limits for a longer period on a rolling cycle. The NHS has been a particular beneficiary of that approach because, following the publication of the Wanless report in 2002, and the linked decision to raise public spending on healthcare in England to a percentage of the nation's gross domestic product comparable with the (then) European Union average, the resource limits for health, but for health alone, were set for the period of two CSR cycles – until 2008. That unprecedented period of clarity about forward spending plans, combined with a commitment to raise expenditure as a share of the national cake, has had a number of interesting consequences.

There are obvious advantages in the ability to plan ahead, but for them to be fully realised the internal distribution mechanisms within the Department of Health and the NHS need to work to a similarly long-term planning horizon. That means having clear plans for the resources across the whole of the period, not just the next year or two, and that has not always happened. There is also a commensurate inflexibility, in that there are no opportunities to go back to ask for more funds if plans change, and so everything must be managed within the totals set over the 6-year period – a particular problem when new ideas and attractive initiatives not even imagined back in 2002 come along in the course of the following years.

Against that must be set the advantage of the removal of the risk that the enthusiasm behind a 2002 commitment to growth in the NHS might, under the more usual arrangements, have been overtaken by other governmental priorities in the meanwhile, and certainly there is little sympathy from other public services for the plight of health services, which have consistently done better than them in terms of their share of public funding in recent years.

More ominously within this lurks a kind of financial hubris. First, there is now much greater political and public interest in how much and how well money is being spent on health services, and accounting for and explaining that is a far from straightforward task. Second, we have become used to both stability and growth in health service resources, but beyond 2008 the overall financial circumstances in which publicly funded health services operate will probably change significantly. That would indeed be all the more worrying if the resources had not been used to best advantage in the meanwhile, but had instead bred a sense of false comfort and even complacency.

The recent widely reported financial strains on the NHS – 2 years before the end of the period of growth – have, whatever the facts of the case, brought those points into sharp focus, and they will be an inevitable part of the background to any debate about the resources publicly funded healthcare should enjoy, and where they might come from. Whatever the outcome of that debate, it is unlikely that there will be a period of financial growth and stability in the 6 years following 2008 equivalent to that preceding it.

How are resources distributed?

The bulk of funding for health services is distributed by the Department of Health to local primary care trusts (PCTs). The sum given to each is based on a formula which starts with population served and adjusts for various factors to take account of morbidity – principally the age and sex structure, but with refinements added over the years as both data improve and research tells us which others have most influence on health need. Nevertheless, the process is not straightforward, even the measure of population being a subject of major debate. The source for population data has been the census administered by the Office for National Statistics (ONS). This has the obvious limitation of only occurring every 10 years, and so allocations can be based only on estimates in the intervening period. Different methods of estimation can give substantially different results, particularly when applied to relatively small areas (such as those served by PCTs). In London, for example, the Greater London Authority's estimates of population growth in certain localities (which take into account new house-building) differ by as much as 20% from ONS estimates over the same period. Both in any case remain only estimates, but which more accurately reflects the likely requirement for the funding of health services, and which will be more nearly correct? This has implications for the formulae which determine the level of resourcing.

Census estimates are based on resident population by geography, which has advantages particularly when planning (and funding) jointly with local authorities, as mental health services do. PCTs, however, are responsible for the population registered with their general practitioners (GPs), and some of that population may not live in the precise geographical locality for which the PCT is nominally responsible, especially, as is often the case in urban areas, where there are practices straddling PCT boundaries. Adjustments can be made to deal with that, and often the impact goes both ways and the net effect is insignificant, but there is a more fundamental concern about whether GP lists are a better way than census data of determining the overall population for the purposes of allocating health resources.

That debate was given particular prominence by the concerns about under-enumeration in the 2001 census. Some local authorities (for which census-based estimates are also very significant in determining resource allocation) have argued successfully with the ONS that their populations were significantly under-counted by the 2001 census, for a variety of reasons. The PCT argument goes that the registered populations of general practices are a more reliable indicator (in some areas at least) than census data, and that it makes for a more coherent system overall, as practice population is already the basis for some payment arrangements under the GPs' contract, and will become of even greater importance once commissioning budgets for health services are devolved to practices under practice-based commissioning (PbC) (discussed below). There are two important caveats: first, not all people in a given area are, or are even necessarily entitled to be, registered with GPs and so there will always be some inherent under-counting in such a system; and second, it depends critically on GP lists being accurate and up to date. There are now many more mechanisms for ensuring that is the case, but it remains a challenging task, particularly in areas of high population mobility, and can lead to overstatement of the population served. A relatively overstated population in one area in a system distributing a fixed amount of resources is inevitably disadvantageous to areas where it is more accurately stated.

For the time being, however, the ONS estimates remain the basis for the allocation of resources from national to PCT level; but history, too, is a factor. In any health system, there is always a pattern to which resources have traditionally been distributed, which may fall out of date as demography and methods of estimating need change. National allocations are always a compromise between that inheritance and the 'correct' distribution as determined by the rational model for allocation of the moment.

Rather than having dramatic shifts each time the measurement of need changes, each PCT is determined to be 'above' or 'below' their target level of resources, and adjustments are made over time, usually by differentiating the rates of growth – or 'movement towards target' – of individual PCTs depending on whether they are over or under their target allocation. That tends to soften the impact of swings in fortune arising from the development of the allocation formulae or revised population estimates, but it also means that many PCTs are not quite at their 'correct' overall level of resourcing at any given time, and their own internal judgements will have to reflect that.

While resources distributed to PCTs in this way form the bulk of health services expenditure, they do not constitute all of it. The other significant categories are: resources allocated to support the costs of training staff for the NHS; resources allocated to support the costs of research and development taking place in NHS services; and a small number of highly specialist services which are funded directly by the Department of Health.

The first category is the largest by value, and includes substantial funds which support contracts with universities for undergraduate and postgraduate nursing and other professional education, and a proportion of the costs of all postgraduate medical education, including training-grade posts and continuing professional development. The resources are administered by strategic health authorities and deaneries. They are not allocated through PCTs, but are one of the few areas where strategic health authorities have direct control over resources. Because training is dependent on the NHS's academic partners, which are distributed in no particular relation to population or health need, the resources are kept separate from those allocated for direct care provision.

The same is true of resources for NHS research and development. These are, on the whole, not for the direct funding of research projects, but to reflect the additional costs borne by NHS services where significant amounts of research and development take place. They go from the Department of Health directly to trusts. They are concentrated in the main academic centres – particularly teaching hospitals and trusts associated with the principal postgraduate institutes for the main specialties – but this is also largely historic, without any tested correlation between, for example, funding and research output of importance to the NHS. A new research and development strategy for the NHS (Research and Development Directorate, Department of Health, 2006) is designed to review that distribution and overhaul the current allocation processes for NHS research and development funding to make it more transparent and to improve its impact in supporting research efforts that are of direct benefit to the NHS as a whole. Needless to say, there is frequently lively debate about the fairness of the distribution of both training and education and research and development resources, given that some trusts are more active in one or both fields than others.

The number of services subject to national commissioning arrangements is kept deliberately small; such arrangements are generally confined to those which are provided in only a few locations nationally, or which are fledgling services at an early stage of their development. In mental health they relate principally to secure services for adolescents, although it could be argued that the arrangements for the commissioning of services from the high secure hospitals amount to the same thing. In both cases, however, there is a relationship with the allocation made to PCTs on the basis of their populations. The funding for specialist services is a precept or a 'top-slice' on their allocations, either on a pro rata basis or, in the case of the high secure hospitals, based on a rather out-of-date account of actual usage.

How do PCTs allocate their resources?

In recent years the pattern has been for PCTs to negotiate service-level agreements with a range of providers of services to meet the healthcare needs of the populations they serve, through a process known as commissioning (the nature and effectiveness of which is the subject of constant and, to date, inconclusive debate). Those service-level agreements set out in detail how PCTs allocate their resources. There was, in theory, wide discretion to change matters to meet the needs of a given population, and most PCTs tried to use analysis by the local public health department to shape what share of their resources should go to different groups. In practice, of course, the existing pattern of provision had already developed in the light of local needs, and there were very few instances of attempts to make radical change. Moreover, PCTs have found themselves increasingly required to commission to meet national performance targets, by augmenting the capacity to meet access targets for elective surgery or for accident and emergency care, for example, or by funding the development of specific new services to meet the requirements of National Service Frameworks.

The PCTs are required to set out their intentions each year in a local development plan and these plans are checked to make sure that national priorities are being met before local objectives are considered. This has had the benefit of ironing out some of the inconsistencies between different local services which had grown up over time. On the other hand, it means that, in practice, PCTs have had fairly limited scope to change how they allocate their resources, except in so far as that corresponded with national priorities. As a result, the proportion of their overall resources that PCTs spend on different care groups varies – in mental health it ranges nationally from around 10% to approaching 20% of the total. Most of that variation is in reality historic, but that does not mean that it is wrong. A substantial part of it can be explained by various factors influencing population need, and a number of formulae have been developed to analyse and explain it, with significant levels of success (McCrone & Jacobson, 2004; McCrone *et al*, 2006).

Changes to the process of resource allocation by PCTs to providers following 'system reform'

The whole process set out above is due to change significantly with the advent of two important new developments, which stand to have a major impact on the practice of any clinician or manager providing services to the

NHS. It is as well to be aware of them. The first is PbC and the second is payment by results (PbR). Both are part of a wider programme of changes to the underlying structures and processes of the NHS known as 'system reform'.

At their heart these changes take a stage further the distinction between commissioning (or purchasing) services and providing them, which was started in 1991, influenced, in part, by the work of Enthoven in the United States (Enthoven, 1985). This led to the establishment of NHS trusts as distinct and 'independent' providers of services, operating within a quasi-market in which they competed to provide services to GPs, growing numbers of whom became 'fund-holders', with direct control over the resources used to pay for a range of (but never all) forms of secondary care, with the opportunity to reinvest any resources saved to improve the services offered by their own practices. For those GPs who chose not to become fund-holders, and for those services that were not within the scope of the fund-holding scheme (which always included most of mental healthcare), district health authorities established contracts with providers. They were also responsible for allocating the budgets to fund-holding GPs and, rather nominally, held them to account for how they were spent.

In practice, only limited change followed the 1990s' reforms. The 'market' was always substantially restricted, in terms of both the overall levels of resources available and the numbers of new entrants as providers. There was little scope for major movement of work in most parts of the country, apart from a few densely populated areas. The new NHS trusts essentially competed with one another for broadly the same amount of money/work, and while there were some relative winners and losers among these nominally independent organisations, they all remained accountable to the Secretary of State for Health, who was, thus, still responsible for what happened across the totality of the public health system, including the fate of individual provider NHS trusts if they got into difficulties. The most significant changes tended to be around the boundaries between primary and secondary care, but these were often small in scale and patchy, and so criticism grew about the variation in services available from locality to locality – the so-called 'postcode lottery'. This largely referred to the new variability; there remained many more long-standing variations in practice, availability of services and patterns of treatment, going back well before the 1990s.

When the Labour government took power in 1997, GP fund-holding was abolished, but the distinction between purchasing and providing was retained. Much stronger measures were put in place at a national level to tackle the problems of variability, in particular the establishment of national standards for services (National Service Frameworks), interventions and treatments (under the auspices of the National Institute for Health and Clinical Excellence – NICE) and finally through the establishment of a national body for the inspection of publicly operated health services – the

Commission for Health Improvement (CHI), since incorporated into the Healthcare Commission.

In the meantime, the PCTs were created to replace health authorities. The PCTs have a much more explicit interest in the systematic development of primary care. More recently the White Paper *Our Health, Our Care, Our Say* indicates the wide scope that is seen for the development of the functions of primary care itself (Department of Health, 2006).

The establishment of that framework has resulted in the policy to establish PbC as a means of increasing the scope and accountability of GPs in exercising direct control over the resources allocated to secondary care for their practice populations. The mechanisms for this were still being determined at the time of writing, but in essence the extent of secondary care under the control of practice-based commissioners will be substantially greater than that covered by fund-holding, while the accountability arrangements, including those for the reinvestment of savings in practices themselves, will be tighter. The whole process, though, still takes place under the regulatory regime that has developed since the 1990s. There is one other crucial difference – under fund-holding, much of the negotiation between a practice and a provider was about the price of a service, and providers might well seek to offer additional capacity at the margin, knowing that their costs would be marginal too. The weakness of that was that much of the interaction tended to focus on price rather than on quality or indeed effectiveness. The new system removes any discussion of price or cost from the local discourse by setting national tariffs to be used by all practice-based commissioners and all providers – this is payment by results (PbR).

Payment by results

Although PbR is in its early days, and indeed it is not intended to cover any aspect of mental health services until at least 2008, its significance extends well beyond its technical details. First of all, it marks a decisive shift away from the traditional compromise struck between the historic pattern of distribution of resources to a given population or service and the corresponding rationally derived 'correct' allocation. The tariff is based on a nationally determined formula – at first just an average – and while there are some adjustments made to reflect the differing costs of premises and salaries around the country, after that the tariff is what a provider gets paid for a particular service. If in practice it costs less actually to provide it, than the provider can keep the difference; if it costs it more, then the provider must (very quickly) find savings to cover the difference, or stop providing a service it cannot afford to run, or go out of business. This creates a system which has the potential to be much more volatile than traditional arrangements, and not just for providers.

The relationship between the volume of activity and resources becomes paramount, in a way that has never been the case hitherto. More work means more income for a provider, less work less income. The opportunity for marginal costing has not, in practice, been entirely abolished, for thresholds have already been set for the upper limits of anticipated growth in emergency admissions, beyond which full-cost payment under the tariff is tempered. That has come about because of the impact of PbR on commissioners. Once work is undertaken it has to be paid for. There is no negotiation other than perhaps about exactly which category – currently set out in a series of 'healthcare resource groups' (HRGs) (see 'Payment by results in mental health', below) – a particular intervention falls into, and therefore which tariff is applied, and whether the activity was properly coded and notified. That obviously presents a problem for commissioners – they are liable for the bill, yet they have relatively little scope to control demand.

The NHS used to rely on waiting lists to manage demand, but the scope for that has been removed in the case of elective surgery by the advent of national standards progressively reducing maximum waiting times. This in turn has created a requirement for additional surgical interventions (though at the end of that process – ominously also in 2008 – there is likely to be significant surplus elective surgical capacity). Also, emergency admissions to hospital are less easy to control and have in practice risen – partly, some speculate, because it is now much easier to be seen quickly in a hospital accident and emergency department than to arrange for an appointment to see a GP. Again, the bill goes to the commissioners, and they have to pay up.

That is why PbC is such a critical part of system reform: because, it is reasoned, the best possibility of shaping the actual use of secondary care services rests at the level of general practice. There the decisions are taken that result in referral. Also, there resides the potential for making alternative interventions that may prevent recourse to secondary care, or limit it, or allow for speedier discharge back to primary care. It is also one reason why there is now growing interest in the management of 'long-term conditions', chronic ill health which results in repeated use of secondary care services, and which may lend itself to better, more coordinated care outside hospital. This must sound familiar to anyone involved in the provision of mental health services over the past 10 years and, indeed, it is a refreshing change for some of the central principles of our approach to be held up as a model to general acute care, rather than our having to adapt rather awkwardly to a model developed with elective surgery in mind!

All this may sound superficially very attractive to providers, especially if they have a high degree of confidence in obtaining ever-growing amounts of work to be undertaken – and that has rarely been a problem in the past. It is a very short-sighted business, however, which delights in seeing its major customer go bankrupt, especially if it only has one of them, and the NHS will continue to operate within a fixed overall allocation. Nevertheless,

75

it is the intention of this change to the mechanism of resource allocation to health service providers that they should be encouraged to behave more like businesses, and in particular to focus on the relationship between the amount of work they do and their income. It creates incentives for them to look at how they measure their own productivity, how to improve it and how it compares with that of other trusts. It makes them pay attention to the factors that may sway patients, where they have a choice, in favour of or against using their services rather than those of another trust. The latter factors comprise a complex list, ranging from friendliness of staff, the availability of car parking and the quality of the environment, to hospital-acquired infection rates and the publication of outcome data.

Payment by results in mental health

All these mechanisms make most sense when viewed from the point of view of acute elective surgery, and that has indeed been the paradigm behind much of the thinking. How then might they be applied to mental health services? There are a number of very important points that have been for some years central to mental health policy that need to be reconciled with a PbR regime. The first concerns the incentives created. As applied in general acute services, PbR creates an incentive to increase the consumption of hospital-based intervention, tempered only to the extent that practice-based commissioners are able to manage demand, either by not referring or by providing alternatives to referral. Mental health services have been developed to encourage secondary services to support people outside hospital, with the aim of minimising the need for admission where possible. That is all the more important in view of the existence, uniquely in mental health services, of the possibility of compulsion in treatment, specifically, for the moment, linked to admission to hospital. That, more than anything, means that notions of 'patient choice' need to be carefully thought through.

In any case, the majority of resources in mental health services are spent on patients who are in treatment for relatively long periods of time and whose care is often funded by both health and social care agencies. It has been a central tenet of recent policy to accelerate the degree of integration between health and social care. Eligibility for social care resources, provided by locally elected authorities through the council tax (although admittedly substantially augmented by a wide range of central government grants), is dependent on being a local resident, or on a locally established responsibility for care. While it is the case that local authorities are very experienced – arguably much more so than PCTs – at commissioning residential services from providers, including those outside their own area, nevertheless it is almost axiomatic that if people are being cared for in their own homes they are unlikely to be receiving that care across a wide variety of geographical locations, and so community-based case management is likely to take place with limited scope for movement from one provider to another.

That is not to say that there are no aspects of mental health services which are not amenable to the acute-hospital model of PbR, rather that the bulk of mental health resources are committed to a different model of care. A relatively small but important part of mental health has some similarities with the 'elective' care approach. Out-patient-based episodic treatment – for example, cognitive–behavioural therapy for anxiety disorders or depression and possibly psychotherapy – can readily be accommodated within the established model: a standard tariff could be developed for a particular course of treatment in relation to a particular disorder. There is, though, a widely acknowledged inadequacy of supply against the potential demand for such services, and so access is constrained. In such circumstances, it is beneficial to create incentives to increase the consumption of interventions. There are no critical features of the service that tie potential patients to a particular geography or provider – they could go to wherever the waiting time is shortest, the location and timing most convenient for them, and perhaps where the outcomes, if published, are best.

For the most part, however, something different will have to be designed if there is not to be a major disjunction between established mental health policy and system reform policy. It is perhaps why many other countries which have introduced a tariff-based system of distributing resources to providers have abandoned the attempt in the case of mental health services. In England, the Department of Health has made it clear that it intends to press on with this aspect of system reform. Indeed, there is a major problem for mental health services generally if PbR proceeds without a mental health element. This problem is already manifesting itself during the transition period between acute services adopting PbR and its planned introduction in 2008 for mental health services. PCTs have an obligation to pay a fixed rate for each episode of treatment they commission, but they have in practice – and certainly at this stage – little real control over the amount of work done. Nevertheless, they have to operate within a fixed overall allocation, and so the obvious option open to them to balance their books is to reduce the amount of resources they allocate to that part of their portfolio *not* subject to PbR, especially where there is no established relationship between funding and activity.

There are already examples of PCTs, faced with growing bills from acute providers undertaking more work covered by the tariff, having made reductions in services which have no tariff – mainly mental health services and their own directly provided community services. That is why it is important that an appropriate system for PbR that suits the needs of mental health services is developed.

How might this work in practice? At the time of writing, no final formulation had been agreed, but a possible approach, for 'non-elective' mental health services, is a tariff based on secondary providers undertaking case management of an individual patient for a period of time for a sum determined by an assessment of the patient's needs. There would not be payment for specific interventions – care by a community team, treatment in a day centre or admission to hospital – but it would be up to the provider (and it would be its financial risk) to manage care as appropriate. That would avoid the problem of creating incentives to admit patients to hospital unnecessarily, and deal to some extent with the difficulty of compulsion, although it would be important to ensure that a perverse incentive was not created which discouraged admission when it was necessary. It would also mean that secondary mental health services would be rewarded for caring for people in a community setting, but there would be incentives for practice-based commissioners to encourage people to return to the care of their GP, and possibly to enhance the resources available within general practice to support that. It would also establish a strict relationship between resources allocated to a provider and the numbers of people on their case-load – increasing resources if case numbers rise and vice versa.

The system would depend critically on how patients were allocated to different tariffs to reflect their likely consumption of resources throughout the period of their care, and that obliges us to look very closely at the factors which really influence resource use in mental health services. The main feature of PbR as it has been developed so far is the use of HRGs to determine resource use, and these are largely based on diagnosis.

One of the problems encountered in the various international attempts to develop tariffs in mental health is the unreliability of HRGs or their antecedents as predictors of resource use in mental health. There are a variety of reasons for that, but at its heart it is because diagnosis is a much less reliable predictor of resource use in mental health care than it is in acute medicine. Even where it is clinically straightforward, two patients with ostensibly the same diagnosis may be much more or less likely to require admission to hospital, to need much more or less intensive levels of care and coercion in their treatment and to remain admitted for greater or lesser periods of time, depending on whether they have supportive relatives or carers, whether they have had contact with the criminal justice system, whether they have their own accommodation, and whether they have legal entitlement to residence, benefits or housing in the UK, never mind whether there is any comorbid substance misuse or other form of dual diagnosis.

The full impact of these various non-diagnostic factors on an individual's resource use in mental health services has yet to be fully quantified, although the resource allocation models used to explain variation in population resource distribution go some way to identifying the significant factors at the wider level. While we do not yet know which are the most significant items on the list – or indeed if we even have the right list yet – it is striking how many of these factors do already play an important part in care planning and the care programme approach (CPA) process more widely. There is an opportunity, therefore, to try to ensure that factors in resource allocation have at least some relationship to routine clinical processes.

If this system is adopted, it means that in future the needs assessment at the inception of the CPA will determine the level of resources allocated to the provider trust against the care of a particular patient. The bill will be paid by the PbC budget of the referring GP, who, of course, has the opportunity to participate in the CPA itself. Thereafter, the financial risks of managing the patient – whatever treatment he or she requires – will rest with the trust, until it is agreed that the patient should be transferred back to the care of the GP. It is, of course, possible to reassess a patient's needs at any point during the course of treatment through the usual CPA review process, and that might have an effect on the tariff and so adjust resource allocation. The tariff itself would be likely to be calculated on the basis of the average resource use of patients from a particular level of need – some would require more intensive treatment than average, others less, but overall it should average out. A problem would arise for the provider if its approach to treatment was more extravagant of resources than average, as it would not be funded to support it.

Productivity in healthcare

This brings us to the critical issue of productivity. Measures of productivity in the NHS have historically been very primitive, and improvements have been driven largely by the shift between in-patient and day surgery. A more convincing overall measure would relate to the improvement of health status of the population achieved by the NHS, but measures are difficult to devise, and it is hard to disentangle that improvement consequent on social factors and that achieved directly by the NHS itself. Nevertheless, for the individual provider trust an understanding of its productivity will be crucial to its survival in future, and the formulation of productivity will derive in large part from the construction of the tariff.

It is important not to confuse productivity with cost. For example, if a ward with a cost per day that is 5% higher than a comparator nevertheless achieves an average length of stay 10% lower, it is more productive, and the additional investment is worthwhile. That is one of the attractions of the tariff-based system for providers – it moves away from a system geared to managing to a fixed budget whatever the amount of work undertaken to one in which the benefits of effective investments can be much more clearly delineated and realised. Even so, if the tariff is initially set at an average, then half of all providers will need to improve their productivity in order to be able to break even, and the effect of their doing that will be to lower the average for the tariff in the following year.

For that reason there has been considerable debate about who should be responsible for setting the tariff. Whoever it is will clearly have considerable influence over the allocation of resources and their adequacy for effective care. There has already been consideration of the extent to which the tariff should take account of NICE guidelines, building into its cost assumptions the latest evidence of best practice. That is most straightforward in relation to the advent of some new drug related directly to treatment in a given HRG – it becomes more complicated the more elaborate and extended the guidance. It does, however, remove the scope for any argument over whether a particular treatment has been funded or not. Equally, though, because of the potential of the tariff to shape the balance of financial risk between PCTs and trusts, it is increasingly tempting for the tariff to become the means by which attempts are made to bring some sort of resolution to financial problems across the NHS as a whole. It is much harder to predict the consequences of such adjustment across a wide range of HRGs (and to anticipate the impact of the incentives and disincentives so created) on the care and treatment of individual patients, and on the financial plight of individual organisations.

Foundation trusts

It is perhaps time to look at the significance of foundation trusts in the wider context of the resources outlined above. It is arguable that the advent of foundation trusts by themselves is of much less significance than PbR and PbC. They are, however, integral to the whole system reform process, and they are in part necessary to enable providers to function effectively in the new world. They convey a degree of autonomy that enables providers to react, within the terms of their authorisation as foundation trusts, to the circumstances they face under a tariff regime. They will need to assess which of the services they provide cover their costs under the tariff and which do not; those that do not will need to improve their productivity to the point where they do, or their future will be in question. A foundation trust which persists in providing services at a loss will rapidly attract the attention of the independent regulator – Monitor – and it is not a tenable position in the long run.

In turn, it will be seen that setting the tariff simply at an average is not tenable in the long run, as half of all providers will inevitably be in difficulty each time the tariff is adjusted. Part of the policy rationale for introducing this regime is to encourage a more pluralistic market of provision for publicly funded health services – not just relying on NHS trusts as the only source of NHS provision. This has attracted attention most controversially in the case of the independent sector treatment centres introduced for acute elective surgery as an alternative to NHS trusts. Paradoxically, there is already much more plurality of provision in mental health services than in acute surgery – the Healthcare Commission registers many more independent providers of mental healthcare than of surgery. It is possible that there will be some new entrants to the market of local mental health services. It is more likely, however, that the current trend for subcontracting elements of a system of care to other parties will be continued. Many trusts, for example, subcontract the provision of day services to voluntary sector organisations, which can often be more flexible in their approach and can build stronger links with other local community resources than the trusts themselves might find possible.

In the future, if other bodies are able to provide an element of service more cost-effectively or more productively than the trust itself, then it is likely to consider whether to ask them to do it – to subcontract within the tariff. There is no reason why that should not extend to in-patient services, but it is very unlikely while independent sector providers charge by the bed-day – a system which creates incentives which militate against prompt discharge. If, however, an independent sector provider were to offer a fixed-price package for an admission, irrespective of the actual length of stay, that might well be attractive to a trust as a form of subcontract.

Decisions on these sorts of question will need to be made in the light of the overall requirements on foundation trusts in relation to the use of resources. They are expected to make a surplus on their operating activities in order to be able to invest it in improving their overall effectiveness. This requirement to make a surplus is novel to the NHS. Expectations of efficiency, however, are not new to the NHS, even if the precise form they take in the foundation trust regime brings an explicitness and clarity that had not always been evident.

If we return for a moment to the way in which resources are allocated to the NHS as a whole, each year there is an assumption for inflation factored into the calculation, based on knowledge of pay agreements and estimates of the increases in costs of drugs, energy and other consumables. From this is subtracted a percentage for improved efficiency, so that in a particular year inflation might be calculated as 6.5% and the efficiency gain at 2.5%, and so the net uplift becomes 4%. This is transferred down to the service-level agreements between PCTs and providers, and in future into the calculation of tariffs, which means that, each year, all services will have to find ways of improving their efficiency or productivity.

Efficiency underpinned the calculations of the Wanless report, which assumed improvements in productivity of between 1.5% and 3% per year in the three scenarios it constructed for the future of the NHS (Wanless, 2002). The ability to realise this improvement in productivity will be critical for providers. In part it will require them to examine very critically the skills they deploy to operate a particular service, and to ask whether they could do it more cheaply with the same result; they will also need to look at the effectiveness with which the work is organised, and so skills in service redesign will be important. Outcomes should also play a part, for if an intervention has a better outcome there is less likelihood of it needing to be repeated, and so wasted. Accordingly, it will be important to understand what the intended outcomes of a particular intervention are and to become much more adept at constantly refining practice to improve it (see Chapter 15).

Accounting for resources

Once a trust has resources, it must be accountable for the use of them, either as a PCT distributing them through service-level agreements or PbC, or as a provider. The boards of trusts have a statutory duty to break even and while there is some scope to manage that duty across succeeding financial years, it is increasingly limited. If a board does not respond to its responsibilities in that regard it is likely to be replaced by one that will – more or less rapidly, depending on the scale of the problem.

In addition to the overall responsibility on boards, there are specific duties upon the chief executive and finance director. Every NHS chief executive is also the 'accountable officer' for the trust – accountable, that is, to Parliament (through the Public Accounts Committee) for the use of public money in their organisation. That accountability extends not just to probity – tackling fraud, corruption and extravagance – but also to ensuring that resources are used efficiently and effectively, and not exceeded. 'Accountable officer' status is conferred by the chief executive of the NHS, and if trust chief executives are deemed not to have discharged their responsibilities properly, they can have the status withdrawn, which effectively prevents them from continuing in the role at that or any other trust.

Finance directors have a professional duty to the accounting body of which they are a member (and they must be a qualified accountant) to ensure that the financial position of the organisation is properly represented. In both cases, therefore, it is possible for a chief executive and a finance director to be placed in a position where the board will not act as they consider it should to tackle the financial problems facing a trust. In such circumstances, they have a duty (and to some extent powers) to make sure that their advice is clearly minuted and communicated to the Department of Health.

In foundation trusts the position is similar, although they do have more flexibility to manage their finances over time. The ultimate recourse is to Monitor, and the evidence to date suggests that it takes a much closer operational interest in finances. A key measure is a foundation trust's EBITDA (earnings before interest, taxation, depreciation and amortisation), which is essentially a test of whether its underlying position is one of making or losing money on its operations in relation to its income.

Foundation trusts, precisely because their finances are independent of the rest of the NHS, are much more exposed to the requirement to manage their cash. In real life, we are all familiar with the need to manage our cash flow – to make sure that we do not run out of money before the end of the month – and with the need from time to time to borrow cash to manage large investments or projects. Historically, the NHS has relied on one part of the system borrowing from another, and so cash management has never been at the forefront of consideration. As each component organisation becomes more autonomous and if, as seems to be the case, the system as whole becomes more indebted, then cash management becomes a real issue if trusts are to be able to pay their suppliers and their staff. For that reason, foundation trusts are required to have the facility to borrow cash if necessary to continue to function; it is therefore all the more important to anticipate and correct financial problems which may lead to their becoming effectively insolvent. If the underlying position of a trust is that it costs more for it to conduct its operations than it recoups in income, then even though one-off items, like the sale of property, may mean that it breaks even in a given year, unless it takes more fundamental corrective action, it will sooner or later run out of cash.

Trust boards have the help of internal and external auditors to give them a proper grasp of their financial standing and of the reliability of their financial systems. External auditors must approve the trust's published accounts and can be directed by the Audit Commission (which, for NHS trusts, appoints them) to undertake work which assesses value for money. Often this compares a number of trusts, and it can be useful as a means of benchmarking areas in which an organisation might look for improvement. Trusts are required to establish a board audit subcommittee, at which auditors can give advice, and also to publish an annual 'audit letter' from the external auditors, advising the board of its financial standing. External auditors also have the power to produce a report 'in the public interest' if they are sufficiently concerned about the position of an organisation.

The other significant aspect of resources which a trust board will need to consider is capital investment. Each trust has a small local allocation for small schemes and maintenance. Larger projects traditionally used to be achieved by bidding against a regional pot of 'strategic capital'. The bid involved putting forward a business case which demonstrated that the scheme was affordable – either because it was cheaper to run than the existing arrangements, or because there was agreement to the investment to fund the improvements envisaged. That approach has largely been overtaken by the Private Finance Initiative (PFI) for bigger schemes (over £30 million), under which a consortium of builders and lenders finances and constructs a facility (and perhaps continues to maintain and service it); in exchange the trust pays a charge over a long period of time, typically 25–30 years.

Hindsight is bringing some clarity to the debate about whether this gives better value for money than traditional procurement, and it is clear that PFI schemes restrict the flexibility to change services as circumstances dictate. You need to have a high degree of confidence that you will need to use a building intensively for the duration of the contract before entering into a PFI scheme. That helps to illustrate the overriding considerations in looking at any form of capital investment: What is the value that it brings? Can the costs of the capital be afforded, whether they are represented as capital charges (the costs of depreciation and an interest payment charged on traditional NHS capital investment), PFI charges, or the cost of borrowing capital commercially? Is there the flexibility to cope with changing circumstances?

Does mental health get the resources it requires?

This is not an easy question to answer. International comparisons tend to suggest that mental health services in the UK do relatively well – the percentage of total health expenditure devoted to mental health (at 12%) is the second highest in the EU after Luxembourg, with only five states above 8% (Commission of the European Communities, 2005). With mental health services in particular, however, the definition of the scope of mental health resources is critical to the validity of such calculations. For example, in some parts of the UK as much as 25% of the total expenditure on mental health services will be associated with the care of mentally disordered offenders, whereas in other countries they may well be managed within the criminal justice system. There are other key boundaries that can make all the difference depending on where they are set, often very specific to national cultures, for example with social welfare and benefits expenditure, housing and education.

This brings us to perhaps the most important point of all in considering the allocation and use of resources in mental health services. It is generally considered from the standpoint of overall health expenditure, and it is a commonplace that it tends to come low down the list of health priorities. If one looks instead at expenditure on mental healthcare and promotion as an investment – the 'pay-back' from which is not limited to improvement in health outcomes for individuals and populations but also extends to wider social benefits – then it has an important bearing on a number of subjects which are high on a wider governmental agenda.

Taken even more broadly, this has led to mental health being drawn directly into the heart of considerations previously the province of economists. In his book *Happiness*, Professor Richard Layard explores the limits of equating changes in the happiness of a society with changes in its purchasing power, as economics has traditionally done, and turns instead to better ways of understanding, ordering and achieving society's priorities, drawing specifically on psychology and neuroscience, as well as sociology and philosophy (Layard, 2005). If we were to take happiness seriously, he concludes, then we should:

'spend more on tackling the problem of mental illness. This is the greatest source of misery in the West, and the fortunate should ensure a better deal for those who suffer. Psychiatry should be a top branch of medicine, not one of the least prestigious.'

Improvements in educational attainment, greater social cohesion, reduced levels of offending and addiction, wider participation in work, and greater personal independence are all areas in which good mental health services can make a difference. There are now pilot projects being established to extend the availability of cognitive–behavioural therapy to enable people on incapacity benefit with anxiety disorders and depression to get back into employment. The savings are not in health expenditure but in the benefits budget – the province of the Department of Work and Pensions – and there are economic benefits as a greater proportion of the population participates in employment.

And that is where the most fruitful discussion of resources and mental health will be in the next few years. The past habit of simply struggling to attract as big a share of the health pot as possible will serve us poorly in a world in which productivity and effectiveness will count for much more. But when good mental health services are viewed in their wider social context, beyond the traditional confines of health expenditure, and their benefits can be demonstrated, there is strong case for investment.

References

Commission of the European Communities (2005) *Improving the Mental Health of the Population. Towards a Strategy on Mental Health for the European Union* (COM(2005) 484 final). CEC.

Department of Health (2006) *Our Health, Our Care, Our Say: A New Direction for Community Services*. The Stationery Office.

Enthoven, A. C. (1985) *Reflections on the Management of the National Health Service*. Nuffield Provincial Hospitals Trust.

Layard, R. (2005) *Happiness – Lessons from New Science*. Allen Lane.

McCrone, P. & Jacobson, B. (2004) *Indicators of Mental Health Activity in London: Adjusting for Sociodemographic Need*. London Health Observatory.

McCrone, P., Thornicroft, G., Boyle, S., *et al* (2006) The development of a local index of need (LIN) and its use to explain variations in social service expenditure on mental health care in England. *Health and Social Care in the Community*, **14**, 254–263.

Research and Development Directorate, Department of Health (2006) *Best Research for Best Health. A New National Health Research Strategy*. The Stationery Office.

Wanless, D. (2002) *Securing our Future Health: Taking a Long Term View*. HM Treasury.

CHAPTER 7

Planning for the medical workforce

Sally Pidd

General overview of workforce planning for medicine

Long-term planning for the medical workforce has never been an easy task. Doctors take a long time to transform from aspiring entrants to medical school into fully trained hospital specialists or general practitioners. Many become highly specialised early on in their careers and their ability to change track to meet varying service demands is very limited. There are numerous points in the career pathway where even small changes can affect the final overall pool of appropriately qualified applicants for consultant posts. Matching supply to demand is a tricky business.

Allowing too many to train for too few eventual consultant vacancies leads to disappointment, discontent and possibly to a loss of doctors to the workforce, whose training costs to the Exchequer have been huge. A recent example of that occurred in obstetrics and gynaecology, when too many doctors completed their higher training ahead of the anticipated consultant expansion.

There is strong central control at some points in the pathway. Places at medical schools are carefully regulated and the recent increase in student numbers has been planned to meet projected future requirements, and to reduce to a considerable extent the dependence on overseas graduates to fill training scheme places at the levels of senior house officer (SHO) and specialist registrar (SpR).

At SHO level for many years there has been a virtual freeze on the creation of new posts, although during 2003/04 there was some relaxation in order to try to relieve the bottleneck in some specialties between the SHO and SpR grades, by altering the ratio of SHO to SpR posts. It is at the SpR level, though, that central control has existed in the most comprehensive way, with the aim of ensuring that any new training opportunities, via additional national training numbers (NTNs), are given to the specialties with the greatest need to expand their particular consultant workforce.

The aim of all this control from the point of view of the four UK health departments is to ensure that the correct balance between supply and demand is maintained, with the emphasis mainly on not training too many. However, on the demand side of the equation, more service work exists than can be covered by those in these regulated training grades. So the past decade has seen a huge growth in the numbers of non-consultant career-grade doctors, recently renamed SAS doctors (staff and associate specialist grades). This is a response to market forces and individual employers' perceptions of service needs, developments and available funding. How many of these doctors will eventually find their way by one route or another into consultant posts is hard to predict.

Overview for psychiatry

The problem for psychiatry with this model of control, aiming for supply and demand to stay in balance, is that, as a specialty, we have never managed to get anywhere near the training targets set, either by central government or as a profession, to generate sufficient fully trained psychiatrists to fill even established posts. Census data from both the health departments and independently from the Royal College of Psychiatrists over many years have shown a high level of consultant vacancies (at the time of writing, the overall figure was in excess of 11%). These are much higher in some sub-specialties and some geographical areas (Royal College of Psychiatrists, 2002).

The reasons behind this failure to match supply to demand are complex. Psychiatry has never attracted enough UK graduates to fill existing training posts at SHO level. Medical schools vary in their ability to generate the next generation of psychiatric SHOs, but consistently the overall figure is stuck at around 4–5% of graduate doctors choosing psychiatry (Goldacre *et al*, 2005). The slack, therefore, has to be taken up by overseas graduates, whose career pathways may be more difficult to predict, and whose initial aptitude for the subject may be harder to gauge if their exposure to psychiatry before coming to the UK has been limited. We have also struggled to retain in the specialty those who have been recruited. Too many fail to make the expected transition along the career pathway, so all the factors that play a part in retaining staff need careful examination.

Workforce planning not only for doctors but for all staff within the National Health Service (NHS) has gained a higher profile in recent years. This is partly because of the need to translate the aspirations of government initiatives (e.g. in England the NHS Plan and the various National Service Frameworks), to drive up standards and modernise services for the 21st century, into care being delivered by the right staff with the right training, in the right place at the right time – in short, a workforce 'fit for purpose'.

Many questions remain to be answered about how to do this:

- What is the 'right' number of doctors for a specialty?
- Where will they come from?
- How will changes to training and working practices affect this?

87

- How can we achieve the right balance between central control and the autonomy of local services to recruit as many (or as few) doctors as they feel are necessary?

The remainder of the chapter, after a brief historical review, looks at the current developments which may provide some of the answers.

Historical background to workforce planning

The history of what used to be called manpower planning, now workforce planning, has been marked by a number of landmark initiatives as successive governments have grappled with the problem of the imbalance in medical staffing. Four of the key initiatives deserve particular mention, as they have shaped the way that central control has increasingly been exercised over the medical workforce.

(1) Achieving a Balance

Achieving a Balance (Department of Health and Social Security, 1986) set out the basic principle that far more care for hospital patients should come from consultants, and hence the numbers of senior registrars should be tailored to the expected consultant expansion needed to achieve this. This meant, in the medium term, planning for consultant growth at around 2% per year while progressively reducing the numbers of career registrars. A new staff grade was introduced in 1988 to plug the gap in service needs for employers and originally a ceiling was set so that numbers could not exceed 10% of the total number of consultants in that specialty.

(2) Joint Planning Advisory Committee (JPAC)

This was given the task of advising on the total number of training posts needed in each specialty from 1985 onwards. Psychiatry was a beneficiary of this annual process, which allowed for increasing numbers of what were then called senior registrar posts. Sub-specialties were aided in their development by these JPAC allocations.

(3) The Calman report

The next significant impact on training and staff numbers came with the need to embrace the changes brought about by the freedom of movement granted to all citizens of the member states of the European Community. Because the length of specialist training was longer in the UK than in the rest of Europe, there was a need to achieve a degree of harmonisation. The reforms came to be known as the Calman proposals because the committee's chair was Sir Roy Calman. The reforms aimed to bring the UK in line with Community legislation on specialist medical training.

The report (Calman, 1993) endorsed five key principles, which are still in force today:

1   Through structuring programmes, overall training times would be reduced.
2   At the end of training, doctors would obtain a UK Certificate of Completion of Specialist Training (CCST) on the advice of the relevant faculty or college.
3   CCST holders would then be eligible for consultant appointment.
4   A unified training grade combining registrar and senior registrar levels would be introduced so that training would comprise basic specialist training – SHO level and higher specialist training, at SpR level.
5   A new system of NTNs was to be introduced, with each specialty having a fixed but annually negotiable quota, which had to be competed for. Progress in higher training became subject to the RITA (record of in-training assessment) process to ensure there were no significant delays in people progressing to CCST and thus blocking the release of an NTN for another doctor.

(4) Medical Workforce Review Team

In England, the Specialty Advisory Workforce Group took over responsibility for the annual review of NTNs for each specialty in 1999. It used computer modelling to predict the likely growth in consultant numbers if variables on the input side changed. Colleges, postgraduate deans and health departments all had the opportunity to influence this modelling process with any evidence they were able to muster as to the particular needs and circumstances of their specialty. It was renamed the Medical Workforce Review Team in 2001.

During 2004, the remit of this team was broadened to cover other grades and other professional groups as well, and this has been reflected in a change of title to the Workforce Review Team.

Current key issues for workforce planning: the national context

Medical school numbers

The number of places at UK medical schools has increased dramatically, from 3749 in 1998 to an expected 7000 by 2010. The increase has come about by introducing new 4-year graduate entry programmes, establishing four new medical schools, and adding places to existing schools. It will take several years for these numbers to translate into extra doctors, but the aim is to reduce some of the excessive dependency on overseas doctors to fill training-grade posts.

The feminisation of medicine

Over the past 40 years the number of women entering medicine has increased dramatically. Over 50% of medical school places are now occupied by women and in some schools the number exceeds 60%. Of the Royal College of Psychiatrists' membership, 40% of UK and Irish graduates are now women. This raises interesting questions about their likely future career paths and demands for flexible training, as well as about how many doctors will be needed to staff services if or when traditional full-time working through most of a career ceases to be the norm. Funding of flexible training has always been subject to short-term decisions and the lack of adequately protected budgets for this growing group of doctors (which clearly includes men as well, but in far lower numbers) means delays to the completion of training programmes and so further unpredictability in the time it takes to gain a certificate of completion of training (CCT) and eligibility for consultant posts.

The Postgraduate Medical Education and Training Board (PMETB)

In September 2005, the PMETB took over responsibility for standards and quality assurance of all postgraduate education, training and assessment in medicine and dentistry. One of its responsibilities is to assess eligibility for specialist registration under new EU legislation (articles 11 and 14). In brief, this means many doctors both outside and within the UK who were previously unable to get on to the specialist register (and hence be available for consultant appointments) may be able to do so by an alternative route. This is based on their experience and demonstrated competence, rather than on their having obtained MRCPsych and a CCT, the 'current standard' route onto the register. This is likely to have a very significant short- to medium-term effect on the numbers of doctors able to be considered for consultant appointment. Psychiatry will be one of the main beneficiaries of this change, but the numbers involved are unknown as yet.

Modernising Medical Careers (MMC)

MMC is an initiative developed from Professor Liam Donaldson's proposals to reform the SHO grade (Department of Health, 2002). In February 2004 the four UK health departments endorsed the importance of care being based on effective interdisciplinary teamwork and flexible training pathways, tailored to meet service and personal development needs.

The first change came in August 2005, after extensive piloting since 2003; this was the replacement of 1 year of pre-registration house officer training with a 2-year integrated foundation programme, focusing on generic competencies and the management of acute illness. This will act as a bridge between undergraduate and specialist medical education, and full registration with the General Medical Council (GMC) will come after successful completion of the first of the two 'foundation years' (FY1 and FY2). Psychiatry figures in both the FY1 and the FY2 programme, with likely 4-month slots and a very different training emphasis to current initial SHO posts. All the assessment in FY2 will be workplace based and the four methods chosen are likely to continue throughout specialist training, as listed in Box 7.1.

Beyond foundation training comes selection for run-through training in one of eight broad specialties, which include psychiatry. The College has a competency-based curriculum approved by the PMETB to cover the 6 years of run-through training in all the current CCT specialties. Work-based assessments of performance and competencies will be key. How selection for the programmes will work out, and the part formal examinations like the MRCPsych will have in this new world, are questions still to be answered. By 2012, though, training will look very different, with a curriculum running through from FY2, run-through training and lifetime continuing professional development (CPD).

The unknowns for all this in terms of workforce planning are how many FY2 slots will be granted to psychiatry and whether they will come from the existing SHO stock. One alternative has been to use some of the nearly 500 extra unfunded SHO posts released in England during 2003/04 which had been intended as a means of improving the ratio of SHO to SpR posts in psychiatry. There is agreement generally that getting psychiatry firmly established in FY2 is crucial. Given the relative reduction of the time allocated to psychiatry in many undergraduate curricula, giving large numbers of young doctors a positive education and professional experience of the subject in FY2 is vital if we are to improve the recruitment figures for UK graduates into the specialist run-through programmes. Overseas doctors will have the opportunity to compete for the schemes as well and may have access to some of the FY2 posts.

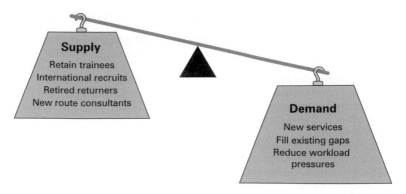

Fig. 7.1 Balancing the supply of and demand for consultants in psychiatry.

This has led to three specific initiatives which, although not only applicable to psychiatry, have been of particular relevance in looking at improving the overall workforce position:

1   international recruitment
2   post-retirement options
3   new ways of working.

International recruitment

The Department of Health in England ran an International Fellowship Programme from 2003 until 2006, designed to recruit overseas doctors to fill vacant NHS consultant posts. The stated intention was to enable overseas doctors to take up appointments for 2 years to broaden their own experience. This programme has recruited more psychiatrists than all other specialties put together (124 out of 202 by the end of 2004) and in some areas it has been seen as a great success, with both Fellows and local services deriving benefit. There have been considerable anxieties expressed, though, at the ethics of taking fully trained staff from countries that can ill afford to lose them. Despite attempts to encourage applicants from countries with an oversupply of doctors, most came from the Indian subcontinent, and widespread concerns exist about taking so many doctors away from the developing countries which have trained them. It is also impossible to predict how many will stay beyond 2 years and for how long. So, another uncertainty in the supply of consultants for the permanent workforce has arisen (Goldberg, 2004).

During 2006, another major change was brought in by the government: 'permit-free training' for international medical graduates was abolished, which meant that such doctors had to obtain work permits before they could take up positions. Those work permits can be issued only if posts cannot be filled by either UK graduates or graduates from member states of the

European Economic Area. This change to the regulations is likely to have a major impact in specialties like psychiatry which have historically had large numbers of international medical graduates in training schemes. How this will affect the future shape of the workforce is not yet clear.

Post-retirement options

Research from the CIPTAC studies (Mears *et al*, 2002) showed the mean planned retirement age for consultant psychiatrists was 60. As many psychiatrists now in their 50s have 'mental health officer' status, which can be an encouragement to retire early (from 55 onwards), there is a potential pool of experienced consultants who could return or continue in the workforce after retirement. The flexible careers scheme of the Department of Health made it much easier and more attractive for doctors to be retained, perhaps in part-time and also different roles, but funding for that came to an end in 2006 and it is too early to say how attractive this type of approach is going to be for trusts to employ. However, persuading more senior consultants to return after retirement will have the quickest and most positive effect on overall consultant numbers, as the computer model clearly demonstrates.

New ways of working

Consultant dissatisfaction with their jobs, workload pressures and changing expectations of mental health staffing for new teams led to a great deal of work on what has come to be known as 'new ways of working' for psychiatrists (Department of Health, 2005). The essence of this approach is to enable those with the most experience and skills to work face to face with those with the most complex needs, freeing up time to supervise and support other staff undertaking less complex or more routine work. Allowing consultants to move into a more consultative style of working and challenging some of the traditional boundaries about what has been felt only consultants can do clearly has implications for the rest of the mental health workforce. They, in turn, are exploring new ways of working for themselves.

To enable these changes to occur, other things have had to happen.

GMC guidance

Agreement needed to be reached with the GMC on the limits of consultant responsibilities and that was done in a statement regarding accountability in multidisciplinary and multi-agency mental health teams, produced by the GMC's Standards and Ethics Committee, and was made available on its website (General Medical Council, 2005). This makes it clear that the responsibility for the care of patients is distributed among the clinical members of a team; consultants retain oversight of patients allocated to their care and are responsible for providing advice and support to the team. They are not accountable for the actions of other clinicians within the team.

Changed and extended roles

Other mental health professionals have had to be willing to embrace new and extended roles. For existing staff such as nurses that has included taking on supplementary and independent prescribing roles. Mental health pharmacists have become more fully integrated into clinical teams, bringing their expertise with them. A third example is that of occupational therapists and dietitians who have worked together on programmes targeted on healthy living and weight control where appropriate for patients.

Introduction of new workers

New types of workers have been created, such as STR ('support, time and recovery') workers, promoting social inclusion and recovery for patients with severe and enduring mental illness. Others, like graduate workers, offer short-term interventions in primary care as part of a move to increase capacity to deliver more treatment outside the framework of the care programme approach (CPA), freeing up members of the community mental health team to focus on people who are more severely ill.

Job descriptions and College norms

Job descriptions for both new and replacement consultant posts need to be drawn up after a careful review of what the expectation was of the part they would play in the overall team or service. To aid this process, two specific initiatives have been pursued as part of the whole 'new ways of working' agenda. The first was to agree joint guidance on the employment of psychiatrists between the College, trust employers and mental health chief executives. In this, the emphasis shifted from having rigid norms for consultants (such as one consultant in old age psychiatry per 10 000 population over the age of 65) to looking at how the whole of the multidisciplinary team, including consultants, could deliver the service required by a defined patient group.

The second initiative was the development of the 'Creating Capable Teams Toolkit', which is due to become available after extensive piloting in early 2007. This enables teams to reflect on their function, the needs of service users, the current workforce structure, their capabilities and how they can deliver a team workforce plan for the short and medium term. Where psychiatrists fit into that is seen as key to the aim of using them to carry out the most complex work while also having time to supervise and train more effectively.

New Mental Health Bill for England and Wales

The changes to the Mental Health Act in England and Wales, still to be finally ratified, envisage new roles of responsible clinicians and approved clinicians for detained patients, who can be professionals other than doctors. So the traditional and familiar responsible medical officer may change for consultants.

Prospects

All this adds up to a time of flux and change, which, added to the MMC agenda, makes predicting future workforce requirements very challenging. The implementation of the new consultants' contract, in the view of many employers, has been too costly to allow for any further significant expansion of consultant numbers. The growth of foundation trusts in mental health will allow more local decision-making on the workforce, which almost certainly will be finance-led as well as service-driven. The assumption that all CCT holders will be able to move into the type of consultant posts we are familiar with now is being openly questioned and debated.

Conclusion

The basic workforce question – how many psychiatrists do we need in the UK to deliver appropriate services for the 21st century? – probably cannot be answered. Some more pragmatic questions always seem to take precedence:

- How many psychiatrists can we afford?
- How many posts can we fill?
- What is the quality of the post-holders?
- How can we address the cost and quality issues around locums to cover existing vacancies?

The next few years will see huge changes in the way medical training, from undergraduate through to CCT, is delivered and assessed as a result of MMC. In the medium term, planning for the medical workforce may become even more problematic than in the past. Keeping pace with the changes and trying to take advantage of them to recruit and retain more psychiatrists will remain a major challenge for the profession.

References

Academy of Royal Medical Colleges (2004) *Curriculum for the Foundation Years in Postgraduate Education and Training.* Academy of Royal Medical Colleges. http://www.mmc.nhs.uk/download_files/curriculum-for-the-foundation-years-in-postgraduate-education-and-training.pdf

Calman, K. (1993) *Hospital Doctors: Training for the Future. The Report of the Working Group on Specialist Medical Training.* Department of Health.

Department of Health (2002) *Unfinished Business – Proposals for the Reform of the Senior House Officer Grade.* Department of Health.

Department of Health (2005) *New Ways of Working for Psychiatrists: Enhancing Effective, Person-Centred Services Through New Ways of Working in Multidisciplinary and Multiagency Contexts. Final Report 'but not the end of the story...'* Department of Health.

Department of Health and Social Security (1986) *Achieving a Balance: A Plan for Action.* HMSO.

General Medical Council (2005) *Accountability in Multi-disciplinary and Multi-agency Mental Health Teams.* See http://www.gmc-uk.org/guidance/current/library/accountability_in_multi_teams.asp

Goldacre, M. J., Turner, G., Fazel, S., *et al* (2005) Career choices for psychiatry: national surveys of graduates of 1974–2000 from UK medical schools. *British Journal of Psychiatry,* **186**, 158–164.

Goldberg, D. (2004) The NHS International Fellowship Scheme in Psychiatry. *Psychiatric Bulletin,* **28**, 433–434.

Mears, A., Kendall, T., Katona, C., *et al* (2002) *Career Intentions in Psychiatric Trainees and Consultants.* Research Unit, Royal College of Psychiatrists. See http://web.archive.org/web/20040727211209/www.rcpsych.ac.uk/cru/complete/CIPTAC+final+report.pdf

Royal College of Psychiatrists (2002) *Annual Census of Psychiatric Staffing 2001* (occasional paper OP54). Royal College of Psychiatrists.

Sainsbury Centre for Mental Health (2005) *Scoping the Current Problems and Solutions Relating to Consultant Psychiatric Vacancies, Consultant Recruitment and the Use of Locums in England.* NIMHE/SCMH Joint Workforce Support Unit.

CHAPTER 8

Multidisciplinary teams

Frank Holloway and Carolyn Chorlton

Since the rise of the asylum, mental healthcare has involved staff with different backgrounds and roles working together in a formal organisational structure. The mental hospital is traditionally understood to have been dominated by doctors, in particular the medical superintendent. In reality, although much formal authority was vested in the doctors, absolute power over the welfare of the patients rested in the hands of senior nurses. Nurses both controlled information flows between the doctors and the patients and the daily routine of care. In the best hospitals, doctors, nurses and other staff worked to advance patients' interests; in the worst, they colluded in regimes that combined financial economy with neglect. A series of scandals resulted in systematic investigations into the determinants of good and bad quality of care within hospital settings (Martin, 1984). Poor standards of care tended to develop in institutional settings where medical and other professional leadership was lacking, training was poor, staff groups worked in isolation and there was no effective external lay or managerial oversight.

Healthcare has changed enormously in the 40 years since the hospital scandals began to emerge. Management structures have evolved. We are now in an era of community care, to the extent that the readily available texts on multidisciplinary teamwork in mental health focus exclusively on community teams (see, for example, Øvretveit, 2001; Onyett, 2003; Burns, 2004). There is much more emphasis on the accountability of health and social care professionals, both to society at large and to service users. However, we ignore the hard-won lessons of the past at our peril.

Multidisciplinary working implies that individuals from different professional backgrounds (and increasingly, as the support worker role expands, without a professional qualification) come together in the common enterprise of meeting patient and carer need and societal demand. The vast majority of staff in mental health services now acknowledge that they are working within one or more multidisciplinary teams, rather than functioning as an independent practitioner ('nurse', doctor', 'occupational therapist', 'social worker', 'welfare benefits advisor', 'support worker'). They contribute their personal and professional skills to the common enterprise. Professionally and personally, one of the worst things that can happen to a psychiatrist is to lose the confidence of the team. Although consultant psychiatrists no longer possess the level of authority and control they once had, or believed they had, within mental health services, they continue to play a pivotal role and require a sound understanding of the nature of leadership and how to foster effective team functioning (Harrison & Gray, 2003).

There is a paradox inherent in the current emphasis on teamwork, particularly within community mental health teams (CMHTs). Referrers, service users, carers, practitioners and the psychotherapy literature all emphasise the importance of the individual relationship, often sustained over the long term, in therapeutic outcomes. The bedrock of effective mental healthcare lies in the work of each practitioner.[1] Teams are a means of providing structure for and enhancing the quality of this work. The particular value of the multidisciplinary team is that it brings together individuals with diverse approaches to understanding mental health problems and a range of professional expertise not available from any single discipline, in a more effective way than referral on to a separate service.

This chapter is written from the perspectives of a consultant psychiatrist and a CMHT practitioner manager with a nursing background; both authors are enthusiastic about the benefits of effective teamwork. The aim is to provide ways of looking at teamwork and practical advice to psychiatrists about how to work effectively as a member of a multidisciplinary team. General adult psychiatry, within which both authors work, lies towards the middle of a spectrum of psychiatric specialties within which the specific medical role is acknowledged. Neuropsychiatry, liaison psychiatry, old age psychiatry and substance misuse quite clearly require the expertise of doctors (although in the last case largely as prescriber and manager of physical comorbidity). The law's traditional reliance on the 'medical man' as expert legitimises the forensic psychiatrist. Psychiatrists working in psychotherapy, child and adolescent mental health and intellectual disability have for many years had to defend and define their specific role within their respective services.

Teamwork in mental health

Kinds of teams

Teamwork is defined in the *New Shorter Oxford English Dictionary* as 'the combined action of a team of players or a group of people especially when

---

1 Psychiatrists in England are being encouraged to abandon their individual therapeutic role to act as 'consultants' to teams (National Steering Group, 2004). They do so at their professional peril.

effective and efficient' or, alternatively, 'co-operation'.[2] In the organisational literature, teams are defined as 'social entities embedded in organisations, performing tasks which contribute to the organisation's goals' (West *et al*, 1998, p. 2). Effective work groups tend to contain between 4 and 20 members. Øvrevteit (2001) identifies five types of team commonly encountered in mental health services:

1   In a *case manager's team*, people are brought together in an *ad hoc* fashion to organise and coordinate services for a client, as in a multi-agency care programme approach (CPA) meeting.
2   A *network team* allows exchange of information and referral, for example when primary and secondary care services join together to review shared cases.
3   In a *formal service-delivery team*, such as a CMHT or in-patient ward, a defined range of services is provided to a specific population.
4   *Project teams* are brought together to undertake a defined task in a limited period, for example to review or develop a service or an operational policy.
5   A *management team* will be collectively accountable for service delivery.

The effective psychiatrist needs to be able to recognise and operate within all these kinds of teams, and other groupings that come together to achieve shared aims, such as consultants' committees and training committees. This chapter focuses on how to work within a *formal service-delivery team*.

A typology of mental health teams

Contemporary local mental health services comprise a complex network of teams. By way of an example, Box 8.1 sets out the 24 individual staff teams responsible for service delivery identifiable at the end of 2006 within the Croydon Integrated Adult Mental Health Service, which is responsible for an urban catchment area with a population of 330 000.

There has been a startling lack of clarity about the precise tasks of the mental health team and how these are to be performed. This has only recently and partially been addressed by the development of service descriptions and fidelity scales (Department of Health, 2001, 2002; Burns and Firn, 2002; Burns, 2004). As an aid to understanding how mental health teams work, Øvretveit (2001) has set out four ways in which teams may differ: accountability of the team; team membership; decision-making processes; and management tasks and structures. These differences

---

2   This is by analogy with the original meaning of a team, which related to horses or oxen yoked together to provide motive power. Although the occupational psychology literature emphasises that effective teams have a sense of autonomy, the contemporary delivery culture seeks to revert to the original meaning.

Box 8.1 Types and numbers of teams operating within the Croydon Integrated Adult Mental Health Service

Residential services

- Acute wards (3)
- Psychiatric intensive care ward
- Women's (residential) unit
- Crisis residential unit
- Rehabilitation ward
- Continuing-care ward

Community teams

- Community mental health teams (5)
- Assertive outreach team
- Recovery and rehabilitation team
- Early-onset psychosis team
- Crisis resolution/home treatment team
- Forensic community mental health team
- Mother and baby community mental health team

Other services

- Psychological therapies service
- Liaison service
- Day care service
- Telephone helpline
- Homelessness assessment team

Croydon Integrated Adult Mental Health Service is under one management structure but is funded from both health and social care budgets. It includes both health and social care teams: all the core community teams are fully integrated.

It is worth noting that the above teams are dependent on the functioning of many other (unidisciplinary) teams within the wider organisation that provide the vital infrastructure for direct service provision, for example information technology, finance, human resources, pharmacy, works and estates, as well as a local management team, which is itself a multidisciplinary team.

(discussed below) are gradually being eroded in the contemporary National Health Service (NHS) as a consensus emerges about how services should work, although the new orthodoxy envisioned in *New Ways of Working for Psychiatrists* (Department of Health, 2005) has not yet been fully described in the literature and may well change again.

For Øvretveit, the mental health team may be a group of staff either who have a collective accountability for meeting the needs of a defined population or who are, as individual professionals, collectively responsible for the welfare of the population but without any shared responsibility for clinical decision-making.

Accountability within multidisciplinary teams

The issue of responsibility is a very vexed one for consultant psychiatrists, who will generally feel personally responsible for the outcomes, good or bad, of all patients under the care of the teams within which they work.

This view is now being challenged and *New Ways of Working for Psychiatrists* spells out the current view of the General Medical Council on accountability in multidisciplinary and multi-agency mental health teams (Department of Health, 2005, pp. 15–16). Contemporary mental health teams should have clear accountability within a management and clinical governance structure, and doctors are required to clarify with their employer any uncertainties and ambiguities they experience. Individual members of staff are responsible for their own actions, and professionals face both managerial and professional sanctions should their performance fall below standard.

Team membership

Teams differ in terms of membership. For example, the traditional in-patient ward team comprised the qualified and unqualified nurses on the establishment, perhaps expanded to include clerical and housekeeping staff, an occupational therapist and the ward doctor. A minority of teams are unidisciplinary (for example within Croydon the nurse-led women's service, the helpline and the day care service).

Teams can be defined in terms of a 'core' membership, those who devote all or the majority of their working week to the team, and an 'extended' membership, of individuals whose involvement with the team is only an element of their work. In the contemporary era of integrated health and social services, 'core' staff within a CMHT will generally include nurses, occupational therapists, social workers, support workers and administrative staff. There are differences internationally with regard to the skill mix and function of professionals within CMHTs: in the United States and Germany, for example, social workers commonly perform the case management role, whereas in the UK this is most often done by nurses (Burns & Lloyd 2004).

Consultant psychiatrists and clinical and counselling psychologists have traditionally fallen into the category of 'extended' membership. Despite their prominent role within the team, consultants have tended to have multiple areas of responsibility, rendering them part time wherever they work.

There are moves to change this pattern, with the development of 'specialist' consultant roles within general adult psychiatry, covering, for example, in-patient services, psychiatric intensive care, CMHTs and the 'functional' mental health teams required by the NHS Plan (assertive outreach, crisis resolution/home treatment and early intervention in psychosis) (Department of Health, 2005). These specialist roles have the advantage of allowing consultants to become more closely identified with a particular team, although there are consequent disadvantages in further fragmenting an increasingly fragmented system of care.

Decision-making processes

Decision-making processes vary between mental health teams. The 'care pathway' for any service includes a number of obvious key decision points: defining the patient group; accepting a patient for assessment; taking an individual on to the case-load or diverting to another service; allocating responsibilities for provision of treatment and care; managing crises that present; reviewing outcomes; and discharge from care.

Some teams have little or no control over who comes onto the case-load, for example the acute in-patient ward. Other, more specialist teams have absolute control over whom they take on: these teams tend to have higher prestige and less stressed staff, even if their client group is recognised as more difficult. Within teams some professionals, most notably psychologists, may have more control over their case-load than others, and operate a parallel referral pathway. In principle, these decisions are subsumed under the overarching care programme approach (Department of Health, 2000), within which decisions about specialist mental healthcare are agreed and coordinated. Day-to-day practice is less clear cut and teams need to develop local agreements (within an operational policy) about how the 'care pathway' is managed.

Management tasks and structures

Mental health teams operate in uncertain and unpredictable policy and practice environments, undertake complex tasks and use treatment technologies that are themselves uncertain and unpredictable. An effective team will not only carry out its task-related objectives but also cater for the well-being and development of its members and be viable in the long term (Onyett, 2003). Mental health teams require adequate numbers of good-quality staff, who have a clear, agreed task and are well managed. Too often either overall or local management is poor and the task blurred.

Øvretveit (2001) sets out eight key management tasks for mental health teams: drafting job descriptions; interviewing and appointing staff; induction; assigning work to staff; reviewing work; appraisal and setting objectives; ensuring quality, training and professional development; and engaging in disciplinary procedures. Traditionally, professionals within teams worked to line managers in their own profession, each of whom was messily responsible for some or all of these management tasks. The allocation of work within a team has frequently fallen between managerial stools.

Management structures for mental health services have evolved rapidly. As recently as the 1980s, only 10% of CMHTs had a manager (Onyett,

1997). Now the norm is for team leaders/managers (ward managers in in-patient settings) to have overall managerial responsibility for all staff within the team, with a degree of professional accountability and supervisory responsibility being held by service-wide professional heads. Currently, it is often only the doctors within teams who remain separately accountable, through a line from the consultant to the clinical director and ultimately the medical director.

Difficult issues for the contemporary mental health team

Mental health services are moving rapidly towards prescriptively structured teams that are highly accountable to local management and responsible for delivering nationally determined targets, for example the implementation of guidelines issued by the National Institute for Health and Clinical Excellence (NICE). There are clear tensions within this framework that affect all professional staff, who have traditionally valued their autonomy, and the organisational literature strongly suggests that staff work best when they experience a degree of control over their workload and working environment.

Handy (1981) warns against excessive monitoring of staff in the pursuit of increased effectiveness. He suggests that pressure by control is demotivating, because of the implied lack of confidence and trust in staff.

The *Mental Health Policy Implementation Guide* from the Department of Health (2002, p. 18) asserts that 'CMHTs function best as discrete specialist teams comprising health and social care staff under single management'. There is potential for conflict between the team leader/manager, who generally now has clear managerial accountability for service delivery and wide-ranging responsibilities for the work of staff within the multidisciplinary team (including who does what), and that of the consultant psychiatrist, who has authority over non-consultant doctors. Team leaders/managers have a key role in allocating work to individual team members and managing the overall case-load. The consultant will generally have strong (and hopefully well-informed) opinions about the needs of patients in contact with the service, as well as a clear idea about the functioning of team members. Team leaders/managers are responsible for meeting external targets that reflect trust and NHS priorities, about which the consultant may be ignorant or dismissive. The consultant falls outside the team management structure but will also feel responsible for the performance of the team: neither the psychiatrist nor the team leader/manager has the authority to constrain the activity of each other. Mutual understanding and respect are the key to a productive relationship between the team leader/manager and consultant; this needs to mirror working relationships higher up the organisation.

Integration of health and social care brings a further challenge for psychiatrists and other healthcare staff, who must now work within altered parameters. The integrated team must adhere to the eligibility criteria for social services, catering for the needs of vulnerable adults as well as of people with a defined mental illness. Statutory responsibilities include assessments under the NHS and Community Care Act 1990, with subsequent provision of appropriate social care. Failure to discharge this responsibility can result in judicial review.

Managing demand

One particular difficulty for many teams is the management of demand, which for all health and social services continually threatens to overwhelm available resources. Doctors, both general practitioners and consultants, have traditionally taken a leading role in this, using mechanisms that have been far from transparent from the public (or the Department of Health). Writing about the covert rationing of healthcare, New (1996) identified some well-worn strategies employed to control workload (see Box 8.2).

Box 8.2 Strategies for managing excessive demand

Deterrence
- Service charges
- Gate-keeping by primary care
- Unfriendly staff
- Inconvenient appointment times
- Poor-quality care environments

Deflection
- Passing referrals to other agencies – shifting between health and social care, primary and secondary care, mental health and intellectual disability services

Dilution
- Thinly spreading service provision
- Adopting minimal standards of care
- Reducing skill-mix in a nursing team

Delay
- Waiting lists (which for psychological treatments can become infinitely long)

Denial
- Not providing a treatment or service at all
- Using eligibility criteria

Recent developments in health policy have sought to block off some of the routes operated in community mental health services to manage demand by, for example, bearing down hard on waiting lists, removing the health–social care divide and demanding written protocols defining the responsibilities of services. The contemporary emphasis in healthcare is on services using strategies that ensure a rapid flow of patients through the metaphorical care pathway, retaining in secondary care a deserving few who will be in receipt of clearly defined and regularly reviewed 'packages of care'. Doctors in all specialties no longer have the same degree of control over their workload and that of the teams within which they work, this role now being shared in psychiatry with the bed manager and the team leader/manager.

The doctor and the multidisciplinary mental health team

What do mental health teams do?

Services at the front line of mental healthcare, such as generic CMHTs and acute in-patient wards, often feel overwhelmed by the extent and diversity of the tasks they are required to undertake. In the contemporary era of 'functional' mental health teams, tasks are becoming more clearly specified. However, even the most privileged of the new 'functional' mental health teams is faced with a very complex set of problems to address in meeting the needs of their patients/clients and those of their carers. Readers will be fully familiar with the manifold nature of the tasks facing mental health services. Fig. 8.1 provides a highly simplified description of the needs of adult patients and their carers. These go far beyond traditional medical areas of expertise (i.e. the assessment, diagnosis and treatment of disease).

The contemporary jargon for the set of tasks to be undertaken by a service is the 'care pathway'. Looking at the care pathway allows one to identify the tasks to be undertaken by the team to achieve the required outcomes. From this flows an understanding of the competencies required to achieve these outcomes. Staff roles flow from the required competencies.

There are multiple tools and exercises available to help services or individual teams map out the care pathways that are in operation (e.g. NHS Institute for Innovation and Improvement, 2005).

Roles of team members

All members of a multidisciplinary team experience difficulties in defining their roles within the team *vis-à-vis* staff from other disciplines. Increasingly, particularly in community teams, job descriptions emphasise the required competencies over the discipline of the post-holder. Accordingly, there have been repeated attempts over the past two decades to establish a generic mental

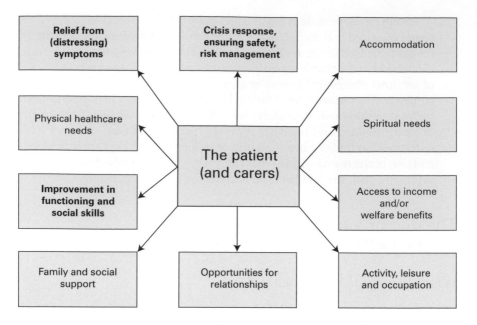

Fig. 8.1 Needs of people with a mental illness – an illustration. Needs in bold are specific to people with a mental illness and will be provided by mental health services. Other needs are common to everyone but people with a severe mental illness may require additional support to meet them.

health worker role. Throughout healthcare, tasks that were traditionally the exclusive province of doctors, such as prescribing medication, have been successfully undertaken by non-medical staff (although evaluation of this delegation of responsibility has focused on relatively routine tasks).

All professions are potentially threatened by the rise of genericism. The College of Occupational Therapists has advised its members that the majority of their case-work should involve specialist occupational therapy interventions (Craik *et al*, 1998). A study by Harries & Gilhooly (2003) explored the way in which occupational therapists function within CMHTs; some were described as 'satisfied genericists', others as 'satisfied specialists', while the largest cohort were described as 'aspiring specialists'. These staff wanted to increase the amount of time spent using occupational therapy skills, but felt pressurised into adopting a more generic case management role.

Social workers may experience particular difficulties within the team, related to role conflict and role ambiguity (Carpenter *et al*, 2003). The dissonance between the 'medical model' and social work ethos can lead to social workers feeling isolated and devalued. Mental Health Act assessments can be a particular challenge for integrated teams; many approved social workers feel the independent nature of their role is compromised by working closely with medical colleagues. There may be justifiable fears regarding an erosion in patients' rights. The proposed changes to mental health legislation will take services further down this route, with other team members, including community psychiatric nurses, acting as approved mental health professionals.

However, within many mental health teams a degree of generic working is enthusiastically embraced, as are the special skills and conceptual frameworks that individuals with a specific personal and professional background bring with them. Tyrer (2000) advocates a 'skill share' model, whereby professionals retain expertise in their core skills but share them sufficiently with colleagues from other disciplines to enable them to be utilised appropriately.

The consultant's role

Doctors retain a special role within mental health teams, to an extent that can on occasion be an embarrassment and irritation to experienced and overburdened consultants. Currently, consultants are by far the most expensive members of any team (although now almost matched by clinical psychologists of equivalent experience). Quite what makes them so special is at times unclear, although as responsible medical officers they retain a specific legal role under the Mental Health Act 1983 (which is to be replaced by a 'responsible clinician' drawn from any mental health profession when the Act is amended).

The extensive education, practical experience and training provided to a doctor who becomes a consultant offer the opportunity for the development of a wide range of personal and professional attributes ('competencies'), of which the most obvious are in diagnosis and formulation, psychopharmacology, the management of comorbid physical disorder, and dealing with urgent, life-threatening situations. The effective consultant needs to combine both very significant technical expertise (oddly, rather easier for the super-specialist than for the generalist) and a range of personal qualities (less required by the specialist than the generalist).[3]

Power, leadership and management

Power and multidisciplinary working

The organisational literature emphasises the roles of power, influence and authority in making any complex organisation work (Onyett, 2003). For Handy (1981, pp. 111–144), power can: be *physical*, as in the bully; lie in the

---

3 Perhaps unsurprisingly, specialist posts, in many ways less demanding and certainly much more prestigious, are more competitive than generalist posts.

control of *resources*; be related to a particular *position* within the organisation; be inherent in some form of *expertise*; or be purely *personal*, flowing from individual charisma. The final source of power that Handy identifies is *negative* power – the capacity to ensure that any initiative does not succeed.[4] In professionally dominated organisations, such as the NHS, professionals, particularly doctors, wield considerable negative power.

Handy goes on to describe how these forms of power can be used to influence the actions of others – which is the key issue for an organisation – by means of *coercion*, the application of *rules* or *procedures*, *bargaining* (as in a *quid pro quo*), *persuasion* (appealing to the other's rationality and professional values) or *altering the work environment*. Hunter (1999) suggests that when managing in the public sector it is more effective to take on the role of 'servant leader', supporting and guiding staff rather than exerting status and power. This may not sit well with some consultant psychiatrists, but may provide an indication of how to lead more effectively.

The culture of the team

Teams work best when the members agree on the common cause rather than merely function according to power relationships. The key issue for members of a team that is functioning well, once its task is clarified, is how to achieve their common objectives. Here persuasion is the most effective form of power. Other forms of power become relevant when there is no agreement about team objectives or methods. Consultants may then have to resort to bargaining and appealing to relevant rules and procedures to ensure that the work is done. (It is also valuable for their credibility within the team if consultants can influence the allocation of resources, even in a small way: this will depend crucially on their skills at working within the larger organisation.) The consultant will be anxious to foster a team culture that is healthily focused on appropriate tasks and outcomes. Changing an established unhealthy team culture is one of the most difficult of management tasks.

Leadership and the multidisciplinary team

Psychiatrists commonly take on management and leadership roles, and much of this book is devoted to describing these roles. There are subtle distinctions between the two terms, and a moment's reflection on past experience will confirm that not all managers are leaders, and not all leaders are designated managers. A variety of leadership styles have been identified, including

---

4 Effective medical managers regularly use all these techniques, apart from bullying, which is not only morally wrong but does not work. Negative power should be deployed only sparingly.

Box 8.3 The NHS leadership framework – 15 leadership qualities

Personal qualities
- Self-belief
- Self-awareness
- Self-management
- Drive for improvement
- Personal integrity

Setting direction
- Broad scanning
- Intellectual flexibility
- Seizing the future
- Political astuteness
- Drive for results

Delivering the service
- Leading change through people
- Holding to account
- Empowering others
- Collaborative working
- Effective and strategic influencing

Available at http://www.NHSLeadershipQualities.nhs.uk (accessed 22 October 2006).

---

the *laissez-faire* style (which might be described as hands-off), *transactional* leadership (getting the job done) and *transformational* leadership, where the overall vision counts most (Harrison & Gray, 2003). The contemporary NHS is much taken by the last (e.g. Modernisation Agency, 2003), which is summarised in Box 8.3. Transformational leadership is obviously most required when there is a need for change, for example when a team or service is under-performing (as, by implication, the Modernisation Agency believed was the case for the entire NHS).

Important though the transformational style may be, there are some often highly prosaic managerial tasks that have to be undertaken to ensure that teams can function (Reynolds & Thornicroft, 1999). These tasks are outlined in Box 8.4. Few consultants would wish to undertake all of them for the teams within which they work, but all should be willing and able to contribute their expertise to ensure that the tasks are carried out effectively.

Emotional intelligence

One currently influential paradigm which is highly relevant to leadership and team-working is the concept of emotional intelligence (Goleman,

111

Box 8.4 Key leadership tasks in mental health teams

Managing change
- Motivation of staff
- Managing anxiety and opposition to change
- Breaking down change into achievable steps

Managing staff
- Recruitment
- Producing job descriptions
- Managing staff performance
- Supervision
- Assessing and meeting training needs
- Dealing with conflict

Managing budgets
- Producing budgets
- Interpreting budget statements
- Implementing financial controls
- Managing under-spends and over-spends

Managing the team
- Maintaining service quality
- Enhancing communication within the team
- Producing and interpreting information
- Delegation of responsibilities

Work with stakeholders
- Managing team boundaries
- Working within the larger organisation to achieve local and shared goals
- Accessing resources
- User and carer involvement
- Working with primary care and commissioners

Anticipating the future
- Awareness of key organisational drivers (e.g. targets, star ratings)
- Awareness of policy and practice trends

Adapted from Reynolds & Thornicroft (1999).

1996). The central thesis is that to be successful in most walks of life one has to have an understanding of oneself and others. Components of emotional intelligence include: knowing your emotions; managing your own emotions; motivating yourself; recognising and understanding other people's emotions; and managing the emotions of others. Developing emotional intelligence may improve a consultant's ability to work within and provide leadership to the team.

Box 8.5 How psychiatrists can succeed within a multidisciplinary team

- High degree of technical competence
- Specialist expertise
- Effective response to crisis
- Respect from patients and carers
- Meeting (time) commitments
- Getting through the required work
- Respect for other members of staff
- Genuine interest in other professional roles (ask questions!)
- Listening to others' opinion
- Making (good) decisions
- Clear communication
- Availability
- Politeness
- Consistency
- Taking responsibility
- Acknowledging error
- Learning from mistakes
- Praise – specific rather than generalised
- Supporting the team with management
- Evidence of strategic vision

Conclusion: how to succeed and how to fail in team-working

Increased emphasis is being given to formal management training for doctors, and all senior trainees and newly appointed consultants need to develop a good grasp of how the healthcare system works and how to work effectively as a senior professional within a team. Some knowledge can be acquired through formal training courses and reading, but experience of good-quality teamwork and personal reflection when things go wrong are likely to be much more informative. Psychiatrists should cultivate an interest in how teams work and an understanding of the complexities surrounding leadership roles within a team.

There are some obvious ways for the doctor to be effective as a member of a multidisciplinary team (Box 8.5). Equally, although rarely acknowledged, there are ways for the doctor to fail (Box 8.6). Broadly speaking, a consultant's success within a team depends both on a modicum of technical competence and a range of interpersonal skills and abilities. Outright failure with a team is almost always due to a lack of interpersonal skills, particularly a failure to manage emotional responses to irritations and difficulties and to accommodate, at least minimally, the emotional needs of colleagues.

Box 8.6 How psychiatrists can fail within a multidisciplinary team

- Rudeness to patients, staff and carers
- High-handedness
- Inconsistency
- Favouritism within the team
- Not listening to staff, patients and carers
- Bullying team members
- Unwillingness to take responsibility
- Blaming others when things go wrong
- Refusal to make decisions
- Unavailability generally and in crises
- Poor time-keeping
- Poor technical competence
- Undermining the team leader
- Disliked/ignored by management and consultant peers
- Failure to learn from mistakes
- 'Pigeon-holing' other professions – holding outdated/inaccurate views about their role

---

Rightly, the consultant will feel responsible for how well the team is working. Our experience is that teams ebb and flow. There will be in the best of services times of excellent functioning and times when the team is going through a difficult period. Difficulties can be due to external or contingent factors, such as seemingly unreasonable demands from management, funding problems, staff turnover or some demoralising adverse event. They can also be due to factors internal to the team, of which the most obvious are lack of agreement about what the team is supposed to do, poor leadership and personal or professional conflicts between team members. The effective consultant will support the team leader/manager in ensuring that the key management tasks required to maintain good team working are undertaken, and will beware when the predominant task becomes one of transformation.

References

Burns, T. (2004) *Community Mental Health Teams*. Oxford University Press.

Burns, T. & Firn, M. (2002) *Assertive Outreach in Mental Health*. Oxford University Press.

Burns, T. & Lloyd, H. (2004) Is a team approach based on staff meetings cost-effective in the delivery of mental healthcare? *Current Opinion in Psychiatry*, **17**, 311–314.

Carpenter, J., Schneider, J., Brandon, T., *et al* (2003) Working in multidisciplinary community mental health teams: the impact on social workers and health professionals of integrated mental healthcare. *British Journal of Social Work*, **33**, 1081–1103.

Craik, C., Austin, C., Chacksfield, J., *et al* (1998) College of Occupational Therapists: Position paper on the way ahead for research, education and practice in mental health. *British Journal of Occupational Therapy*, **61**, 390–392.

Department of Health (2000) *Effective Care Co-ordination in Mental Health Services. Modernising the Care Programme Approach.* Department of Health.

Department of Health (2001) *The Mental Health Policy Implementation Guide.* Department of Health.

Department of Health (2002) *Mental Health Policy Implementation Guide. Community Mental Health Teams.* Department of Health.

Department of Health (2005) *New Ways of Working for Psychiatrists: Enhancing Effective, Person-Centred Services Through New Ways of Working in Multidisciplinary and Multiagency contexts. Final Report 'but not the end of the story…'* Department of Health.

Goleman, D. P. (1996) *Emotional Intelligence.* Bloomsbury.

Handy, C. B. (1981) *Understanding Organizations.* Harmondsworth.

Harries, P. & Gilhooly, K. (2003) Generic and specialist occupational therapy casework in community mental health teams. *British Journal of Occupational Therapy,* **66**, 101–109.

Harrison, T. & Gray, A. J. (2003) Leadership, complexity and the mental health professional. A report on some approaches to leadership training. *Journal of Mental Health,* **12**, 153–159.

Hunter, D. (1999) *Managing for Health: Implementing the New Health Agenda.* Institute for Public Policy Research.

Martin, J. P. (1984) *Hospitals in Trouble.* Blackwell.

Modernisation Agency (2003) NHS leadership qualities framework. Available at http://www.NHSLeadershipQualities.nhs.uk (last accessed March 2007).

National Steering Group (2004) *Guidance on New Ways of Working for Psychiatrists in a Multi-disciplinary and Multi-agency Context.* Department of Health.

New, B. (1996) The rationing agenda in the NHS. *BMJ,* **312**, 1593–1601.

NHS Institute for Innovation and Improvement (2005) Process mapping, analysis and redesign. Available at http://www.institute.nhs.uk/Products/ImprovementLeaders GuidesGeneralImprovementSkills.htm (last accessed March 2007).

Onyett, S. (1997) The challenge of managing community mental health teams. *Health and Social Care in the Community,* **5**, 40–47.

Onyett, S. (2003) *Teamworking in Mental Health.* Palgrave.

Øvretveit, J. (2001) The multidisciplinary team. In *Textbook of Community Psychiatry* (eds G. Thornicroft & G. Szmukler), pp. 207–214. Oxford University Press.

Reynolds, A. & Thornicroft, G. (1999) *Managing Mental Health Services.* Open University Press.

Tyrer, P. (2000) The future of the community mental health team. *International Review of Psychiatry,* **12**, 219–226.

West, M. A., Borrill, C. S. & Unsworth, K. L .(1998) Team effectiveness in organizations. In *International Review of Industrial and Organizational Psychology, Volume 13* (eds C. L. Cooper & J. T. Robertson), pp. 1–48. Wiley.

CHAPTER 9

The development of community care policies in England

Koravangattu Valsraj and Graham Thornicroft

Mental health services are in a process of transformation in England at the start of the 21st century. The main aim of this chapter is to highlight the development and content of current community care policies in English adult mental health. The chapter focuses on the building blocks of government policy and guidance for mental health services. We present a brief overview of the recent policy and legal changes that constitute key milestones in the development of community and hospital care policies for the National Health Service (NHS) (Table 9.1).

The NHS and Community Care Act 1990

This 1990 Act was the culmination of the series of reports listed in Table 9.1. In 1985, the House of Commons Social Services Select Committee, under the chair of Renée Short, produced an authoritative review of community care provisions (the 'Short report'); it made 101 recommendations and concluded with the message that community care 'cannot be and should not be done on the cheap'. The NHS and Community Care Act aimed to bring greater coordination to the provision of community care by the health and social services. The Act requires local social services and health authorities to jointly agree community care plans for vulnerable psychiatric patients with long-term, severe disorders; these must be needs-based, individual care plans, with clear indications of how they can be implemented locally. The key objectives of the Community Care Act are listed in Box 9.1.

A key role that has been defined in the Act is that of the care manager. 'Care management' needs some clarification. The term was introduced in 1991 as a variation of the term 'case manager', which had been used for the previous decade in the USA. 'Care manager' describes the role of qualified social workers, who assess the needs of service users and who then purchase direct care services from other providers. It is different from the role of health service 'key workers', who assess needs and who then also provide direct care. The Act makes the following statutory requirements of care managers:

Table 9.1 Key stages in the development of community care policy

Year	Policy development
1975	Ministry of Health White Paper *Better Services for the Mentally Ill*
1983	Mental Health Act
1985	House of Commons Social Services Select Committee report on community care
1986	Audit Commission report *Making a Reality of Community Care*
1988	Report by Sir Roy Griffiths, *Community Care: Agenda for Action*
1990	National Health Service and Community Care Act
	Department of Health guidance on the 'care programme approach'
1992	Department of Health's *Health of the Nation*, in which mental health was a key area
1994	Ritchie report into case of Christopher Clunis
	House of Commons Health Select Committee report *Better Off in the Community*
	Introduction of supervision registers
1995	Seito Trust report *Learning the Lessons*
1996	Mental Health (Patients in the Community) Act
	Supervised discharge
	NHS Executive report *Spectrum of Care*
1999	National Service Framework for Mental Health
2000–03	NHS Plan: policy implementation guidelines on various services from the Department of Health, including:
	• early intervention
	• home treatment
	• crisis intervention
	• community mental health teams
	• suicide prevention strategies
	• women's mental health
	• Black and ethnic minority mental health

Box 9.1 Key objectives of the NHS and Community Care Act 1990

- To promote the development of domiciliary, day and respite services, to enable people to live in their own homes wherever feasible and sensible
- To promote the development of a flourishing independent sector alongside good-quality public services
- To coordinate social care through the 'care manager'
- To allow for proper assessments of need
- To provide services on the basis of needs assessments
- To clarify the responsibilities of agencies and so make it easier to hold them to account for their performance
- To secure better value for taxpayers' money by introducing a new funding structure for social care
- To ensure that service providers make practical support for carers a high priority

Where it appears to a local authority that any person for whom they may provide or arrange for the provision of community care services may be in need of any such services, the authority (a) shall carry out an assessment of his needs for those services and (b) having regard to the results of that assessment, shall then decide whether his needs call for the provision by them of any such services.

This distinction is now less clear cut, as many social workers are members of community mental health teams as 'care coordinators', a term that was introduced in the 1999 revised version of the care programme approach (CPA), and this role effectively replaces the roles previously referred to as 'case manager' and 'key worker'.

The care programme approach

The government instructed mental health and social services to implement the CPA in 1991 (Department of Health, 1991). The CPA is still a central part of the government's mental health policy and was brought in following concern that, after discharge, many service users did not have a named member of staff to contact, or a defined care plan.

The CPA is the central process to be applied to adults in contact with specialist mental health and social care services, the aim being an integrated approach across health and social services. The key guiding principles in developing the CPA were the following: to specify an approach focused on the service user, appropriate to the needs of the individual; to provide a framework to prevent service users falling through the net; to recognise the role of carers and the support they need; to facilitate movement of service users through the healthcare system according to need and service availability; to put into effect the full integration of health and social services; to copy to service users their care plan; and to include risk assessment and crisis contingencies in care planning.

In 2000 the three levels of the CPA were simplified into two types of the CPA, 'standard' and 'enhanced'. The key features of these two current levels of the CPA are listed in Box 9.2 (Department of Health, 2000b).

Importance of the care programme approach

The CPA represents a managed process of care and remains the cornerstone for all aspects of policy for services for adults with a severe mental illness. The limitations of the CPA also need to be recognised, as it does not in itself contribute to the active therapeutic content of direct face-to-face treatment and support. There remain considerable local variations in how far the CPA has been implemented. The importance of the CPA is that it is designed to target resources to those who need them most, to ensure that vulnerable people do continue to receive the care they need, and to coordinate the delivery of such care (Bindman et al, 1999).

Box 9.2 The two levels of the care programme approach

Standard CPA
- Patient requires the support or intervention of one agency or discipline
- Patient is more able to self-manage his or her mental health problems
- Patient has an informal support network
- Patient poses little danger to him- or herself or others
- Patient is more likely to maintain contact with services
- No specific CPA paperwork is required

Enhanced CPA
- Patients who fulfil the criteria for section 117 of the Mental Health Act 1983 for after-care will automatically be included on the enhanced CPA (i.e. patients who have been detained in hospital under sections 3, 37, 37/41,47/49 or 48/49 of the Mental Health Act 1983)
- Patient has a diagnosis of severe and enduring mental illness (see Department of Health, 1995)
- Patient requires multi-agency involvement and coordination
- Patient has a history of repeated relapse of illness owing to a breakdown in medical and/or social care in the community
- Patient has severe social dysfunction, or major housing difficulties, as a consequence of the illness
- Patient has a history of serious suicidal risk, or self-harm, severe self-neglect, violence or dangerousness to others consequent on the illness
- Patient should receive a written copy of the care plan
- Patient should have a care coordinator allocated, with clear responsibilities and tasks agreed in the care programme
- Patient should have regular reviews for as long as deemed appropriate

---

Supervised discharge

Supervised discharge was introduced on 1 April 1996 following the implementation of the Mental Health (Patients in the Community) Act 1995. The 1995 Act amends the Mental Health Act 1983 to introduce this new provision. It provides a legal framework for the supervision of after-care in the community. Supervised discharge applies to the limited number of patients who, after being detained in hospital for treatment under the Mental Health Act 1983, need formal supervision in the community to ensure that they receive suitable after-care. It reflects the principles of the CPA and is intended to be operated as an integral part of it for the patients concerned. Supervision is for 6 months and is renewable in the first instance for 6 months, and thereafter for periods of up to 1 year (Bindman *et al*, 2000).

Box 9.3 Defining the client group for 24-hour nursed care

Twenty-four-hour nursed care is for people with severe and enduring mental illness who need:
- daily mental state monitoring
- frequent monitoring of risk
- supervision of medication
- assistance with self-care and daily living
- support to access with day care/rehabilitation
- skilled management of challenging behaviour
- ongoing evening and weekend active support

NHS Executive report on 24-hour nursed care

Launched in 1996, at the same time as the 'Spectrum of Care', the NHS Executive report on 24-hour nursed care focused on the needs of the 'new long stay' group. Possibly numbering 5000 or more in England and Wales, these people include many who respond only partially to acute treatment and who remain substantially disabled. They usually require transfer to longer-term, high-intensity treatment and support, without which they often remain for too long in acute psychiatric beds. The NHS Executive report makes clear that when service users require facilities which offer 24-hour nursing care, this is an NHS responsibility, as it was in the days when many more long-stay wards in psychiatric institutions were provided (see Box 9.3).

The likely client group for this service are people who are severely socially disabled by mental illness; many similar service users in previous decades would have become long-term in-patients in psychiatric institutions. The development of these new services now requires in each local area a residential care strategy that is carefully coordinated and costed by health and social service purchasers.

National Service Framework for Mental Health

A central element of current policy is the National Service Framework for Mental Health (NSFMH). Discussed in greater detail in Chapter 5, the NSFMH covers health promotion, primary care services, local mental health and social care services, those with mental health problems and substance misuse, and more specialised mental health services, including all forensic mental health services. This framework therefore encompasses a wide range of service activities, including those provided by local authorities and health authorities, and it draws on a review of the vast array of relevant evidence, including related information from other countries (Thornicroft, 2000).

The NHS Plan

In relation to mental health, the NHS Plan (also discussed in Chapter 5) added more specific detail than the NSFMH in describing which services should be provided in each local area (Department of Health, 2000*a*). In particular, it required the provision of early intervention teams, assertive outreach teams and crisis resolution teams.

Early intervention teams

One objective of the Plan was to reduce the period of untreated psychosis in young people, in order to prevent initial problems and improve long-term outcomes. Fifty early intervention teams were to be established by 2003, to provide treatment and active support in the community to these young people and their families. By 2004, all young people who experience a first episode of psychosis should have been receiving the early and intensive support they need. Some teams are now being progressively implemented throughout England.

Assertive outreach teams

A further 50 assertive outreach teams were due to be established over the next 3 years in addition to the 170 teams in place by April 2001. By 2004, all 20 000 people estimated to need assertive outreach were due to be receiving these services. Services to provide assertive outreach and intensive input 7 days a week are required to sustain engagement with services, and to protect patients and the public. The assertive outreach teams are now also being implemented nationwide.

Crisis resolution teams

Crisis resolution teams respond quickly to provide assessment and treatment to people wherever they are. By 2004, 335 teams were to have been established, and all people in contact with specialist mental health services were to be able to access crisis resolution services at any time. The teams will treat around 100 000 people a year.

Progress on targets

The NSFMH and the NHS Plan targets were conceived as a 10-year programme to improve mental healthcare in England. At the mid-way point (i.e. 5 years after implementation), the government published its own assessment of progress towards the targets (Department of Health, 2004). This internal evaluation concluded that substantial progress had been made towards the targets set and that in the 2005–09 period the key areas to be addressed were:

- social exclusion in people with mental health problems
- improving their employment prospects
- opposing stigma and discrimination
- services for ethnic minorities, abolishing inequalities in care and earning the confidence of people from minority communities
- the care of people with long-term mental disorders
- setting out a new model of mental healthcare in primary care
- the availability of psychological therapies
- better information and information systems
- workforce redesign, with new roles for key staff.

Key government documents and guidelines on mental health

In the context of the NSFMH and the NHS Plan, several key mental health policy guidelines have since been published, as given below, and together these constitute the current adult mental health policy framework for England for 1999–2009 (Department of Health, 1999, 2000a, 2001, 2002).

Mental health policy guidelines

- The NHS Plan
- The National Service Framework for Adult Mental Health Services
- The National Service Framework for Older People
- The National Service Framework for Children
- The Journey to Recovery: The Government's Vision for Mental Health Care
- Cases for Change: A Review of the Foundations of Mental Health Policy and Practice 1997–2002
- Positive Approaches to the Integration of Health and Social Care in Mental Health Services: Briefing for Directors of Social Services on the Integration of Mental Health Services

Mental health policy, implementation guidance and information

Acute in-patient care

- *Mental Health Policy Implementation Guide: Adult Acute Inpatient Care Provision.* See http://www.dh.gov.uk/PublicationsAndStatistics/ Publications/PublicationsPolicyAndGuidance/ PublicationsPolicyAndGuidanceArticle/fs/en?CONTENT_ ID=4009156&chk=hdBfGn

- *Mental Health Policy Implementation Guide: National Minimum Standards for General Adult Services in Psychiatric Intensive Care Units (PICU) and Low Secure Environments.* See http://www.dh.gov.uk/PublicationsAndStatistics/ Publications/PublicationsPolicyAndGuidance/ PublicationsPolicyAndGuidanceArticle/fs/en?CONTENT_ ID=4010439&chk=XB8C8w
- *Mental Health Policy Implementation Guide: Developing Positive Practice to Support the Safe and Therapeutic Management of Aggression and Violence in Mental Health In-patient Settings*

Asylum seekers

- *Caring for Dispersed Asylum-Seekers.* See http://www.dh.gov.uk/ PublicationsAndStatistics/Publications/PublicationsPolicyAnd Guidance/PublicationsPolicyAndGuidanceArticle/fs/en?CONTENT_ ID=4010379&chk=fsxJo5

Black and ethnic minority mental health

- *Inside Outside: Improving Mental Health Services for Black and Minority Ethnic Communities in England.* See http://www.dh.gov.uk/PolicyAnd Guidance/HealthAndSocialCareTopics/MentalHealth/MentalHealth Article/fs/en?CONTENT_ID=4002020&chk=PFFceH
- *Engaging and Changing: Developing Effective Policy for the Care and Treatment of Black and Minority Ethnic Detained Patients*
- *Delivering Race Equality: A Framework for Action*

Carers

- *Developing Services for Carers and Families of People with Mental Illness.* See http://www.dh.gov.uk/PublicationsAndStatistics/Publications/ PublicationsPolicyAndGuidance/PublicationsPolicyAndGuidance Article/fs/en?CONTENT_ID=4009233&chk=qDc1ps
- *Direct Payments Guidance Community Care, Services for Carers and Children's Services (Direct Payments) Guidance England, 2003*
- *A Guide to Receiving Direct Payments from Your Local Council*
- *London Carers' Charter*
- *London Carers' Guide*
- *London Carers' Handbook*

Community mental health teams

- *Mental Health Policy Implementation Guide: Community Mental Health Teams*

Deaf services

- *A Sign of the Times: Modernising Mental Health Services for People Who Are Deaf*

123

Dual diagnosis and substance misuse

- *Mental Health Policy Implementation Guide: Dual Diagnosis Good Practice Guide.* See http://www.dh.gov.uk/PublicationsAndStatistics/ Publications/PublicationsPolicyAndGuidance/PublicationsPolicy AndGuidanceArticle/fs/en?CONTENT_ID=4009058&chk=sCQrQr
- *Alcohol Harm Reduction Strategy for England*

Early intervention

- *Early Intervention for People with Psychosis Expert Briefing*

Gateway workers

- *'Gateway' Workers: Best Practice Guidance*

Graduate primary care workers

- *Fast-Forwarding Primary Care Mental Health, Graduate Primary Care Mental Health Workers: Best Practice Guidance.* See http://www.dh.gov.uk/ PublicationsAndStatistics/Publications/PublicationsPolicyAnd Guidance/PublicationsPolicyAndGuidanceArticle/fs/en?CONTENT_ ID=4005784&chk=5cCbHf

Mental health promotion

- *Making It Happen: A Guide to Mental Health Promotion.* See http://www. dh.gov.uk/PublicationsAndStatistics/Publications/PublicationsPolicy AndGuidance/PublicationsPolicyAndGuidanceArticle/fs/en? CONTENT_ID=4007907&chk=i2SwWZ

Modernisation

- *Mental Health Pilot: Improvement Case Studies*
- *Modernisation Agency Improvement Leaders' Guides*
- *Redesigning Mental Health: Access and Choice Service Improvement Guide*

Personality disorder

- *Personality Disorder: No Longer a Diagnosis of Exclusion.* See http://www. dh.gov.uk/PublicationsAndStatistics/Publications/PublicationsPolicy AndGuidance/PublicationsPolicyAndGuidanceArticle/fs/en? CONTENT_ID=4009546&chk=BF%2B3ka
- *Breaking the Cycle of Rejection: The Personality Disorder Capabilities Framework*

Social inclusion

- *Community Renewal and Mental Health* (the King's Fund and National Institute for Mental Health in England (NIMHE))
- Mental Health and Social Exclusion

Suicide prevention

- *National Suicide Prevention Strategy for England.* See http://www.dh.gov.uk/PublicationsAndStatistics/Publications/PublicationsPolicyAndGuidance/PublicationsPolicyAndGuidanceArticle/fs/en?CONTENT_ID=4009474&chk=sr1kpe
- *Preventing Suicide – A Toolkit for Mental Health Services*
- *National Suicide Prevention Strategy for England: Annual Report on Progress 2003*

Support, time and recovery workers

- *Mental Health Policy Implementation Guide: Support, Time and Recovery Workers.* See http://www.dh.gov.uk/PublicationsAndStatistics/Publications/PublicationsPolicyAndGuidance/PublicationsPolicyAndGuidanceArticle/fs/en?CONTENT_ID=4006254&chk=hSWweM

Women's mental health

- *Mainstreaming Gender and Women's Mental Health: Implementation Guidance.* See http://www.dh.gov.uk/PublicationsAndStatistics/Publications/PublicationsPolicyAndGuidance/PublicationsPolicyAndGuidanceArticle/fs/en?CONTENT_ID=4072067&chk=uuBKuS

Workforce

- *Mental Health Services – Workforce Design and Development: Best Practice Guidance*
- *New Roles for Psychiatrists – British Medical Association Consultation Report*

NICE guidelines

- *Schizophrenia: Core Interventions in the Treatment and Management of Schizophrenia in Primary and Secondary Care*
- *Eating Disorders: Core Interventions in the Treatment and Management of Anorexia Nervosa, Bulimia Nervosa and Related Eating Disorders*
- *Depression: Management of Depression in Primary and Secondary Care.*

References

Bindman, J., Beck, A., Glover, G., *et al* (1999) Evaluating mental health policy in England. Care programme approach and supervision registers. *British Journal of Psychiatry*, **175**, 327–330.

Bindman, J., Beck, A., Thornicroft, G., *et al* (2000) Psychiatric patients at greatest risk and in greatest need. Impact of the supervision register policy. *British Journal of Psychiatry*, **177**, 33–37.

Department of Health (1991) *The Care Programme Approach*. Department of Health.

Department of Health (1995) *Building Bridges: A Guide to Arrangements for Interagency Working for the Care and Protection of Severely Mentally Ill People*. Department of Health.

Department of Health (1999) *National Service Framework for Mental Health. Modern Standards and Service Models*. Department of Health.

Department of Health (2000*a*) *The NHS Plan. A Plan for Investment. A Plan for Reform*. The Stationery Office.

Department of Health (2000*b*) *The Revised Care Programme Approach*. Department of Health.

Department of Health (2001) Crisis resolution/home treatment teams. In *The Mental Health Policy Implementation Guide*. Department of Health.

Department of Health (2002) *Community Mental Health Teams, Policy Implementation Guidance*. Department of Health.

Department of Health (2004) *National Service Framework for Mental Health: Five Years On*. Department of Health.

National Collaborating Centre for Mental Health (2004) *Depression: Management of Depression in Primary and Secondary Care. National Clinical Practice Guideline Number 23*. NICE.

Thornicroft, G. (2000) National Service Framework for Mental Health. *Psychiatric Bulletin*, **24**, 203–206.

CHAPTER 10

Psychiatry management and legislation in Northern Ireland

Graeme McDonald

Political background

Northern Ireland is a province of some 1.6 million people comprising the six north-eastern counties of Ireland. It was formed in 1921 by remaining in the UK after the partition of the island created the Republic of Ireland. It is presently ruled by the Westminster Parliament, although the devolution proposals embodied in the Good Friday Agreement intended there to be a local assembly with limited self-governing powers, which include health and social services. The Legislative Assembly with devolved powers began its most recent incarnation in May 2007. Health and social care is administered by a single department under the leadership of a local minister and scrutinised by a Health and Social Care Committee. Until now government functions were the responsibility of a Westminster Minister of State, who had control of a number of varied departments within the Province and who reported to the Secretary of State for Northern Ireland (a UK cabinet minister).

Northern Ireland is the only part of the UK with a land border. It would appear reasonable to establish all-Ireland mental health services, to secure economies of scale and offer specialties not readily available to a small population and to allow integrated care across the border. With few exceptions, progress towards such rational provision has been slow and faltering.

During periods of direct rule from Westminster, legislation affecting only the province is most often passed through an Order in Council and without a full debate in Parliament. It is then called an Order rather than an Act. The current mental health legislation is the Mental Health (Northern Ireland) Order 1986 (discussed below).

An annual budget is set for Northern Ireland finances from the central exchequer, using a broad population-based formula. It is acknowledged that this results in funding for health and social services that is significantly below that available in the rest of the UK. The gap is probably rather less than it is believed to be by practitioners, but it is clearly the case that mental health services have not seen the increases in funding associated with the

currently being reorganised and is likely to sit within a government agency responsible for regulation and quality improvement. It is anticipated that specialty training at postgraduate level will become founded on schools for each discipline.

Mental health legislation

The statutory basis for mental healthcare in the province is the Mental Health (Northern Ireland) Order 1986. This allows for the detention of patients with mental disorder, their compulsory treatment, reception into guardianship, treatment of offenders with mental disorder and review by a tribunal comprising a legal president, a medical member and a lay member. The Order is supported by a code of practice and by rules for mental health review tribunals.

Mental disorder is defined as mental illness, mental handicap and any other disorder or disability of mind. The Order contains specific provisions that prevent compulsory admission of patients by reason only of personality disorder, substance misuse, sexual deviancy or immoral behaviour.

Action under the Order is triggered where a person suffers from a mental disorder of a nature or degree that warrants detention in a hospital *and* failure to so detain him or her would create a substantial likelihood of serious physical harm to him- or herself or to another person. This criterion of 'serious physical harm', with no mention of welfare, and the specific exclusion of personality disorder make the conditions for detention the narrowest in these islands.

Compulsory admission to hospital follows an application by a patient's nearest relative (defined according to a hierarchy) or an approved social worker and is founded upon a medical recommendation, which should usually be given by a medical practitioner who has had previous clinical knowledge of the patient. Only in exceptional circumstances should a doctor who is on the staff of the receiving hospital give the medical recommendation. It is not expected that the recommending doctor will be a psychiatrist or a general practitioner with specific training in psychiatry.

On admission the patient will immediately be examined by a doctor. Consultants approved under part II of the Order may detain patients, in the first instance, for up to 7 days for assessment. Should a doctor not approved under part II examine the patient on admission, the initial period for assessment will be 48 h. Further examination and report by a consultant psychiatrist may extend the period of assessment to a maximum of 14 days.

Voluntary patients may be detained in hospital for up to 6 h by an experienced nurse and for up to 48 h by a registered medical practitioner in order to allow an application for assessment to be made.

At any point during the period of assessment the patient may be detained for treatment. In order to proceed to detention for treatment, a consultant approved under part II, usually the responsible medical officer, must report that the patient suffers from mental illness or severe mental impairment.

The definition of severe mental impairment has caused much controversy in recent years. Challenges mounted through the mental health review tribunal sought to define the category in terms of measured 'intelligence quotient' (IQ). Those mounting the challenges have suggested that patients with an IQ of greater than 55 should not be detained under the category of severe mental impairment. In practice, consultant psychiatrists in intellectual disability viewed the legislative definition of severe mental impairment as a broad concept measuring patients' global functioning. The Royal College of Psychiatrists has produced a consensus statement, endorsed by the Council of the College at a meeting on 24 January 2005, reflecting the views of the profession locally that IQ measurement of itself is not the definition of severity of impairment and that evidence to tribunals should include factors which may cause a global estimate of impairment to be substantially different from measured IQ. At present, the outcomes of tribunal hearings continue to show that those who drew up the 1986 Order did not foresee this debate.

Reception into guardianship requires recommendations by two medical practitioners, one of whom should be a consultant psychiatrist, and an approved social worker. An application may be made on the grounds that a patient suffers from mental illness or severe mental handicap and it is necessary in the interests of the welfare of the patient that he or she should be so received. Guardianship allows the receiving trust to require patients to reside at a specified place, to require them to attend for treatment and to have access to their residence at any time for any medical practitioner or approved social worker. It is most commonly used by intellectual disability services and has proven a valuable protection for those at risk of exploitation and abuse. There is no real sanction against patients who are disinclined to facilitate a trust's legal powers under guardianship.

Patients, or in some circumstances their relatives, may apply to a mental health review tribunal for discharge from hospital or guardianship at prescribed intervals. Treating trusts are required to refer patients to the tribunal at prescribed intervals (at least every 2 years). The tribunal is composed of a legal member, who presides, a medical member (an experienced consultant psychiatrist) and a lay member (recruited by open advertisement), supported by a civil service secretariat. The Northern Ireland Mental Health Review Tribunal has consistently taken the view that it was for the treating trust to prove that the patient should remain detained or subject to guardianship. A recent legal challenge demonstrated that there was not legal authority for this approach and so the legislation was amended to provide such authority.

The medical member of the tribunal performs an examination of the patient before the hearing and reports the findings to the tribunal. Representatives of patients have questioned the apparent dual role of the medical member in both giving evidence and decision-making. It is presently believed to be compliant with European human rights legislation, provided the content of the examination is disclosed to both parties.

The Order defines three groups of treatments for the purposes of consent:

1   the treatments that require the patient's consent and a second opinion are psychosurgery and the implantation of sex hormones
2   treatments that require either the patient's documented valid consent or a second opinion include electroconvulsive therapy and the administration of medicines by any means after the elapse of 3 months from the first dose
3   all other treatments may be administered to detained patients without either their consent or a second opinion.

Treatment provided urgently to save life, to prevent deterioration or to prevent danger to the patient or others is exempt from the consent provisions.

The courts may, on conviction, order treatment in hospital with or without restriction. The Secretary of State for Northern Ireland may, on receipt of reports by two medical practitioners, direct the transfer to a psychiatric hospital of sentenced or remand prisoners who suffer from mental disorder. In practice, such transfer directions are likely to take effect to the medium-secure unit at Knockbracken Healthcare Park on the south-eastern outskirts of Belfast.

The Mental Health Commission for Northern Ireland has statutory responsibility to keep under review the care and treatment of patients. In discharging this duty it scrutinises legal forms, makes announced and unannounced visits and enquires into cases where it believes there to be evidence of ill treatment or deficiency of care. The Commission appoints medical members by interview following open advertisement.

Several problems are evident with current mental health legislation. Patient groups have expressed concern that an apparently large proportion of patients who apply to the Tribunal find themselves re-graded to voluntary status before the hearing takes place. The so-called 'Bournewood gap' of patients who are not detained but who are not able to leave hospital is not covered. The only capacity provisions in the legislation relate to property, finance and consent.

Future developments

At the time of writing, two initiatives promise to change the delivery of mental healthcare in the province.

First, the review of public administration (http://www.rpani.gov.uk) has recommended that the delivery of health and social services be concentrated in five trusts, although these are not aligned with local government bodies.

They have recommended the creation of a number of local commissioning groups that will have many of the same functions as are allotted to primary care trusts elsewhere in these islands. It is hoped that the diminution in trust numbers will lead to more efficient care and reduce divisions between practitioners at local level. It is feared that the cumbersome commissioning arrangements will magnify health inequalities and make service planning more difficult at all levels.

Professor David Bamford, Professor of Social Work at the University of Ulster, was asked to lead a major independent review of mental health and intellectual disability policy, practice and legislation with the active involvement of service users and carers. A series of reports have been published and consulted upon. Of particular note was the proposed application of the inclusion agenda to shift the balance of psychiatric care for those with intellectual disability to generic psychiatric services. The reports describe best practice, as derived from local services and other healthcare systems. Time-bound standards have been identified. Government has been asked to identify significant additional resources in terms of finance and workforce in order to deliver these aspirations. The review of legislation is taking account of the absence of capacity legislation and considering a broad-based framework that will permit substitute decision-making for people with impaired capacity by reason of mental disorder in order to intervene in their health and welfare. There is general support for the principles-based approach adopted in Scotland.

Sadly, Professor Bamford died in early 2006. His work has been carried on by Professor Roy McClelland. At the time of writing, the government has been unable to identify any additional resources for the implementation of the Bamford Report. Now professionals of all disciplines, together with users and carers, are united in wishing to see an adequately resourced modern mental health service delivered in a planned coherent manner and supported by sensitive legislation.

CHAPTER 11

Special issues for the psychiatrist in Scotland

Donald Lyons

Since 1999, Scotland has had its own Parliament. Even before then, it had its own system of healthcare and its own legislation relating to mental health. This chapter describes the organisation of Scottish healthcare and the legal and policy context in which psychiatrists operate.

The Scottish Parliament, Scottish Executive and the Health Department

Members of the Scottish Parliament (MSPs) are elected by a system of proportional representation. The Scottish Executive, headed by the First Minister, is responsible to the Parliament for the management of Scottish government. The Parliament's Health and Community Care Committee scrutinises legislation. There are also cross-party groups that involve a variety of stakeholders and can help to shape policy. Within the Executive, there are a number of departments relevant to mental health. In particular, the Scottish Executive Health Department (SEHD) oversees the provision of most aspects of health and community care. The SEHD is responsible both for NHS Scotland and for the development and implementation of health and community care policy.

The Minister for Health and Community Care provides political leadership to the Department. There is also a Deputy Minister, who usually deals with the mental health agenda. A chief executive manages the National Health Service (NHS) in Scotland (NHS Scotland). There are also chief officers (e.g. medical and nursing). The chief executive of NHS Scotland leads the central management of the NHS, is accountable to ministers for the efficiency and performance of the service and leads the Health Department, which oversees the work of area health boards; the latter are responsible for planning health services for people in their area.

The SEHD also has responsibility for:

- NHS 24, which provides 24-hour telephone access to medical advice from clinical professionals

- the Scottish Ambulance Service
- the State Hospital at Carstairs, which cares for patients who require treatment under conditions of special security
- NHS Health Scotland, which promotes positive attitudes to health and encourages healthy lifestyles
- NHS Quality Improvement Scotland, which sets and monitors clinical standards.

The SEHD has a number of divisions, of which the most relevant here is the Mental Health Division. The head of the Division is a civil servant, responsible to the chief executive. The Division oversees mental health policy, planning and service delivery. It has advisory posts for psychiatrists. At present, there is a medical advisor to the Division and a forensic advisor, who is responsible for advice to the First Minister on restricted patients. The Scottish Division of the Royal College of Psychiatrists is in a strong position to influence the Scottish Executive and holds frequent meetings with senior officials.

Health boards

Health boards in Scotland are responsible to the Executive for local planning and delivery of health services. They work in partnership with local authorities to provide a 'joined up' system of health and community care. Much work has gone into this under the auspices of 'Joint Future', a process of better integration of health and social care. This has resulted in some pooling or sharing of budgets and joint management of health and social care.

One of Scotland's problems is that the health boards and local authorities do not all share the same boundaries. For example, one health board and one local authority serve Fife, but Greater Glasgow Health Board relates to several local authority partners, some of which also overlap into other health board areas.

Community health partnerships were created in 2004 and have gone some way to addressing this problem. Scotland abandoned the structure of NHS trusts in favour of integrated health and social care partnerships at local level. These partnerships deliver services for their local populations in accordance with health and social care policies agreed at higher levels. Some partnerships manage specialist services over a wider area. Mental health services may be managed in this way.

Mental health policy

Mental health legislation in Scotland is described later in this chapter. Two other strands of mental health policy deserve special attention.

135

In 2001, Scotland launched a national programme for improving mental health and well-being. This had four key aims:

- raising awareness and promoting mental health and well-being
- eliminating stigma and discrimination
- preventing suicide
- promoting and supporting recovery.

The programme has given rise to a number of initiatives to support these aims, notably the anti-stigma campaign See Me, the suicide prevention campaign Choose Life and the Scottish Recovery Network. There are links to websites for these at the end of this chapter.

Scotland's mental health framework, launched in 1998, was superseded by the mental health delivery plan published in December 2006. Part of a wider 'delivering for health' policy, the plan is concise and has clear priorities, with three key targets supported by 14 commitments. The targets are: a reduction in the annual rate of increase of defined daily dose per capita of antidepressants, reduction of suicides in Scotland and reduction in the number of readmissions within a year. The commitments that support these targets include:

- a focus on recovery, rights and social inclusion
- improvements in assessment and a greater range of evidence-based psychological therapies
- improved assessment of physical health of people with mental disorder
- better training in suicide prevention and improved crisis services
- integrated care pathways for common mental disorders
- better services for younger people, with a reduction in admissions to non-specialist facilities.

The delivery plan is available on the internet. It will have a major influence on the shape of mental health services in Scotland over the 5 years from 2007 to 2112 and all consultants working in Scotland need to be familiar with it.

Clinical governance and regulation

As with the rest of the UK, psychiatrists are responsible to the General Medical Council for their professional standards of conduct and practice. However, Scotland has its own organisations for inspection and governance of mental healthcare.

NHS Quality Improvement Scotland

NHS Quality Improvement Scotland (NHS QIS) was established as a special health board by the Scottish Executive in 2003, in order to act as the lead organisation in improving the quality of healthcare delivered by NHS Scotland. NHS QIS was initially formed through the amalgamation of a number of organisations that worked on improving the quality of healthcare in Scotland.

The role of NHS QIS is:

- to provide clear advice and guidance (based on a thorough review of evidence) to NHS Scotland on effective clinical practice, in order that changes can be made to the benefit of patients
- to set clinical and non-clinical standards of care, to help improve performance (such standards show the public the level of care that they can expect), and to set targets for continuous service improvement
- to review and monitor the performance of NHS Scotland, and to determine how well its services are performing against the targets set (instances of serious service failure within NHS Scotland will also be investigated by NHS QIS and recommendations made to prevent their recurrence)
- to support and encourage NHS Scotland staff in improving services, by running development programmes, publishing best practice statements and organising conferences and events that will aid the sharing of best practice
- to promote patient safety by learning from past experiences and putting arrangements in place that will ensure that patients are safe at all times.

In mental health, NHS QIS is in the process of implementing a new strategy. The aims are:

- to weave together previous initiatives by NHS QIS component organisations
- to learn from experience of previous NHS QIS initiatives in mental health
- to adopt a 'quality improvement' approach which will help mental health services in the implementation of the Mental Health (Care and Treatment) (Scotland) Act 2003 (discussed below)
- to focus on outcomes for individual users, building on the results of an audit project supported by NHS QIS
- to develop an information culture in which up-to-date information is appropriately shared and based on a common data-set
- to accredit the development of locally agreed integrated care pathways.

Mental Welfare Commission for Scotland

The Mental Welfare Commission for Scotland (MWCS) is an independent organisation that works to safeguard the rights and interests of people with a mental disorder. It was established under mental health legislation in Scotland. Under the Mental Health (Care and Treatment) (Scotland) Act 2003 (see below), it has the duties of monitoring the operation of the Act and promoting best practice in relation to its use, including promotion of the principles of the Act. It has various other functions under the Act.

Psychiatrists are likely to have regular contact with the MWCS. An important part of its safeguarding function is to give advice and guidance to psychiatrists on legal and ethical issues. This is not 'legal advice' but it does give psychiatrists an opportunity to discuss difficult legal or ethical problems with an experienced practitioner who has special knowledge in this area. The MWCS can be contacted during office hours by telephone or by email. There is also a website (http://www.mwcscot.org.uk) with up-to-date information and guidance on good practice in using legal interventions.

Psychiatrists can also come into contact with the MWCS in the following ways:

- *Visits to individuals.* The MWCS visits people who are subject to compulsory treatment or guardianship. This may result in recommendations about that person's care.
- *Service visits.* The MWCS visits all mental health hospitals and units to see individual people and hear about their experiences of their care and treatment. It provides reports to services that comment on positive findings and make recommendations for improvement.
- *Investigations and inquiries.* The MWCS may conduct an investigation where it appears that a person with mental disorder may have suffered abuse, neglect or other deficiency in care. It may also inquire into improper detention.
- *Suicides, accidents and incidents.* Psychiatrists are asked to report to the MWCS any suicide or serious incident involving a person under their care. The MWCS will usually wish to see a local report into the incident and may wish to make further inquiry.
- *Requests for independent opinions on treatment.* The MWCS arranges independent opinions from 'designated medical practitioners' when required by the law. Experienced psychiatrists may become designated medical practitioners by undertaking training provided by the MWCS.

Other inspection agencies

The Scottish Commission for Regulation of Care (the Care Commission) regulates social, voluntary and independent care services. The Social Work Inspection Agency (SWIA) inspects social work services in Scotland. There is a move towards joint inspection of services, especially for people with intellectual disability.

Mental health legislation in Scotland

Mental Health (Care and Treatment) (Scotland) Act 2003

The main provisions of the Mental Health (Care and Treatment) (Scotland) Act 2003 came into force in October 2005. It replaced the Mental Health (Scotland) Act 1984. It was the first major overall of mental health law in Scotland since 1960 and was long overdue.

The Act starts with a list of principles that should result in greater respect for the individual. These include giving the person information, encouraging participation and taking account of the person's views. The principles emphasise the importance of patients benefiting from treatment, minimum restriction of freedom and the role of carers. The Act says that anyone providing care should 'have regard' to the principles.

The Act imposes duties on health boards. New duties include appropriate services for younger people and for mothers and babies. An important duty is that of maintaining a list of 'approved medical practitioners' (AMPs). Only AMPs can undertake certain duties under the Act, including being a responsible medical officer (RMO) to someone subject to the Act. An AMP must be either a Member or Fellow of the Royal College of Psychiatrists, *or* have at least 4 years' experience in mental healthcare, *and* have attended a training course on the Act.

A psychiatrist coming to Scotland from another part of the UK, or another country, is not automatically recognised as an AMP under Scottish law. He or she will need to provide evidence of appropriate experience or qualifications and will need to be trained. Undertaking RMO responsibilities for anyone subject to the Act would not be lawful and any action taken in relation to compulsory treatment could be challenged in court.

Local authorities also have new duties under the Act to provide services that support people and promote well-being and development.

One of the biggest changes brought about by the Act is the introduction of the mental health tribunal. This will replace the role of the sheriff court under previous legislation. The tribunal will hear all applications for long-term civil orders as well as reviewing orders and hearing appeals. Tribunals will consist of three people: a legal member, who will act as convenor; a medical member, who will be an experienced mental health practitioner; and a general member, who will have personal experience of caring for someone with a mental disorder, or who will be or will have been a service user. Psychiatrists acting as AMPs will attend tribunals, will provide reports and are likely to be questioned by tribunal members.

It is not within the scope of this chapter to provide a comprehensive description of all the powers available under the Act. Broadly, for a person to be subject to civil orders, medical practitioners need to apply five tests:

- Does the person have a mental disorder?
- Is treatment available?

- Does this disorder impair the person's ability to make decisions about medical treatment?
- Without treatment, would the person's health, safety or welfare, or the safety of anyone else, be at risk?
- Is compulsion necessary?

There are differences in the orders that relate to mentally disordered offenders and those that relate to people who require emergency care. The usual route into civil compulsory treatment will be via a short-term order. An AMP must consider it likely that the above five tests are met. Long-term compulsory treatment orders can grant a variety of powers and do not need to stipulate detention in hospital.

There are welcome new provisions of the Act. Many of these are intended to give people more rights, such as the right to appoint a 'named person' who can receive information about the patient's treatment and can make applications to have orders revoked. Neither this person, nor any relative, can make applications for compulsory treatment or give consent to an order. Only a social work 'mental health officer' can do this. The Act gives everyone with a mental disorder the right of access to independent advocacy. Further, it is possible to appeal against conditions of excessive security and 'de facto detention'.

Another important new provision is the right to make an advance statement. If capable of doing so, a person can set out how he or she would or would not wish to be treated if subject to compulsory treatment under the Act. Anyone providing treatment must have regard to the statement. It is possible to give treatment that conflicts with the advance statement, but reasons must be recorded in writing. This record goes to the patient, named person and the MWCS.

The Act has various levels of safeguards for medical treatment. These cover neurosurgery for mental disorder, deep brain stimulation, electro-convulsive therapy, transcranial electromagnetic stimulation, vagal nerve stimulation, artificial nutrition, drug treatment to reduce sexual drive and, after 2 months, any other medication for mental disorder.

Another new part of the Act concerns communications and security. Previously, it been unclear whether patients could be searched, and whether they could be stopped from having certain items with them, from having visitors or from using the telephone. The new Act sets out regulations to make sure that any of this is done with good reason and recorded and reported. It is essential to consult regulations before restricting the person's communications, searching him or her or insisting on samples for drug and alcohol testing.

Adults with Incapacity (Scotland) Act 2000

The Adults with Incapacity (Scotland) Act 2000 was one of the first major pieces of legislation passed by the Scottish Parliament. It replaced fragmented legislation, some of which dated from the 16th century. Built on a clear set of principles, it provides a legal framework for financial and welfare interventions for adults who lack capacity. This Act has several important implications for psychiatrists.

The Act defines incapacity as being incapable of acting, or making decisions, or communicating decisions, or understanding decisions, or retaining the memory of decisions. All medical practitioners should be able to assess capacity. Psychiatrists may need to provide assessments when capacity is in doubt or where the Act specifically requires an opinion from an AMP.

This Act changed the law on powers of attorney. It is possible to appoint an attorney for welfare and/or financial matters. There are new provisions for simple financial transactions. The Act covers management of residents' funds in hospitals and care homes. Psychiatrists will need to provide appropriate certification of incapacity and, along with managers, follow best practice in using an incapable person's money for his or her benefit.

The Act clarifies the law on medical treatment where the person lacks capacity. Except in an emergency, treatment is authorised by a certificate of incapacity. This can be accompanied by a treatment plan to cover complex treatment packages. There are some safeguarded treatments, including electroconvulsive therapy and drug treatment to reduce sexual drive. The interface between this Act and the 2003 Act is complex. Treatment for physical illness is covered by the 2000 Act alone. For mental disorder, the 2000 Act can be used for informal patients who are incapable of consenting but who do not resist or object.

For some interventions, it may be necessary to apply to the sheriff court for an intervention order or a guardianship order. These can be for welfare and/or financial matters. They require two medical recommendations, one of which must be from an AMP. Guardians and attorneys may have the power to give proxy consent to medical treatment on the person's behalf. There is a mechanism to resolve a dispute if the proxy disagrees with the proposed treatment.

General points about working as a psychiatrist in Scotland

It is important that psychiatrists working in Scotland familiarise themselves with their local health board, local authority and community health partnerships. They may be expected to adhere to approved care pathways and so should make sure they know these and understand the standards expected.

Psychiatrists from outside Scotland should get to know Scottish mental health and incapacity law as quickly as possible and find out about the next available training course. The Mental Welfare Commission gives advice on best practice under the law for those who are unsure.

For experienced psychiatrists, there are opportunities, in addition to local management roles, to broaden their experience. These include:

- being a medical member of a mental health review tribunal
- taking an advisory role with NHS QIS
- assisting the work of the Scottish Division of the Royal College of Psychiatrists
- providing independent opinions as designated medical practitioners at the request of the MWCS
- taking an advisory role within the Scottish Executive.

Further reading

Mental Health (Care and Treatment) (Scotland) Act 2003. See http://www.nes.scot.nhs.uk/mha/
Adults with Incapacity (Scotland) Act 2000. See http://www.scotland.gov.uk/Topics/Justice/Civil/16360

Other useful internet resources

Choose Life (suicide awareness/prevention): http://www.chooselife.net
Mental health delivery plan: http://www.scotland.gov.uk/Resource/Doc/157157/0042281.pdf
Mental Welfare Commission for Scotland: http://www.mwcscot.org.uk
NHS Quality Improvement Scotland: http://www.nhshealthquality.org
Scotland's health on the web: http://www.show.scot.nhs.uk
Scotland's Mental Health First Aid: http://www.healthscotland.org.uk/smhfa
Scottish Executive: http://www.scotland.gov.uk
Scottish Recovery Network: http://www.scottishrecovery.net
See Me (anti-stigma campaign): http://www.seemescotland.org.uk

CHAPTER 12

Policy, strategy and operational development of mental health services in Wales

Richard Williams and Stephen Hunter

This survey of mental health services in Wales and their strategic management provides an insight into policies in Wales that, in certain values-based strategic and practical aspects, we think are diverging increasingly from those for England. We take it as axiomatic that the client groups are broadly similar and, therefore, have similar needs. However, Wales has very high levels of deprivation. As we know that deprivation maps strongly onto the prevalence of psychiatric disorder and need for mental health services, need in Wales is, predictably, high. The leadership and management tasks facing mental health professionals and practitioners, general managers, managers of the professions and policy-makers at all levels are also similar. None the less, the different political climate in Wales imposes a different range of circumstances and solutions on all of these parties and, therefore, on people with mental health problems and mental disorders who need to use those services, and stakeholders who wish to participate in their design, commissioning and delivery.

The historical background

The dominant driver for change in mental health services in the Principality through the early 1990s was the *All Wales Mental Illness Strategy* (Welsh Office, 1989). That brief document identified ten client groups, covered all ages and was developed from local debate coupled with extraction of the principles that underlay the changes that were taking place in mental health services in England. Community mental health teams (CMHTs) in mental health services for adults were identified as the cornerstone of service provision. The strategy called for expansion of services for older adults, and improved work across agencies by enabling better relationships between the health and local authorities and the voluntary sector. The, then, Welsh Office ring-fenced the revenue and capital assets of Welsh mental health services in order to underpin the developments and made available recurring top-sliced monies from 1990 to 1994.

The Welsh National Health Service (NHS Wales), under the direction then of John Wyn Owen, had a deserved international reputation for health-care strategy, including its series of documents on the strategic intent and direction of healthcare. This type of strategic thinking is still evident in publications from Wales (e.g. Warner & Williams, 2005). His experience with parallel initiatives, including the All Wales Learning Disability Strategy, resulted in a permissive governmental approach that engaged clinicians, recognised the importance of joint working and endeavoured to protect non-acute services from the burdens falling on secondary care.

Implementation of the Strategy was overseen by a series of Secretaries of State for Wales, who made a point of emphasising their 'one nation' Conservatism. Arguably, this took into account the political situation in Wales, which meant that, after the general election in 1987, they were *de facto* governors imposed from Westminster on a substantially politically hostile Principality. However, judging by events, they appeared to be seeking to distance themselves from the reforming zeal shown elsewhere in the cabinet at that time.

As a consequence, Wales was spared much of the controversy that surrounded the publication of the White Paper *Working for Patients* (Department of Health, 1989) and implementation of the changes proposed in it consequent on the NHS and Community Care Act 1990. The first NHS trust in Wales was created in Pembrokeshire in 1992. Thirteen trusts were established a year later, some 3 years after similar developments began in earnest in England. During that time, many of the early vicissitudes of the new self-governing arrangements had been worked through. As a consequence, mental health services in Wales were largely spared exposure to the initial impacts of the 'internal market'.

The Mental Illness Strategy was successful in so far as it was implemented. The Strategy did enable: successful reprovision of the North Wales Hospital, a former asylum, into community and district general hospital services in Gwynedd, Conwy and Wrexham; the closure of Parc and Pen-y-Fai Hospitals in Bridgend, with the reprovision of those services into district and community hospitals; the closure of Pen-y-Fal Hospital in Abergavenny, together with the partial decommissioning of St Cadoc's Hospital in Newport; and the development of a number of dispersed, self-contained community facilities throughout the county of Gwent.

There was also considerable additional investment in the voluntary sector, which became a major provider of care in the community, particularly supported community housing in Newport, Cardiff, Swansea, Bridgend, the Valleys and North Wales. As a result, the voluntary sector developed considerable expertise through, particularly, the services provided by Wales Mind and in a number of specialist mental health housing associations.

However, the Strategy and ring-fencing of assets and revenues did not survive the appointment of John Redwood as Secretary of State for Wales in 1993. Local government was reorganised in 1995, which removed the co-terminosity that had existed between the mental health and community NHS trusts and the local authorities.

After 1993, the overwhelming majority of mental health services were managed in a growing number of community and mental health trusts in the Principality, with the exception of Bridgend and Merthyr, where services were managed by integrated general trusts.

Policy and strategy since 1997

The election of the New Labour government in 1997 brought a major change in the arrangement of trusts. In 1999, community and mental health services across Wales were merged into a much smaller number of generic NHS trusts that now deliver acute, community and mental health services.

Governmental devolution was implemented from 1999. An early action of the new Welsh Minister for Health and Social Services was to require a review of commissioning arrangements, which had, hitherto, been the responsibility of five area health authorities. That review resulted in the establishment of 22 local health boards, their co-terminous status with local government, and substantial local government and public representation on these boards.

Initially, it appears that few people realised that the National Service Framework (NSF) for Mental Health (see Chapter 5) did not apply to Wales and, therefore, that funds to support modernisation of services were not available in Wales. An NSF for adults of working age in Wales was subsequently published in 2002. That NSF was reviewed and a second version was published in 2005 (see below).

Arguably, the most striking strategic developments of mental health services have been in child and adolescent mental health services (CAMHS). Work began on the government's strategy for CAMHS in 1999. The confirmed policy programme, *Everybody's Business*, was published by the National Assembly for Wales in 2001. It envisaged a four-tier approach to commissioning and providing services through primary care (Tier 1), secondary care in the community (Tier 2), more specialised secondary services delivered at centres or as outreach activities from them (Tier 3) and very specialised tertiary care (Tier 4). We have been told that this was one of the formative influences on the new 10-year strategic model for healthcare in Wales, *Designed for Life* (Welsh Assembly Government, 2005b), not only for mental health services, but for all health and social care. Thus, in future, NHS and social services contributions to mental health services for adults in Wales will be expected to be mapped onto the four tiers in that strategy.

Looking back, it appears that the elision of mental health services with acute, community and other secondary care health services has had variable effects across the Principality. In some areas, it has resulted in much closer working across departments (e.g. in CAMHS and community and hospital paediatric services, and between mental health services for older adults with geriatrics). In other areas, by marked contrast, it is undoubtedly the case that mental health services have become more disadvantaged. Whether there is a direct relationship is not proven, but there have been serious concerns raised about clinical governance problems in a number of services and facilities in Wales, and some major adverse events.

Behind this analysis of the circumstances within Wales lies an increasingly different political and cultural approach to healthcare in Wales in comparison with England. Those differences are becoming more marked with the passage of time. Arguably, they are most evident in the attitudes of the National Assembly for Wales (in effect, Wales' parliament) and Welsh Assembly Government and NHS Wales to:

- competition and market approaches to commissioning services
- choice
- involving the private and independent healthcare sectors
- providing public sector capital.

Designed for Life, for example, comes with substantial earmarked investment of public capital across the Principality over a 10-year period that includes the potential for reprovision of a number of mental health facilities and services. They might well have been replaced as a consequence of the 1989 strategy, if it had run its true course, although some were not. Similarly, the Welsh NSF envisages a distinctly different approach to mental health services for adults compared with that being taken in England, with continued emphasis being given to enhancing the role and functionality of CMHTs rather than adding additional stand-alone services.

Service design and the agenda for change

Designed for Life (Welsh Assembly Government, 2005b) identifies three periods for redesigning and redeveloping NHS Wales. They are:

2005–08, Strategic Framework 1: Redesigning Care
2008–11, Strategic Framework 2: Higher Standards
2011–14, Strategic Framework 3: Ensuring Full Engagement

Designed for Life states that 'The next three years will be amongst the most challenging and critical for the service in Wales'. As regards the first 3 years, *Designed for Life* states:

'The following targets provide a broad but selective view of those milestones listed to indicate the areas to be tackled. The targets represent a first stage in the process – and will prompt a sharp shift towards:

- Preventing problems rather than waiting for them to occur;
- Improving access to all elements of health and social care; and

- Better designed, better delivered services in key priority areas – cancer, coronary heart disease, chronic disease and long-term conditions, mental ill health and services for children and young people and for older people.'

That strategy promises that mental health services 'will be remodelled over the three years to meet any new legislative requirements, the adults of working age mental health National Service Framework and the Mental Capacity Bill'. Also, 'There will be significant capital investment in modernising mental health services over the next three years'.

It is plain that there is much to be done to deliver this aspect of the Welsh Assembly Government's policy. As regards CAMHS, the agenda for service development has been set by *Everybody's Business*, the Welsh NSF for children, young people and maternity services launched for consultation in 2004 and confirmed in 2005, and a variety of Welsh health circulars. The agenda for mental health services for older people is being set by the NSF for older adults in Wales.

The agenda for mental health services for adults of working age can be derived from reading three reports that were published on World Mental Health Day in October 2005. These are: *Under Pressure*, a review of services (Wales Collaboration for Mental Health, 2005); *Adult Mental Health Services in Wales*, a baseline review of service provision (Auditor General for Wales, 2005); and *Raising the Standard* (Welsh Assembly Government, 2005a), a revised version of the original NSF, *Adult Mental Health Services* (Welsh Assembly Government, 2002).

As readers will see, these documents form a considerable body of recommendations for change and development. None the less, more recently, the Welsh Assembly Government has commissioned a strategic review of mental health services for adults and a separate review of forensic mental health services, including, specifically, secure mental health services. Both are due to report in 2007. In addition, the Wales Audit Office and the Healthcare Inspectorate for Wales (which has a broadly similar role to the Healthcare Commission in England) are working together to review all of CAMHS in Wales in 2007 and their report is expected in 2008.

Under Pressure

Under Pressure, the risk and quality review of NHS mental health services for adults, was conducted in 2004 by the Wales Collaboration for Mental Health (WCMH). The WCMH is a voluntary body, created in 2003, that brings together patients and service users with the voluntary sector, professionals and managers from mental health services, board-level strategists from NHS trusts, local health boards and local authorities, and researchers and teachers from the institutions of higher education in Wales. The Welsh Assembly Government appointed the WCMH to conduct its audit. The WCMH concluded that 'The two major indicators of pressure on the system are … Over-occupancy of inpatient units – at times exceeding 100%; and the high workload of community mental health services'. The WCMH further observed that its findings were 'remarkably consistent across Wales, and indicate a service system under great pressure, despite the efforts of many dedicated, committed and creative staff'. Consequently, the WCMH made 24 recommendations that aimed to reduce the serious risks which it saw. These included:

- the quality of patient care being compromised
- an increased likelihood of high-profile incidents in which the safety of the public would be jeopardised
- a further reduction in staff morale.

Adult Mental Health Services in Wales

Adult Mental Health Services in Wales: A Baseline Review of Service Provision (Auditor General for Wales, 2005) summarises the baseline position as in 2005 against the standards set by the NSF of 2002. The Wales Audit Office recommended that the Welsh Assembly Government should:

- ensure that funding mechanisms support long-term service development and that efficiency savings in the health sector are ploughed back into services
- develop guidance on joint commissioning of adult mental health services by NHS bodies, local authorities and Health Commission Wales (which is responsible for commissioning certain very special services on an all-Wales basis)
- issue more detailed guidance in a number of key areas to service planners, commissioners and providers, who should:
  - develop a whole-system approach to mental health
  - increase initiatives that focus on mental health promotion and early intervention
  - remodel services to provide more community-based care and to support and improve training for general practitioners.

In addition, the Wales Audit Office provided a more detailed critique in four topic areas and a checklist for action to aid remedying the shortcomings. It concluded that:

1   There are significant gaps in key elements of service delivery that are currently preventing full implementation of the NSF:
    - There has been a limited focus on mental health promotion, tackling stigma and early intervention.
    - Mental health services in general practices are often under-developed;
    - There are key shortages of community-based services that act as an alternative to hospital admission, that support safer and

more prompt hospital discharge and that support well-being and recovery.

- Modernised, fit-for-purpose in-patient services and facilities are not in place in all parts of Wales.

2   There is scope for greater integration and coordination of adult mental health services across different agencies and care sectors:

- Community mental health teams provide important multi-disciplinary assessment, support and treatment, but few teams are fully integrated and there are gaps in out-of-hours cover.
- A change in working practices and culture is needed if the care programme approach is to be fully implemented.
- The transition between child and adolescent and adult mental health services is problematic and gaps exist in services for adults with early-onset dementia.
- There is scope for better coordination of care between mental health services and other specialist services, such as criminal justice and drug and alcohol services.
- An integrated approach to workforce planning across health and social care is generally not in place to help address variations and shortfalls in staff resources.

3   The approach to empowering and engaging service users and carers varies considerably:

- Access to information and advocacy services can be a problem for many service users, and the extent to which users and carers are involved in the development of their care plans varies significantly.
- The extent to which service users and carers are involved in assessing services and planning improvements varies considerably across Wales.

4   Current planning and commissioning arrangements do not fully support the development of whole-system models of care:

- Mental health services are not always seen as a local priority.
- The effectiveness of local multi-agency planning groups varies across Wales and some areas have limited capacity to stimulate, drive and implement change.
- Explicit multi-agency visions of future mental health services are generally not in place and whole-system service development is made difficult and complex by fragmented commissioning arrangements.
- There are key gaps in the information that is available to support planning and commissioning, and performance management arrangements are underdeveloped.
- The way in which mental health services are currently funded does not facilitate effective long-term service planning and development.

Raising the Standard

Raising the Standard is the revised mental health NSF for adults of working age and it provides an action plan for Wales. It is based on the same four key principles as the first version of 2002: equity, empowerment, effectiveness and efficiency. The Welsh Assembly Government says that its NSF now takes account of *Designed for Life*, the reports from the WCMH and the Wales Audit Office as well as a number of other reviews and investigations when reviewing its NSF and coming to its action plan.

The NSF has eight standards, relating to:

1   Social inclusion, health promotion and tackling stigma
2   Service user and carer empowerment
3   Promotion of opportunities for a normal pattern of daily life
4   Providing equitable and accessible services
5   Commissioning effective, comprehensive and responsive services
6   Delivering effective, comprehensive and responsive services
7   Effective client assessment and care pathways
8   Ensuring a well-staffed, skilled and supported workforce.

There are 44 key actions through which the Welsh Assembly Government intends to achieve the standards.

The NSF and *Designed for Life* establish the following service components or functions as priorities (but with no particular ranking) for improving mental health in Wales and they are consistent with recommendations made by the WCMH and the Wales Audit Office:

- perinatal mental health
- liaison psychiatry
- work entry programmes
- day activity services
- tackling substance misuse
- court diversion
- psychological therapies
- comprehensive rehabilitation facilities
- risk management skills
- primary care
- workforce reconfiguration
- low-secure services
- eating disorder services.

In addition, Strategic Framework 1, Redesigning Care (2005–08) (in *Designed for Life* – see above), requires more prevention, better access and better services. The NSF also proposes that priority be given to undertaking a review to consider whether a move to regional mental health service organisations will improve standards and services for patients.

Operational leadership and management

Shooter & Lagier (2005), a psychiatrist and a senior commissioning manager in Wales, have provided a commentary on the roles, functions and management of CAMHS in an era of change. They identified ten aspects of poor operational practice. Arguably, their observations apply rather more universally and do not relate solely to CAMHS. Where the matters they identify occur, considerable leadership, management and support for staff at the level of delivering services are required if progress is to be made. These 10 aspects are:

1 vague service aims
2 lack of management
3 confusion of roles and responsibilities within multidisciplinary teams
4 weak internal communication
5 poor record-keeping
6 idiosyncratic clinical practice
7 indecisive service remit
8 unclear referral pathways
9 audit aversion
10 precarious commissioning.

Shooter & Lagier also identified ten contemporary pressures for change:

1 increasing demand
2 changes in allied services
3 political imperatives
4 reassessment of roles and values
5 empowerment of users and carers
6 incidents, complaints and investigations
7 external reviews
8 trust reconfigurations
9 risk management
10 patterns of commissioning.

Interestingly, they went on to offer ten processes for handling these drivers for change and risks for poor service delivery. They, too, apply to many services. The first three stages of that process are aimed at establishing the ownership of change by the staff:

1 listening to staff
2 agreement on a rationale
3 laying down a strategic plan.

The next four relate to the strategic service management that is required to translate policy into better operational services, with good service design, strategy, commissioning, operational management and, particularly important, clinical leadership as the intermediary processes. They are:

4   needs assessment
5   assessment of resources
6   reforming structures and protocols
7   auditing outcomes.

Finally, they describe three interpersonal matters that are vital to success:

8   monitoring staff's feelings
9   working round resistance
10 helping staff who become 'casualties'.

Developing the workforce in Wales

The workforce challenges that face mental health services in Wales are similar to those that face all mental health services across the UK. They include recruitment of trainees and achieving sufficient numbers of senior staff in all disciplines. However, just as the recent history of mental health services is particular to Wales, so, too, is some of the workforce history.

Academic psychiatry in the Principality, for example, has undergone a sea change during the past 20 years. By the 1980s, there were several large and strong rotational training schemes for psychiatry in South Wales. The Huntington's gene had been discovered in Cardiff, from DNA obtained in extended family cohorts from the Gwent Valleys. A new professor appointed to the University of Wales College of Medicine (as it then was) brought with him the specialty of psychiatric genetics from the Maudsley Hospital. He established a psychiatric genetic research laboratory which has since become one of the largest and most productive in the world. A North Wales offshoot of the department was also developed. Appointees in that department have revolutionised psychiatric training in the Principality, established a masters programme and recruited a number of senior trainees and research fellows from all around the UK. In addition, there has been a rapid increase in investment in research on mental health services conducted by a variety of disciplines and in related teaching made by a number of other universities in Wales in the past decade.

In part, this has helped to spare Wales from the worst of the workforce problems that beset psychiatric services in the UK through the 1990s and into the millennium, but it has not been sufficient. So, at times, and in some parts of Wales, workforce shortages have proved far more resistant to resolution than elsewhere in Britain.

It is clear that large numbers of junior doctors want to undertake training in psychiatry in Wales and senior house officer (SHO) appointments have been very sharply contested over several years. Also, the basic and specialist registrar (SpR) training schemes have not struggled to retain trainees in psychiatry and this is strikingly different from the situation in England. However, gaps in psychiatric staffing across the UK have attracted senior trainees from Wales when they have completed their training. More recently, though, there have been signs of greater preparedness of senior trainees to move into Wales for consultant appointments. Moreover, it appears that the Welsh Assembly Government has been persuaded of the need to invest in expanding postgraduate training in psychiatry. At the time of writing, those efforts were beginning to bear fruit.

Designed for Life identifies the key areas for workforce development across the NHS:

- recruitment and retention
- equality and diversity
- pay modernisation
- workforce development
- modernising the local human resources, training and learning infrastructure
- building leadership and management capacity and capability.

Over the 3 years to 2008, it expects the National Leadership and Innovations Agency for Healthcare (NLIAH) in Wales to help with:

- redesigning the workforce
- bringing service improvement
- embedding innovation
- securing leading-edge practice
- building leadership.

To this end, the Welsh Assembly Government has established a national workforce development and education unit based in the NLIAH to provide strategic leadership and action.

In *Designed for Life*'s Strategic Framework 2: Higher Standards (2008–11), the Welsh Assembly Government intends to increase the pace of change and to create a strong emphasis on making workforce development critical to improving standards, through a workforce design initiative, to which there will be five core elements:

1 creating a sustainable workforce that will be well educated and well trained, thereby contributing to the economic and social fabric of Welsh society
2 supporting the development of new clinical professional roles
3 progressively improving the qualifications of care managers and staff under the National Minimum Standards for Social Care
4 continuing to deliver the leadership capability and capacity which will be needed at all levels to sustain the change agenda
5 establishing flexible career options, as work–life balance becomes an increasingly important factor.

This agenda signals that 'new ways of working' in mental health will become policy for mental health services for adults in Wales, as in England (Department of Health, 2005). Already, 'new ways of working' is policy for CAMHS in Wales and local initiatives are under way in a number of mental health services. In particular, the NLIAH has been funded by the Welsh Assembly Government to take forward in 2006–2007 initiatives in workforce development, including promoting New Ways of Working in Mental Health of mental health services for people of all ages.

Finally in this section, late in 2005 the Wales Office for Research and Development awarded contracts for three new research networks in Wales that are concerned with: mental health; dementia and neurodevelopmental disorders; and intellectual disability. Two of these successful bids were prepared on behalf of the WCMH and there is cross-representation of co-applicants across all three. The intention is that they will work closely and in parallel with equivalent networks in England. We hope that they will contribute to developing the workforce and improve the involvement of service users and carers in Wales.

Conclusion

While Wales' mental health services have 'a long way to go' (Auditor General for Wales, 2005), the problems that are to be tackled are similar to those found elsewhere in the UK. A summary of the nature of the strategy and its application to mental health services in achieving what is required is provided from a Welsh source and orientation by Warner & Williams (2005). Previous initiatives, dating back to 1989, had positive effects until they were curtailed. Now, there is little argument between policy-makers, managers and professionals about the developments that are required. The questions are about the will, dedication, consistency and resources required to move from policy to practice.

Also, the reports about services that we have discussed recognise that Wales' mental health services are fortunate in having a dedicated, committed and creative staff. Skilled leaders and high-quality managers are required to take forward a challenging agenda and to harness the dedication and creativity of the staff. Thus, we come back to the lessons from Shooter & Lagier (2005) and from Heginbotham & Williams (2005). The former drew a parallel between the notion of the 'good enough' parent and the 'good enough' leader and manager who should 'shepherd those in their charge through the phases of healthy development'. High-calibre leaders and managers should engage the staff of our mental health services in the excitement as well as the difficulties of change and help them to take progressively more responsible roles in the process.

References

Auditor General for Wales (2005) *Adult Mental Health Services in Wales: A Baseline Review of Service Provision.* Cardiff: Wales Audit Office. See http://www.allwalesunit.gov.uk/index. cfm?articleid=1921 (last accessed March 2007).

Department of Health (1989) *Working for Patients*. HMSO.

Department of Health (2005) *New Ways of Working for Psychiatrists: Enhancing Effective, Person-Centred Services Through New Ways of Working in Multidisciplinary and Multiagency Contexts. Final Report 'but not the end of the story ...'*. Department of Health.

Heginbotham, C. & Williams, R. (2005) Achieving service development by implementing strategy. In *Child and Adolescent Mental Health Services: Strategy, Planning, Delivery, and Evaluation* (eds R. Williams & M. Kerfoot), pp. 63–80. Oxford University Press.

National Assembly for Wales (2001) *Everybody's Business – Child and Adolescent Mental Health Services Strategy Document*. National Assembly for Wales.

Shooter, M. & Lagier, A. (2005) Child and adolescent mental health services – roles, functions and management in an era of change. In *Child and Adolescent Mental Health Services: Strategy, Planning, Delivery, and Evaluation* (eds R. Williams & M. Kerfoot), pp. 487–500. Oxford University Press.

Wales Collaboration for Mental Health (2005) *Under Pressure: Risk and Quality Review of NHS Mental Health Services*. Welsh Assembly Government.

Warner, M. & Williams, R. (2005) The nature of strategy and its application in statutory and non-statutory services. In *Child and Adolescent Mental Health Services: Strategy, Planning, Delivery, and Evaluation* (eds R. Williams & M. Kerfoot), pp. 39–62. Oxford University Press.

Welsh Assembly Government (2002) *Adult Mental Health Services: A National Service Framework for Wales*. Welsh Assembly Government.

Welsh Assembly Government (2005a) *Raising the Standard: The Revised Adult Mental Health National Service Framework and an Action Plan for Wales*. Welsh Assembly Government. See http://www.wales.nhs.uk/sites3/page.cfm?orgid=438&pid=11071 (last accessed March 2007).

Welsh Assembly Government (2005b) *Designed for Life: Creating World Class Health and Social Care for Wales in the 21st Century*. Welsh Assembly Government. See http://www.wales.nhs.uk/documents/designed-for-life-e.pdf (last accessed March 2007).

Welsh Office (1989) *All Wales Mental Illness Strategy*. Welsh Office.

CHAPTER 13

Mental health review tribunals

Eve Russell

The inclusion of a separate chapter on mental health review tribunals (MHRTs) in this third edition of *Management for Psychiatrists* reflects the increasing importance of this topic in the day-to-day work of consultant psychiatrists. This chapter is a review neither of the Mental Health Act 1983 (MHA) nor of the increasing wealth of case law in this area. It is written from the viewpoint of a National Health Service consultant with an interest in medico-legal issues. The views expressed are my own and do not reflect the opinion of my trust, the tribunal service or the Mental Health Act Commission (MHAC). It is aimed at specialist registrars and consultants (especially the newly appointed) and is in large part based on discussions with junior colleagues under my supervision as to what they feel they would like to know before facing a tribunal. It is not intended to be used by specialists in the field or medical members of the tribunals and hence does not include detailed information on the Act or references to restricted patients. Although the Act referred to here applies only in England and Wales, the principles of appeal and tribunals are similar across different parts of the UK.

Accessing information about the Mental Health Act

All professionals working with patients with mental health problems should be aware of the content of the Code of Practice (Department of Health, 1999) and the Memorandum of the Mental Health Act (Department of Health, 1998). The Memorandum says what to do and the Code of Practice says how to do it. Recent judgments have made it clear that patients and their carers are entitled to expect professionals to use the Code of Practice and that it should be observed unless professionals have good reason for departing from the guidance therein. If doctors do intend to depart from the Code, it would be sensible for them to seek advice beforehand and essential to document clearly in the notes the reasons.

Almost invariably, at a tribunal, on the table will be a copy of Richard Jones's *Mental Health Act Manual*, often well used and tagged. This book, which is now in its tenth edition (Jones, 2006), has become the bible of mental health law, in spite of its occasionally controversial interpretations of the law. It includes the MHA and discussion of the cases arising from it, the Code of Practice on the Act and the Human Rights Act 1998. The layout is unfamiliar to those used to reading medical texts and the index refers to sections, not pages, but it is clearly laid out and it soon becomes easy to refer to the relevant sections, particularly with a few judiciously placed notes.

There are other important sources of information. Your trust, either directly or through its solicitors, may be circulating updated information on mental health law practice. You also must access training if you are to maintain your status as a section 12 approved doctor. The internet is an excellent source of information. MHAC guidance notes are published from time to time on http://www.mhac.org.uk, which also provides other documents and links to other useful sites. The MHRT has a helpful website (http://www.mhrt.org.uk) and it is likely that your trust's solicitors will have their own website.

Mental health review tribunals and the consultants' workload

There is a widespread perception that the effect of MHRTs on consultant workload has increased over the past few years and in my view there are four major factors which are responsible for these changes.

First, there have been significant changes in the patient mix on in-patient wards. The proportion of patients who are detained under a section of the MHA has increased over the past few years, as has the level of acuity and risk, which psychiatrists have to manage. This, combined with improved systems to facilitate patients accessing tribunals and legal representation, has meant that more patients are exercising their rights to a tribunal hearing. Moreover, because of the complexity of the needs of patients, reports are more difficult to prepare. Hence, even if the amount of work generated by tribunals had not increased, it certainly feels like it.

Second, more general societal changes, intensified by recent high-profile cases involving medical experts, has meant that the medical evidence is more likely to be challenged during the hearings. Patients are likely to be legally represented and increasingly the lawyers instructed are likely to be specialists in mental health law and certainly will be more knowledgeable of the area than the average psychiatrist. Although tribunals were set up to be inquisitorial, without rules of evidence, and, in my view, work best when conducted in this way, they can at times become adversarial. When this occurs, consultants can feel quite challenged and outside the relatively protected position that they held in the past.

Third and fourth are two important changes to the law that have had a significant effect on the management of MHRTs. One was the passing of the Human Rights Act 1998. Article 5 of the European Convention on Human Rights, which is set out in Schedule 1 of the Act, guarantees the right to liberty and security. It states that 'Everyone has the right to liberty and security of person' but it goes on to outline exceptions, which include the 'lawful detention ... of persons of unsound mind'. Article 4 of the Convention states that 'Everyone who is deprived of his liberty by arrest or detention shall be entitled to take proceedings by which the lawfulness of his detention shall be decided speedily by a court and his release ordered if the detention is not lawful.' The key word here is 'speedily' and the previous practice of organising tribunals for dates 8 weeks after the receipt of a section 3 application was found to be unlawful. The tribunal service has set standards to adhere to the wording of the Act. Currently these are that, from receipt of an application, the patient must have access to a tribunal within 7 days if detained under section 2, within 5–8 weeks for section 3 and within 15–20 weeks for restricted cases. Logistically, meeting the targets is extremely difficult for the tribunal service, which organises 13 000 sittings a year, staffed by about 1000 members, who work on a part-time basis and so have to fit their tribunal work around other commitments. Before expressing irritation with the local MHA administrator about the inconvenience of the date of a tribunal hearing, it is worth reflecting on the wider issues around the detention of people who are mentally ill. Although individual psychiatrists may be working for the best interests of their patients, there are societies in which the definitions of mental disorder have been distorted for political ends and rights to a fair hearing have been denied. The checks provided by the MHRT system are essential to ensure adherence to the Human Rights Act.

The other important change to the law that has affected the conduct of tribunals is a shift in the burden of proof to justify continuing detention. Before a decision in 2001 by the Court of Appeal, the burden of proof was on the patient to argue that detention was not justified. This was found by the Court to be incompatible with the Human Rights Act. Subsequently, the burden of proof changed so that the detaining authority now needs to provide the evidence as to why continuing detention is required and if the MHRT is not satisfied that the criteria justifying detention continue to exist it must direct the discharge of the patient. This change to the burden of proof has tended to result in hearings becoming longer. Moreover, as it is now for the detaining authority to demonstrate why continuing detention is necessary, the members of the tribunal are unlikely to suggest after the responsible medical officer (RMO) has given evidence that 'they are sure the consultant is busy elsewhere and would they like to leave'. Consultants are now expected to remain for the full hearing, allowing them to provide further information or clarify points as they arise during the course of the hearing and hence improve the quality of evidence available to the tribunal.

So, things are changing in the tribunal system and busy consultants can feel under pressure. How, then, can doctors work with the tribunal system so that the work involved in preparing for and attending MHRTs can be slotted in with their numerous other commitments?

It is important to recognise that the tribunal is a court dealing with the lawfulness of detaining and treating people against their will. The MHRT Rules 1983 provide for a code of procedure to be followed in proceedings before MHRTs. These 35 rules cover preliminary matters, such as making an application, the appointment of the tribunal, disclosure of documents, adjournments and so on. The set-up is deliberately informal, to ease the stress on patients, but nevertheless the tribunals do have significant authority. Rule 14, which covers evidence, allows the tribunal to subpoena witnesses to appear before it or to produce documents. Not writing a report or not appearing at a tribunal are not options. MHRTs are courts for the purposes of the law of contempt and an application can be made to the High Court for the committal of any party who is in contempt of the tribunal.

The first port of call is the local MHA administrator, who is helpful and knowledgeable and who would have often worked in the National Health Service in another capacity and knows how busy everyone is. Get to know your administrator and understand the pressures they face. If your timetable is relatively constant, it can be useful to plot out the sessions as red/amber/ green or some similar system to represent the relative ease with which you could attend a tribunal. Red sessions might include booked clinics, psychotherapy appointments or ward rounds at another site. It is also useful to include the administrator in the circulation list of memos outlining future absences because of annual or study leave. This sort of proactive approach makes it much easier for your MHA administrator to negotiate potential times for tribunals with the MHRT administration and get back to you sooner with a confirmation of the exact date. The MHRT policy states that hearings have to be listed within 72 hours of receipt of an application, so there is little time for negotiation around dates.

The second general approach is to review proactively which patients may be making an application to the tribunal. This could be done routinely alongside the other legal aspects of delivering care to detained patients, such as assessing the ongoing need for detention, checking documentation on capacity and consent to treatment, and completing section 17 leave forms. Nursing staff are likely to be aware if a patient has requested a solicitor and is about to make an application. There are also some patients, including those who lack capacity to appeal, who are routinely referred to a tribunal (e.g. when a section order 3 is renewed) and it is worthwhile having a system to identify these. Again, the administrator can help you here. Where there is sufficient notice, it may be that a report can be prepared by a higher trainee, by way of a training exercise, as it will allow feedback and revision of a draft. If the application is subsequently withdrawn, the trainee's work is not wasted and, as well as the training opportunity for a junior colleague, the report can be useful in clarifying issues relating to the patient's care.

the general risks associated with the disorder. Risks to the public can include serious persistent psychological harm to others and may also refer to a single individual, not just to the public at large. Again, this will ideally require a detailed knowledge of the patient's history, but if this is not available, then the report may need to include details that may be hearsay. It is important when documenting risky behaviour to be clear about where the information came from and not to represent uncertain information as factually correct; nevertheless, potentially high-risk behaviours should not be left out of a report merely because the doctor has not had the opportunity to confirm the history with a reliable informant. The tribunal is able to examine such hearsay evidence, which would not be admissible in a court. The inquisitorial nature of the tribunal is helpful in looking at the evidence before it and seeking further clarification from witnesses at the hearing.

Neither health nor safety is defined in the Mental Health Act but health is generally thought to include physical as well as mental health. Tribunal members generally are extremely experienced and apply common sense to their decision-making and are helped by clearly written reports. According to the Act, the threshold for continuing detention under section 2 (for which detention is 'justified') is lower than that for section 3 (for which detention has to be deemed 'necessary') and this reflects the situation in practice, where often there is less information about a patient detained under section 2 than section 3.

Where reports have been prepared some time in advance, it is worthwhile examining the patient on the day of or the evening before the hearing. It is then possible to consider the verbal evidence that you wish to present to the tribunal concerning the nature or degree of the disorder. The dialogue with the medical member will be improved if discussions relate to mental state examinations carried out in a similar time frame. A not uncommon scenario is for a patient to improve with treatment such that the disorder is not of a 'degree' that requires detention, but the issues around 'nature' remain unchanged and it is perfectly reasonable to provide such verbal evidence in addition to the evidence presented in the report. In restricted cases, where the mental state of patients may change only slowly and reports can be very lengthy, it is the practice of some RMOs to prepare reports on a regular basis, and not necessarily for a particular tribunal hearing, and for members of the team to present updates at the hearing.

Conduct during the tribunal hearings

In practice, many consultants see patients at a number of sites and the tribunal hearing may no longer be held just along the corridor from their office. Tribunal panels often have to deal with a number of cases in a sitting and there may be considerable delays (e.g. to allow the patient's legal representative to interview the patient). Significant amounts of time can be spent waiting outside tribunal rooms and it is worth identifying with the MHA administrator a room where you can sit and attend to routine work, with an arrangement that you will be called when the tribunal is ready for you.

The tribunal panel is made up of three members: the president (who is a lawyer and conducts the proceedings and writes the decision on behalf of the panel); a medical member (who is a consultant psychiatrist and who will have examined the patient before the hearing); and a lay member. The lay members come from a wide variety of backgrounds and have considerable expertise and experience in the field of mental heath. There may also be other people present, who will be introduced as observers and who do not take part in the proceedings. Examples would include newly appointed members and staff conducting appraisals of the panel. Rule 21 of the MHRT states that the 'tribunal shall sit in private unless the patient requests a hearing in public and the tribunal is satisfied that a hearing in public would not be contrary to the interests of the patient'.

Rule 22 provides that 'any party and, with the permission of the tribunal, any other person, may appear at the hearing and take part in the proceedings as the tribunal thinks proper'. Normally, those present at the hearing, in addition to the panel members and their observers, may include: the patient, the patient's legal representative, the nearest relative and other family members or friends as requested by the patient, the RMO, a nurse from the ward, a social worker and other members of the clinical team as appropriate. You may well know the medical member or other members of the tribunal, but it is important not to breach professional boundaries. The patient needs to know that the tribunal is entirely independent of the hospital, and social chat with the medical member, either on a ward visit or at the start of the tribunal, can be misinterpreted as bias.

The role of the doctor at the tribunal also needs clarification. Are you there as a witness or a representative of the detaining body, or both? You may be asked, albeit rarely, whether you are representing the detaining body. Unless you know exactly what that means and have discussed it with your trust before the hearing, the safe answer is 'no'. Then your role is that of a witness. If the RMO is to represent the detaining authority, then this should have been identified before the hearing and not at the start or during the hearing, which would jeopardise its fairness. If you are asked to represent the authority, it is worthwhile discussing the implications of this with your defence union before agreeing and you may wish to be represented.

Rule 22 gives tribunals considerable discretion as to how they can conduct hearings. Tribunal panels vary in the order in which evidence is taken. All tribunals will start by introducing the members, clarifying who is to be present at the hearing and their roles, and making it clear that the tribunal is independent of the hospital. The medical member will present findings and then may be asked to cross-examine the RMO. This may be followed by the lay member asking questions of the social worker, with other members of the panel being offered the opportunity to ask questions at different points in the proceedings. Lawyers may prefer this approach, as it allows them to answer all the points when they examine the patient towards the end of the hearing, but patients may spend an hour, possibly even longer, hearing things being said about them with which they disagree, which must be extremely difficult. Practice differs nationally and some tribunals may go straight into taking evidence from the patient.

Many consultants are used to taking the lead in managing clinical meetings but this is not their role in a tribunal. Unless you are appearing as a representative of the detaining authority, you do not have the right to cross-examine other witnesses (e.g. an independent witness whose views you may disagree with) and you would need to seek permission from the tribunal to do so. If the patient addresses a question to you, normally the president will take control of the proceedings and explain that the patient will have an opportunity to speak and the solicitor can indicate that he or she is making a note of all the issues the patient is raising, to deal with later. However, if this does not occur and a patient or other member of the team address questions to you it is important to point out that the president is in charge of the tribunal proceedings but that you would be happy to discuss the matter after the hearing. If the RMO shows respect for the tribunal as a court, this is important role-modelling for the patient and other less experienced members of the team.

Giving medical evidence to the tribunal

The RMO will normally be cross-examined by the medical member of the tribunal. There is no need to read out your report but it is helpful to sum-marise your decision in terms of the statutory requirements for continuing detention (as discussed earlier). The tribunal will be making its decision on the balance of probabilities.

The other issue that the tribunal will ask you to consider is the after-care plan and it is important to be able to state what services would be available if the patient were discharged on the day of the hearing. It is the duty of the primary care trust and the local social services authority to provide, in cooperation with relevant voluntary agencies, after-care services for all discharged section 3 and certain other categories of patients. The Code of Practice advises that a care plan should be in place 'at least in embryo'. Tribunal members live in the real world of mental health services and if there is a lack of appropriate provision it is important to state exactly what services are available and what could be offered, however little. The tribunal has the power to discharge immediately, to defer discharge, usually for a period of weeks rather than months, or to make recommendations (e.g. about the provision of services to the patient) and adjourn and reconsider the case at a later date if the recommendation is not complied with by the appropriate authority. The tribunal can request, for example, that the chief executive of the trust or director of social services attend the adjourned hearing to explain delays in the provision of appropriate services for a detained patient.

Conclusion

History has shown us that the way in which societies treat their most vulnerable members, including people who are mentally ill, can be a measure of their civilisation. The UK has adopted the Human Rights Act, which defines the right to liberty and security for all of us. The right of appeal to the MHRTs is important for our patients. I hope that this account will be useful in increasing our understanding of the framework within which tribunals work and help us contribute more effectively to the tribunal service and hence to the care of our patients.

References

Department of Health (1998) *Mental Health Act 1983: Memorandum on Parts I to VI, VIII and X*. HMSO.
Department of Health (1999) *Code of Practice to the Mental Health Act 1983*. The Stationery Office.
Jones, R. (2006) *Mental Health Act Manual* (10th revised edn). Sweet & Maxwell.

R v. *Canons Park Mental Health Review Tribunal ex p. A* [1994] All E.R. 659
R v. *Mental Health Review Tribunal for the South Thames Region ex p. Smith* [1999] C.O.D. 148.

CHAPTER 14

Mental Capacity Act 2005

Jonathan Waite

In April 2005, in the dying moments of the second Blair administration, just before Parliament was dissolved, the House of Commons rushed through the Mental Capacity Act. The Mental Health Bill was not so widely supported and a new Mental Health Act is still not agreed, but the Mental Capacity Act is partly in operation and the remainder will come into force in October 2007. What will this new legislation mean for practising psychiatrists?

For hundreds of years, persons who were incapable of making decisions for themselves were dealt with by the courts, on the authority of Parliament under the principle that the monarch was 'father of the people' (*parens patriae*). In latter years, this principle was incorporated in successive Mental Health Acts. After the 1959 Act, Parliament stopped ratifying the principle and powers to act on behalf of incapacitated people were included under the guardianship provisions of that Act. These were very wide and essentially gave the guardian the powers which a parent would have over a child of less than 16 years. The Mental Health Act 1983 drastically curtailed the powers of guardians, particularly in the field of healthcare decisions, and removed completely any control over people with intellectual disability who were not 'mentally impaired'. This lacuna in the law became apparent soon after the 1983 Act came into force and the Law Society started to consult on what new law was required. This work was taken over by the Law Commission, which in 1995 produced its report on Mental Capacity, as well as a draft Mental Capacity Bill (Law Commission, 1995); the current Act is based on this, with some modifications as a result of public consultation and comments by a joint parliamentary committee.

The Law Commission report and its earlier drafts were widely circulated in legal circles and its recommendations have been very influential on judges and legislators throughout the world. In the interval between the 1983 Act and 2007, the courts have had to fill the gap left by the lack of statutory measures by interpreting the common law; these judgments have been used by bodies such as the British Medical Association and the General Medical Council in producing guidance for doctors. As a result of the incorporation of the concepts of the new Act in common law in that interval, there is no great philosophical or ethical change in the legal basis of medical practice brought about by the new legislation. The effect of the Mental Capacity Act is to codify current good practice and to introduce some new mechanisms to put these approaches into practice. Many of the concepts concerning the treatment of patients who lack capacity will therefore already be familiar to psychiatrists, but there will be some major changes in managing the financial affairs of patients and in making decisions on medical treatment.

The underlying philosophy of the Act is outlined in section 1, 'The principles':

(1) The following principles apply for the purposes of this Act.
(2) A person must be assumed to have capacity unless it is established that he lacks capacity.
(3) A person is not to be treated as unable to make a decision unless all practicable steps to help him to do so have been taken without success.
(4) A person is not to be treated as unable to make a decision merely because he makes an unwise decision.
(5) An act done, or a decision made, under this Act for or on behalf of a person who lacks capacity must be done, or made, in his best interests.
(6) Before the act is done, or the decision is made, regard must be had to whether the purpose for which it is needed can be as effectively achieved in a way that is less restrictive of the person's rights and freedom of action.

A broad definition of capacity is given in section 2, 'People who lack capacity':

(1) For the purposes of this Act a person lacks capacity in relation to a matter if at the material time he is unable to make a decision for himself in relation to the matter because of an impairment of, or a disturbance in the functioning of, the mind or brain.
(2) It does not matter whether the impairment or disturbance is permanent or temporary....

Inability to make a decision is defined (along the lines familiar from the current Mental Health Act Code of Practice) in section 3, 'Inability to make decisions':

(1) For the purposes of section 2, a person is unable to make a decision for himself if he is unable –
 (a) to understand the information relevant to the decision
 (b) to retain that information
 (c) to use or weigh that information as part of the process of making the decision, or
 (d) to communicate his decision (whether by talking, using sign language or any other means).
(2) The fact that a person is able to retain the information relevant to a decision for a short period only does not prevent him from being regarded as able to make the decision.
(3) The information relevant to a decision includes information about the reasonably foreseeable consequences of –

(a) deciding one way or the other, or

(b) failing to make the decision.

Acts made on behalf of a person who lacks capacity will have to be in that person's 'best interests' (section 4). In order to make a decision on best interests, the following factors will need to be considered:

- Is the person likely to regain capacity and if so when?
- How can their participation in the process of decision-making be maximised?
- What are the past and present wishes of the person, what are the person's beliefs and values, and are there other relevant factors?
- The views of carers and other nominated or appointed persons should be sought on the beliefs and so on of the person lacking capacity.

Early drafts of the Bill included a 'general authority to act reasonably', which has been replaced by 'Acts in connection with care or treatment' (sections 5–8), which allows carers to act informally in non-contentious situations.

Enduring powers of attorney (EPAs) will be replaced by lasting powers of attorney (LPAs) (sections 9–14). These will enable people at risk of losing capacity to appoint proxy decision-makers, who will be able to make healthcare and welfare decisions as well as managing matters of finance. The powers of the Court of Protection set out in Part VII of the Mental Health Act will be amended by Part 2 of the Mental Capacity Act. Where patients have not made express provision before the onset of incapacity, the Court will be able to make a ruling (section 15) on whether a proposed action is in a patient's best interests; alternatively, the Court can appoint a deputy (sections 16–21), who will be able to have a role in making decisions on health and welfare matters, as well as in respect of financial affairs, should the court so decide in a particular case. 'Receivers' will be replaced by deputies.

Neither court-appointed deputies nor attorneys will be able to make decisions on treatments for mental disorder covered by Part IV of the Mental Health Act (section 28); some other acts are also excluded (sections 27–29).

Advance directives to refuse treatment will also be given a statutory basis (sections 24–26). For a time, it appeared that patients might be able to make requests for treatment which would be binding on doctors but the judgment of the Court of Appeal in the Burke case (Burke v. GMC, 2005) has confirmed that only refusals of treatment are binding.

Research on people lacking capacity will be regulated by sections 30–34, which will add to the burdens which researchers have to cope with from existing ethical committees.

Many of the proponents of the Mental Capacity Act were keen to see strong statutory measures to ensure the provision of advocacy services for people who lacked capacity. The government was initially reluctant to incorporate these wishes in the statute, but later conceded that placement of people lacking capacity in care homes by health and social services and the provision of certain medical treatments will require prior discussion with an 'independent mental capacity advocate' (IMCA) (sections 35–41). The Department of Health has invited comments on the role of the IMCA but no definite results have emerged from this consultation process.

The Mental Capacity Act will be accompanied by a Code of Practice. Anybody who is employed in providing care for people without capacity will be required to 'have regard' to the Code. The Code is very long, but detailed and easy to read. It offers a great deal of practical guidance on how the Act is to be understood and implemented. It also offers advice on how capacity might be assessed.

A new offence of ill treating or wilfully neglecting a person without capacity is created by section 44.

Part 2 of the Act is concerned with the Court of Protection and the Office of the Public Guardian. The role of the Court of Protection will be enhanced. The Court will sit in a number of regional centres. It is envisaged that the Court will continue to act in a relatively informal manner, without the need for parties to be legally represented. The Public Guardian will be responsible for administering the supervision of LPAs and activities of the Court; the first Public Guardian has already been appointed.

Part 3 relates to technical legal matters.

The decision of the European Court of Human Rights in the Bournewood case (*HL* v. *UK*, 2004) has caused considerable embarrassment for the government; by the time it was published, the Mental Capacity Act was too far through its legislative passage to be amended to fill the 'Bournewood gap'. The 2006 Mental Health Bill contains proposals for authorising deprivation of liberty in a hospital or registered care home, where this is in the best interests of a person lacking capacity to make a decision on their place of residence owing to mental disorder. Authorisations will be issued by primary care trusts for patients in hospital, and by local authorities for care home residents. A psychiatrist or other suitably trained doctor will be required to undertake a mental health assessment. In most cases it is expected that the same individual will assess the person's mental capacity. An approved mental health professional (AMHP) will be needed to assess whether the proposed deprivation of liberty is in the person's best interests. Further training will be required for the professionals involved. Bournewood assessments may become a large part of the work of psychiatrists, particularly those working with older people and people with intellectual disability.

References and further reading

Official papers on the Mental Capacity Act are available on the website of the Department for Constitutional Affairs (http://www.dca.gov.uk) and by following links to 'Legal policy' and 'Mental capacity'. In May 2007 the Department for Constitutional Affairs became part of the new Ministry of Justice (http://www.justice.gov.uk) but the website of the Department for Constitutional Affairs remains as an archive and for information purposes.

Bartlett, P. (2005) *Blackstone's Guide to the Mental Capacity Act*. Oxford University Press.

British Medical Association & Law Society (2004) *Assessment of Mental Capacity: Guidance for Doctors and Lawyers* (2nd edn). BMA Publishing Group.

Greaney, N., Morris, F. & Taylor, B. (2005) *Mental Capacity Act 2005: A Guide to the New Law*. Law Society.

Law Commission (1995) *Mental Capacity*. Law Com 231. The Stationery Office.

Burke v. *GMC* [2005] EWCA Civ 1003

HL v. *UK* [2004] ECtHR Appln No. 45508/99

Part II
Changes and conflicts

CHAPTER 15

Understanding systems

Kate Silvester and Simon Baugh

As doctors are becoming increasingly accountable for their clinical actions, it is vital that they understand how to redesign the system to ensure that they see and treat patients in safe, patient-centred, timely and cost-effective manner. Most management practice is about establishing hierarchical organisational structures with accountability for patient care, but little is done to understand and prevent system failures.

A process view of the system provides greater insight into why an episode of care, despite all good intentions, is poor. Patients do not flow smoothly through the system but can be subject to delays and poor-quality decisions at each step, often because the information does not flow in tandem with the patient. This leads to rework and wasted resources downstream, with frustrated staff blaming each other, and often their patients, for failures in their system.

This chapter considers the process of care from presentation to discharge, in terms of how patients and information flow between the organisational structures and roles within the whole system. The first section outlines the process view and looks at: the high-level view; detailed process mapping; process redesign; and the quality cycle (plan, do, study and act). The next section looks at areas of pathology of processes: bottlenecks; matching demand and capacity, in particular in relation to variation in both (queue theory). The final section discusses how to measure for improvement.

Taking a process view

High-level view

Follow the journey of a 'typical' patient from presentation to discharge in a system. The process map in Fig. 15.1 shows the patient 'journey' for a non-urgent referral from primary care to a typical community mental health service. Note the 15–20 key steps to discharge back to the general practitioner (GP). This helps identify the key, and often unrecognised, staff involved in each step of the process.

173

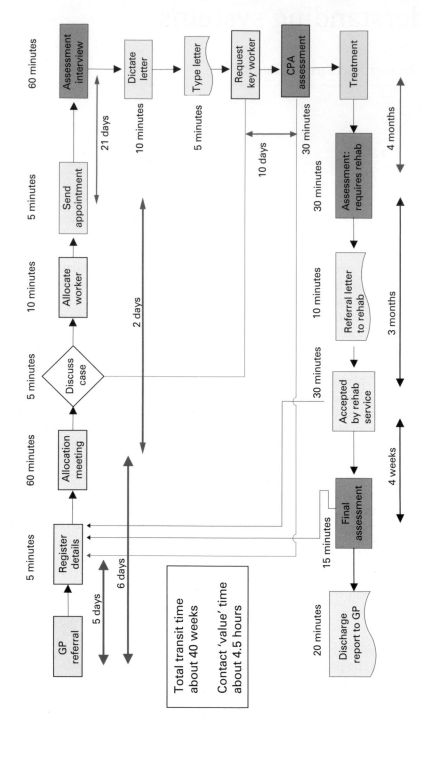

Fig. 15.1 A high-level process map showing the time taken for each step and the waiting times between steps for a community referral. CPA, Care programme approach.

Detailed process mapping

Having carried out high-level process mapping, from presentation to discharge, invite all the staff involved, clinical and administrative, to a detailed process-mapping event. To improve relationships and to assess the likely effect of any changes proposed, extend the 'process net' out beyond one department and into other organisations (e.g. primary and secondary care, social and ambulance services). Be brave and include patients, especially those who use the service frequently, since only they experience the system from end to end.

Before and at the beginning of the process-mapping event, ensure that everyone understands that it is the system that is at fault, not the people. At the event, participants should be 'walked through' the high-level process map to get an overview of the whole system. Everyone must listen, without judgement, as the more detailed steps performed by one role, in one place, at one time are represented by stick-on notes and placed between the key steps on a large sheet of brown paper. Concentrate on what happens to most patients most of the time. Avoid the exceptional cases and anecdotes.

An example of a detailed process map is given in Box 15.1.

Box 15.1 Example for detailed process mapping: a discharge letter

During the clinic, the psychiatrist writes in the notes and put the notes aside for dictation later. The notes are collected up by the clinic staff and left in a basket in the public reception area at the end of the clinic. The secretary collects the basket of notes later in the day and takes it up to her office. She transfers the notes onto a shelf and places a voice recorder next to them ready for the doctor to do the dictation. A week later the doctor does the dictation but is now often unable to decipher the notes or remember the patient concerned. She dictates a letter to the GP. The tape, containing several letters, is placed with the bundle of notes and put on another shelf for the secretary to transcribe. Meanwhile, the patient has been back to the GP for a repeat prescription. The GP or case-worker is now repeatedly interrupting his working day to telephone the secretary via the busy switchboard. The secretary shuffles through piles of notes to see if the letter has or has not been dictated yet. Notes and tapes become scrambled. Then she listens to several long tapes to find this particular patient's letter. She decides to give a verbal report or 'prioritises' this urgent letter. In the brief interludes when her telephone is not ringing, the secretary works her way through the notes and tapes, producing letters that she will attach to the front of each set of notes for the doctor to sign. Meanwhile, the patient is due for another clinic appointment or has turned up in accident and emergency department but no one can find the notes. The filing clerk extracts them from the doctor's office or a new set of notes is made. Several days later, the doctor reads and signs her now out-of-date letters but cannot remember anything about this patient and needs to check the notes. Where are they? Which set of notes comes back from filing now?

Table 15.1 Characterisation of waste

Type of waste	Examples
Transportation	Patients and notes being moved around
Bad quality and defects	Prescription error. Delayed reports. Wrong diagnosis, wrong treatment, wrong telephone number or address
Inappropriate (or dangerous) processing	General practitioners telephoning for appointments. Managing a waiting list. Patients being told to go to assessment units that do not have diagnostic skills or facilities in order to try to 'reduce demand' on accident and emergency services
Unnecessary motion	Staff moving around to find or get things, or to get to meetings. Poor 'ergonomics'
Unnecessary inventory	Inventory in manufacturing is raw material or partly processed 'stuff' hanging about. In healthcare it is supplies but also partly processed or unprocessed patients and incomplete information (notes, letters, films, etc.). A waiting list is inventory
Waiting	When and where patients (at home and elsewhere), staff, equipment and materials sit about just waiting for something to happen
Over-production	Printing off a whole sheet of 21 sticky labels when 4 is the most that is ever needed. Ordering huge batch quantities of information leaflets rather than printing off one when needed. Teams routinely meeting to discuss patients who have never been seen. Slots that are reserved for particular groups of patients but not always used. Annual follow-up visits irrespective of the patient's condition
Untapped human potential	Patients or staff are capable of performing a task but are not 'allowed' or it is not recognised that they could do it
Rework	Doing work twice because it was not right first time. Reassessments for the same problem, sending referrals back because of poor information, more admissions out of hours because the system could not deliver a care plan that covered these times
Customer time	Wasted patients' time – a day off work to attend a brief appointment at 11.20 h
Defecting customers	In the US healthcare system, and in some instances in the UK, patients defect and go elsewhere. Some 'did not attends' are an example of this. Patients find the service so 'non-value-adding' they do not bother to turn up

Looking for waste

One of the key tools for assessing cost-effectiveness is to look for the waste generated by the system. Waste can characterised by type, as illustrated in Table 15.1.

Identify the waste 'hot spots' on the process map and where the patients' key frustrations occur (e.g. delays, communication failures, excuses and rudeness). Do not engage in a debate or make excuses for what the patients are saying, however painful. Staff will share many of these frustrations. The hot spots are where improvement efforts should be focused and the issues form the measures for improvement (see below).

Process redesign

Process mapping quickly identifies the steps that add value, that is, contribute directly to patient care, and those that do not. The more steps and 'hand-offs' between roles there are in a process, the more likely errors, communication failures and delays become. Hand-offs are when the patient or information is passed from one person to another.

Ideas to improve or eliminate steps can be captured by staff and patients during the process mapping and discussed in turn. Often valuable insight from GPs, patients, ambulance staff, clinic clerks, receptionists and secretaries are 'drowned out' by more 'senior' clinicians and managers with the fateful words 'We can't do that because...'. The manager should list *all* possible changes, the roles involved and the measure for improvement.

The quality cycle: plan, do, study and act

Many management initiatives in the National Health Service (NHS) have dictated big changes without those introducing them necessarily under-standing the problem or the effects elsewhere in a complex system. The clinical approach to this uncertainty would be to perform a double-blind, randomised controlled trial comparing a pilot scheme with another unchanged system. This, however, requires the huge assumption that both systems are otherwise the same and not subject to any other change in the meantime. A quicker and safer approach is use Deming's iterative quality cycle of plan, do, study, act (PDSA), in which small changes are tested quickly and built on gradually to change the larger dynamic system (Shewhart, 1986). An example of such process redesign using PDSA is set out in Box 15.2.

To check that improvements are not the result of chance, a different branch of statistics is required to check for statistical significance. Statistical process control (see below) allows a process to be monitored for significant changes in performance in real time, thus avoiding the assumptions in the comparative method used in clinical trials.

Process redesign has, unfortunately, become synonymous with process re-engineering, which is a radical approach to redesigning a process by replacing jobs with information technology (IT) to reduce costs. Of the organisations that re-engineered in the 1980s, and did it for this reason, 75% did not survive 5 years. In contrast, organisations that steadily redesigned and included IT to realise untapped human potential and to improve the productivity of their system did very well. By way of example of the latter case, the secretarial role could shift to take on administration and scheduling of clinics, releasing nurses from administration to add value to patient care.

> **Box 15.2** Process redesign through a series of PDSA cycles
>
> **Plan**. One consultant and her secretary decided to reduce the backlog of letters, to reduce the number of irate calls they were receiving.
>
> **Do**. They tried dictating and transcribing letters in one clinic to see if it could work.
>
> **Study**. To study the impact, the secretary, at the end of each day, plotted the number of notes in her office and the number of calls she had received on a run chart (see under 'Measuring for improvement'). In this case the objective was to reduce the number of all calls, not to achieve a target of zero irate calls. In the study, it is important to avoid setting targets – as soon as a measure becomes a target it becomes subject to 'gaming' and is useless. It is better to find simple measures of the right things and to avoid debate about definitions, which generally result in more time being spent measuring than doing.
>
> **Act**. The secretary marked in the dates on which they had made their various changes on the run chart. This made it possible to see the effects of the new process. The secretary presented the new process and results to the multidisciplinary monthly meeting to check the impact on other staff up- and downstream. The clinic clerks reported that the numbers of missing notes had decreased and the care workers reported that it was much easier to care for patients out of hours when they were carrying a copy of their letter. The consultant pointed out the clinical and confidentiality risks in the old 'batch' production system for the letters and the benefits of the new system. It became difficult for other consultants to ignore the facts (as demonstrated by the run chart) and to resist the benefits and so each consultant gradually adopted the new process through a further series of PDSA cycles, with the manager helping to reschedule several shorter clinics with access to secretaries, computers and printers in the clinic area.

This would also free consultants to spend longer with more difficult cases or to see 'extra' patients to keep the waiting times safe (see below).

The pathology of processes

Process mapping is an excellent way of shifting the focus from blaming people to redesigning the system. However, some understanding of the pathology of processes is useful when assessing changes aimed at improving the timeliness, quality and cost of care.

Bottlenecks

Process bottlenecks

Every process has a rate-limiting step, or process bottleneck. This is the step, performed by one person, in one place, at one time, that takes the longest time to do. The process bottleneck governs flow through the system.

In the redesigned process outlined in Box 15.2, the secretary may have felt that she was 'hanging about' between patients in the clinic. This is because she is not the process bottleneck – in this case it is taking the history and examination of the patient by the consultant. The secretary cannot be expected to go at the same rate as the process bottleneck. Her role now is to work alongside the clinic staff to alleviate the process bottleneck by facilitating the efficiency of the consultant's task in her 'slack' time between patients.

Functional bottlenecks

Another suggestion may be to ask the secretary to look after other tasks that are not immediately consecutive up- and downstream of transcribing and printing letters, for example to file notes, answer the telephone and book appointments. Inevitably, she is going to be asked to do all three jobs at once. Which takes priority? Even though the history and examination by the consultant is still the rate-limiting step, the flow would now be governed by the secretary's ability to juggle competing tasks. Consultant, patients, notes and appointments will all wait their 'turn' at this functional bottleneck. Processes should be untangled to prevent functional bottlenecks and balancing sequential tasks along the process, up- and downstream.

Matching demand and capacity

In order to balance the work along the process, demand and capacity at the rate-limiting step (process bottleneck) have to be matched. It is important to distinguish between demand, activity, capacity and backlog (waiting list, queue).

- The *demand* is all the requests for the service. For a community mental health team, this could be new referrals plus requests for key workers for discharge from the hospital wards. Since it is not routinely measured, it is often confused with activity. Often a clinician will ask 'What is the demand for the service?', to which the usual reply will be 'We saw 151 patients last month', which is a report of activity. The demand was the number of referrals received during that period. Do not fall into the debate about true demand versus unmet need. If there are no requests then there is no demand. Unmet need may turn into demand if the system's dynamics change. So it is important to measure the demand constantly, in this case all the requests (emergency and routine) for a service each week and to note any significant changes in demand using statistical process control (see below).
- *Activity* is what has actually been done. It can be kept artificially high by the waiting list – the same principle of a dam maintaining a steady output. If session utilisation is a misguided measure of system efficiency and staff performance, then there is a perverse incentive to have a queue to demonstrate apparent efficiency, similar to the

secretary's potential discomfort at losing the pile of notes and tapes that keep her busy.

- The true *capacity* of the system is often unknown but it is what the system could do or was planned to do. It may be the total number of slots per week with a community team. Activity is a crude indicator of the effective capacity but it underestimates the true system capacity (see below).

- The *backlog* is the cumulative unmet demand. Where there is a delay in the process, a queue or a waiting list, it is easy to assume that demand exceeds supply and that more resources are required. However, there are two other reasons why there may be a queue: artificially maintaining a queue to give a false impression of efficiency in response to an inappropriate measure of performance (as above); and a mismatch between the variations in demand and capacity.

Consider an example of a referral clinic. Table 15.2 shows the weekly demand (referrals and requests for a service) and the weekly capacity (total number of slots available in the clinics). Fig. 15.2 show the mismatch in the variations of the demand and capacity each week, the pattern of the activity and resulting the backlog (waiting list) at the clinic. The demand for the service (the number of referrals) varies each week. So does the clinic capacity, as staff may be away. Unused capacity cannot be passed on to the following week because it is tied up in a fixed session. However, the unmet demand can be passed forward and accumulates as a backlog (waiting list), which now fills any unfilled clinic slots in the future. Notice how the average weekly demand equals average weekly capacity but the average weekly activity is slightly less (Table 15.2).

The NHS commissioning process is fundamentally flawed. It mistakes activity for demand and it fails to understand the impact of variation – the basics of queue theory. NHS commissioning is based on averages and proceeds to performance manage against the very queue it guarantees! Providers are equally ignorant and conclude that a queue is proof that demand exceeds capacity.

Faced with a backlog, clinical staff have no option but to start prioritising the queue. Hence, yet more precious time and resources are wasted drawing up complicated referral criteria. Slots are reserved for urgent patients but the overall capacity remains unchanged (until the faulty business case for more capacity – based on past average activity and waiting time – is approved). The demand for 'urgent' patients varies each week but the number of reserved slots in the clinic does not. Any unused urgent slots are wasted unless a receptionist, secretary or clerk can find a 'short notice' routine patient to fill it. The queue now starts to churn with patients being seen out of turn. This fuels the debate as to what is and is not an 'urgent' referral. The routine waiting times start to increase (because more capacity is being wasted in the urgent system) but GPs are blamed, wrongly, for making more referrals. In face of the lengthening routine waiting times, the GPs have no option but

Table 15.2 Example statistics for a referral clinic: demand, capacity, activity, backlog

Week	Demand	Capacity	Activity	Unmet demand	Number waiting (backlog)
1	11	5	5	6	6
2	13	12	12	1	7
3	6	9	9	0	4
4	7	11	11	0	0
5	12	14	12	0	0
6	8	15	8	0	0
7	8	11	8	0	0
8	14	5	5	9	9
9	9	6	6	3	12
10	12	13	13	0	11
11	10	8	8	2	13
12	11	9	9	2	15
13	8	14	14	0	9
14	5	10	10	0	4
15	11	13	13	0	2
16	7	7	7	0	2
17	12	6	6	6	8
18	11	6	6	5	13
19	7	11	11	0	9
20	6	15	15	0	0
21	9	11	9	0	0
22	15	9	9	6	6
23	14	7	7	7	13
24	13	5	5	8	21
25	11	13	13	0	19
26	11	12	12	0	18
27	10	9	9	1	19
28	5	9	9	0	15
29	14	15	15	0	14
Weekly average	10	10	9.5		

to refer a greater proportion of patients as 'urgent'. In response to the needs of patients, staff are constantly trying to alter the ratio of urgent to routine slots or to perform expensive and exhausting waiting list initiatives. The problem is impossible to solve this way.

The solution is a system that sees all patients in turn within the response time for the most urgent patient, that is, without any queue. This reduces the clinical risk and avoids wasting resources to perform non-value-adding prioritisation and administration.

There is a strong belief that improving access increases demand. It does not – patients do not fall ill to keep us in business. The evidence is that after an initial peak of unmet demand draining through the system, demand goes

181

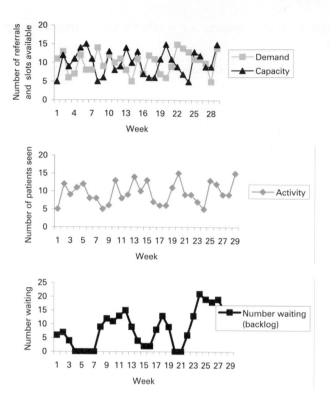

Fig. 15.2 Example charts for a referral clinic: variations in the demand and capacity each week, the pattern of activity and resulting the backlog (waiting list).

down as confidence grows that access is possible when it is required. Hence it is important to measure demand continuously and, more importantly, the variation in demand.

In order to avoid a queue, it is necessary to account for the underlying variation by commissioning an average weekly capacity that is greater than the average weekly demand. The amount of extra capacity required depends on the amount of variation in the system and the acceptability of the waiting time. If there is no variation in either the demand or the capacity, then it is easy to match them and have no queue. If there is variation in both and it is not possible for any patient to wait any time at all (i.e. an emergency system), then the average capacity must be funded to meet the normal peaks of demand. This will result in 'slack' capacity. If patients can wait a short time, then the rule of thumb is to set the average capacity at 80% of the 'normal peaks' in demand (excluding unusual peaks demand or troughs in capacity). In the example above (Table 15.2), average weekly capacity for the service needs to be planned at 13 slots for new patient referrals each week. If this is not affordable, then the only option is to reduce the *variation* in the demand and capacity. Do not fall into the trap of 'demand management', that is, trying to reduce the average demand by adding extra assessment steps to the process or sending it elsewhere. It will come back again.

Since most systems are in balance, as shown by the fact that waiting times are not increasing, then demand must equal capacity. The issue for most services is to reduce the variations in capacity by reducing the amount of 'carving up' of the overall capacity.

Carve-out

Carve-out is where the overall capacity is reserved for particular demands, even though the process that the patient goes through is the same. Examples of this are:

- GPs referring to specific named consultants because they know them personally
- over-specialisation (80% of patients have the 20% of complaints that occur commonly and specialisation does not reflect this) (the Pareto principle; Pareto, 1935)
- the specification of different waiting times (urgent, soon, routine)
- carving up the capacity according to geography or 'sub-sectors', (i.e. specific groups of GP practices).

Reducing carve-out

Since 80% of patients have the 20% of common conditions it is possible to pool all referrals and negate the impact of holidays and study leave. Eliminating 'urgent', 'soon' and routine appointments in favour of just emergency and routine reduces the wasted capacity and administration. This can be enhanced by abolishing fixed session working in favour of flexible systems that allow for 37.5 hours/week annualised over the year.

Variation is compounded

Variation at each step of a dependent process is compounded, so that steps at the end will be subject to greater variation than those at the start. Hence the variation in demand for social or rehabilitation services is greater than the variation in the primary demand upstream, even though the average demand may be the same or less. Hence conversion rates (e.g. ratios of new to follow-up cases) do not work. Demand must be counted at each step and every change must reduce the variation in the system by both removing steps and carve-out of capacity, and eliminating errors and rework from upstream.

Plotting the demand and capacity continuously over time reveals what is normal variation for the system and what are the special causes (e.g. weekends, Easter, Bank Holidays, drug scares). If the variation in demand is predictable, then move capacity appropriately to meet it (e.g. more capacity to meet the deferred demand on Mondays) or eliminate the cause of variation.

Measuring for improvement: statistical process control

To understand the significance of changes, we need to understand the pattern of variation in the system over time. Statistical process control (Shewart & Deming, 1939) is based on the moving range (distance between consecutive measurements) rather than the distance between a complete collection of points and their mean or median. This branch of statistics is not routinely taught on medical or management courses.

The risk of using comparative statistical methods alone to identify the significance of a change is best illustrated with an example. Consider a change that has resulted in a major reduction in waiting time, from an average of 70 days before the change to 35 days after the change, as shown in Fig. 15.3. This may be accompanied by an analysis of the variation to demonstrate a significant statistical shift in the mean (e.g. a t-test). However, plotting the consecutive waiting times over time may have shown three very different scenarios, each suggesting a different interpretation of the effect of the change (Fig. 15.4). In scenario 1, the statistically significant shift in the mean of the variation in the system may have been caused by the change. In scenario 2, the mean is significantly shifted but the run chart implies that waiting times were improving anyway, despite the change. In scenario 3, the link between the cause and effect is more uncertain: whether the change was responsible is not clear and whatever did occur was not sustained. Using a comparative statistical method, all three of these scenarios would have given a similar result. However, plotting the run charts for consecutive waiting times would lead to three very different interpretations of the effect of the change.

The secretary's record of the PDSA cycles (Box 15.2) can serve as a further example, as shown in Fig. 15.5. Even though the secretary sometimes forgot to record the number of telephone calls and notes, the charts clearly show the improvement and amount of time being wasted by telephone calls initially. This is also discussed in Chapter 26.

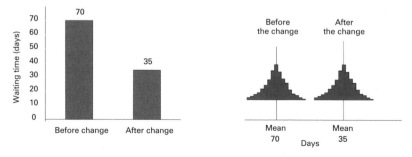

Fig. 15.3 Effect of a hypothetical change on waiting times.

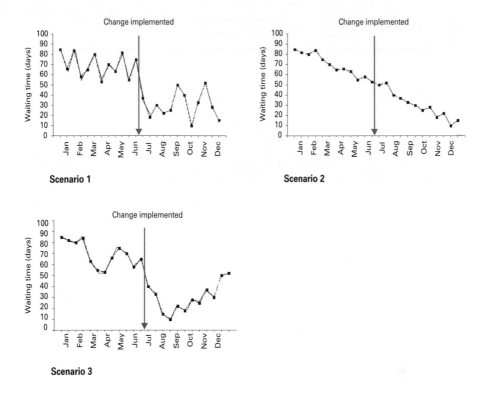

Fig. 15.4 Three scenarios that could produce the effect of the hypothetical change on waiting times.

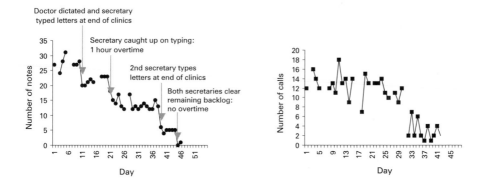

Fig. 15.5 Run charts for a secretary's initiative to reduce the numbers of notes in the office and the number of telephone calls (from Box 15.2).

185

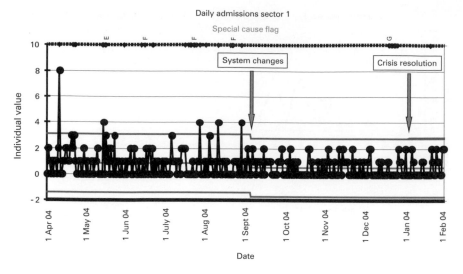

Fig. 15.6 Impact and statistical significance of reducing the 'carve out' in daily admissions.

Provided clinicians and managers give up their 'comparative' approach to understanding the impact of changes to systems, run charts are the most simple and useful way of displaying data. Run charts monitor the process about the median in real time, whereas control charts provide the 'normal' range (i.e. 99% of the process). In order to calculate the estimate of the standard deviation (sigma) the moving range is used (i.e. the distance between consecutive points). Both run and control charts are methods for identifying statistically significant changes to a process in real time.

The control chart in Fig. 15.6 clearly shows the effect and statistical significance of reducing the 'carve-out' in the daily admissions to a sector psychiatric ward. The upper solid horizontal line (upper process limit) shows how many admissions can be expected 99% of the time for this service. Anything above this is 'not likely to be normal' for this process and is termed a 'special cause'. In this example, carve-out was reduced by working as a team not as sub-teams, reviewing patients from any part of the sector concerned and introducing robust case management. As a consequence, the peaks and troughs in admissions were smoothed, since the variations in the capacity caused by consultant availability were eliminated. Introducing a crisis team between 09.00 and 17.00 h in an attempt to reduce the admissions had no effect. This control chart shows that the capacity of the system (free beds at 00.00 h, plus discharges, plus transfers in the following 24 hours) must be equal to 3 in order for there to be a 99% chance of a bed being available for an admission. Previously, 3 beds would not have been enough to guarantee an admission.

There are several excellent texts on the use of run and control charts to monitor variation in systems and thus to measure the effect of changes to improve flow and quality of care.

Conclusion

Taking a process view shifts the blame for poor quality services from the staff and patients to the system. Provided all the roles are represented, the changes to redesign the system and improve care become obvious. However this depends on clinicians and managers understanding how quality at each step causes variation and how this impacts the bottlenecks in system. The objective is to understand the causes of variation and to reduce the impact. Change is possible when clinicians and managers drop the comparative approach for assessing the impact of change and use Statistical Process Control, a branch of statistics not normally used in the clinical or management environment.

References

Pareto, V. (1935) *The Mind and Society [Trattato di Sociologia Generale]*. Harcourt, Brace.
Shewhart, W. A. & Deming, W. E. (1939) *Statistical Method from the Viewpoint of Quality Control*. Graduate School, Department of Agriculture, Washington, DC.

Further reading

Audit Commission (2003) *Acute Hospital Portfolio. Review of National Finding: Outpatients*. Available from http://www.audit-commission/reports
Erlang, A. K. (1909) The theory of probabilities and telephone conversations. *Nyt Tidsskrif for Matematik B*, **20**.
Feigenbaum, A. V. (1986) *Total Quality Control*. McGraw-Hill.
Goldratt, E. & Cox, J. (2000) *The Goal* (2nd ed). Gower.
Murray, M. (200) Patient care: access. *BMJ*, **320**, 1594–1596.
Schonberger, R. J. (1982) *Japanese Manufacturing Techniques: Nine Hidden Lesson in Simplicity*. Free Press.
Schonberger, R. J. (1986) *World Class Manufacturing: The Lessons of Simplicity Applied*. Free Press.
Shewhart, W. A. (1986) *Statistical Method from the Viewpoint of Quality Control*. Dover Publications.
Silvester, K., Lendon, R., Bevan, H., *et al* (2004) Reducing waiting times in the NHS: is lack of capacity the problem? *Clinician in Management*, **12**, 105–111.
Slack, N., Chambers, S. & Johnston, R. (2000) *Operations Management* (3rd edn). Prentice Hall.
Womack, J. & Jones, D. (1996) *Lean Thinking: Banish Waste and Create Wealth in Your Organisation*. Simon and Schuster.

Other useful guides

Carey, R. G. & Lloyd, R. C. (1995) *Measuring Quality Improvement in Healthcare: A Guide to Statistical Process Control Applications*. American Society for Quality. A simple guide to using run charts and control charts in the clinical environment including measuring for quality issues with examples of applications to deaths and errors.

Hart, M. K. & Hart, R. K. (2002) *Statistical Process Control for Healthcare*. Duxbury Thompson. A more detailed guide with case studies of SPC as applied to the clinical environment.

NHS Executive (2000) *A Step-by-Step Guide to Improving Outpatient Services: Variations in NHS Outpatient Performance Project Report II*. Department of Health. http://www.dh.gov.uk/en/ Publicationsandstatistics/Publications/PublicationsPolicyAndGuidance/DH_4008694. A step-by-step guide to improving out-patient services tells you how to start tackling a backlog in out-patients, but the principles apply at a bottleneck anywhere.

Owen, M. & Morgan, J. (2000) *Statistical Process Control in the Office*. Greenfield. A simple guide to applying statistical process control to administrative processes

Wheeler. D. J. (1999) *Understanding Variation: The Key to Managing Chaos* (2nd edn). SPC Press. A brief and excellent introduction to statistical process control and the impact on organisational behaviour.

Wheeler. D. J. & Chambers, D. S. (1992) *Understanding Statistical Process Control*. SPC Press. Definitive text book on statistical process control

Websites

NHS Modernisation Agencys' guides at http://www.modern.nhs.uk/improvementguides. These brief guides are based on the practical experiences of NHS teams and can be downloaded in PDF format.
Series 1
Process mapping, analysis and redesign
Matching capacity and demand
Measurement for improvement
Series 2
Involving patients and carers
Managing the human dimensions of change
Sustainability and spread
Series 3
Building and nurturing an improvement culture
Working in groups
Redesigning roles
Working with systems

Improving patient flow, at http://www.steyn.org.uk, has presentation material, reading lists and models that demonstrate the impact of variation on flow

CHAPTER 16

Leadership

Stephanie Marshall

'High performing leaders ACT NOW to shape the future. They are motivated to take action to achieve a radically different future – one in which health services are truly integrated and focused on the needs of patients.' (NHS Institute for Innovation and Improvement, 2005)

Since the publication of the second edition of *Management for Psychiatrists*, in which the term 'leadership' was not deemed to be a concept warranting unpacking, the world has changed dramatically, as the above quotation demonstrates. Leadership at all levels ('dispersed' leadership), with a concomitant move away from the notion of the heroic leader, is now recognised as important, not only in the private sector, where books such as Collins's (2001) *Good to Great*, Goleman *et al*'s (2002) *The New Leaders*, and Kanter's (2004) *Confidence* have influenced thinking, but also in the public sector. Local government, higher education and the National Health Service (NHS) have all had to rethink the ways in which 'best value', modernisation, effectiveness and efficiency can be delivered. 'Leadership development', as distinct to 'management development', is seen as the key to unlocking everyone's potential – from chief executives to cleaners. This chapter explores the complexity of leadership development and suggests that leadership does, indeed, make a difference, not only to the bottom line but to society more generally, and also to individuals in terms of self-esteem, motivation and commitment to 'the job'.

The previous two editions of *Management for Psychiatrists* emphasised, quite rightly, the importance of managerial skills and the need to have appropriate systems and procedures in place. It hinted at leadership skills, most particularly when referring to the role of consultant psychiatrists and their ability to get things done.

As Kotter (1996, pp. ix–x) notes, leadership is 'the engine that drives change', and it is this notion that is explored here.

Leadership archetypes and qualities

Mayo & Nohria (2005) identify three distinct leadership archetypes: the entrepreneurial leader, the 'leader' and the manager leader. Their studies suggest that the proportions of leaders falling into these three categories are approximately 10%, 10% and 80%, respectively. There is a good chance that people who are effective managers possess a set of skills which provide them with a sound basis from which they can make the transition from manager to manager leader, and then on to 'leader' or entrepreneurial leader. Thus, it seems appropriate, in this edition of *Management for Psychiatrists*, to engage more fully with the concept of leadership, to help consultants to consider the key role they have in setting the tone for the health service. This they can do by:

'using their insights into the broad strategic direction of health and social care to help shape and implement the approaches and culture in their organisation, and to influence developments across the wider health and social care context' (NHS Institute for Innovation and Improvement, 2005).

They could also do so by demonstrating to others the ways in which they would like them to behave and act, to promote shared values and achieve mutually agreed goals.

The NHS leadership qualities framework (LQF) identifies 15 attributes; these cover the personal, cognitive and social domains. The LQF presents these 15 'qualities' as a three by five matrix, as shown in Table 16.1. Each of the 15 attributes is elaborated on in terms of providing level 'descriptors', with each having three to six levels, which are cumulative in terms of behaviours demonstrating their attainment. However, for the purposes of this chapter (and for simplicity!), what follows is a simple stroll through six key attributes of effective leaders as identified by numerous participants on leadership programmes which I have delivered over the years: vision, strategic direction, 'quick wins', inspiring 'followership', negotiating and influencing skills, and role modelling. This 'package' of six attributes is

Table 16.1 The NHS leadership qualities framework

Personal qualities	Setting direction	Delivering the service
Self-belief	Seizing the future	Leading change through people
Self-awareness	Intellectual flexibility	Holding to account
Self-management	Broad scanning	Empowering others
Drive for improvement	Political acuteness	Effective and strategic influencing
Personal integrity	Drive for results	Collaborative working

Source: NHS Institute for Innovation and Improvement (2005), with permission.

what enables individual leaders to be categorised as 'inspirational' and 'authentic' – that is, standing out as 'great' leaders as opposed to 'good' or otherwise. An exploration of what these attributes might mean in the context of one's chosen profession is offered below. It is suggested that to benefit the most from this exploration, readers consider auditing their own skills, attributes and behaviours against those offered, prompted by the 'Reflect' points below.

Vision

'High performing leaders are quickly able to assess a situation and to draw pragmatic conclusions. They are able to switch between the significant detail and the big picture to shape a vision – for their own service, organisation, or across the wider health context ... [and are] receptive to fresh insights and perspectives from diverse sources, both internal and external to the organisation (driven by their values of inclusiveness and service improvement)... [They are also] open to innovative thinking and encouraging creativity and experimentation in others' (NHS Institute for Innovation and Improvement, 2005).

The ability to present a vision for the future of the organisation is not a one-dimensional task: it requires a lot of skill and learning gained over time. As the NHS Institute for Innovation and Improvement (2005) suggests:

'Outstanding leaders are focused on articulating the vision with compelling clarity. They keep up the focus on change by reiterating the modernisation message ... with a strong focus on local needs.'

Beyond this 'compelling clarity' of vision is the need to assist others in picturing themselves in this vision. Without this, leaders do not often gain the 'followership' (see below) required to bring about transformational change. A key question many great leaders are asked and are able to answer succinctly is 'What would success in realisation of this vision look like?' In addition, the mark of a great leader is that followers, similarly, are able to answer this question in terms of themselves and their role in achieving the vision.

Kotter (1996) suggests that one of the factors working against translating the vision into the change process is 'undercommunicating the vision by a factor of 10 (or even 100 or even 1000)' (p. 9). In assuming the role of leader, therefore, regular and varied approaches to communication, with some 'quick wins' (see below), are essential to provide inspiration to the followership, providing them with a constructive and positive view of the future.

- *Reflect.* What is your vision for your role in 3–5 years? The NHS Institute for Innovation and Improvement (2005) suggests that this vision should be part of the modernisation agenda, but also a means of leaving your own distinctive legacy. So, further to your vision, do others share this vision and want to make it happen? If not, how could both you and they be encouraged to embark on, first, an understanding of this vision and, second, an understanding of the key role they will play in achievement of this vision?

Strategic direction

Additional to the ability to articulate and 'paint' a picture of a vision for the future of the service, great leaders possess the ability to determine the broad strategic direction required to realise the vision, as well as the determination to act now to achieve a radically different future. Encouraging others to engage in the strategic planning process has not been a feature of the 'command and control' or 'heroic' leaders of the past (Khurana, 2002). In looking to issues of sustainability and ownership, and, indeed, the gaining of confidence to attain the vision, staff need to be led by a confident, 'can do' leader who understands not only the local culture but also the national context, and who engages stakeholders in exploring the various routes and modes of travel to achieve the clearly identified and articulated vision.

To encourage 'dispersed' leadership, that is, leadership at all levels, inspirational strategic leaders involve others in an inclusive planning process. They help others to take responsibility for delivering the strategy. Great leaders inspire the dispersed leadership to undertake transformational rather than just transactional and incremental change.

- *Reflect*. What strategy do you have in place for planning for the future? Who and what is involved in the strategic planning and analysis process? Do all stakeholders or a subset get involved in strategic planning? And what 'tools' are used (e.g. benchmarking, stakeholder analysis, strategic mapping, data gathering, scenario modelling, risk assessment)?

Quick wins

Quick wins, or some tangible early successes, are essential to provide followership with a sense that the vision is not just some fantasy but something that is, indeed, achievable and attainable. Kanter *et al* (1992) refer to the notion of change being a 'long march'. Kanter *et al* (1992), Kotter (1996) and Kotter & Cohen (2002, p. 125) all refer to the need for 'quick wins'.

'short-term wins – victories that nourish faith in the change effort, emotionally reward the hard workers, keep the critics at bay, build momentum. Without sufficient wins that are visible, timely, unambiguous, and meaningful to others, change efforts inevitably run into serious problems' (Kotter & Cohen, 2002, p. 125).

Part of the leader's strategy for achievement of the vision should be to have parallel strategies – one which outlines the long game, and one that is a series of short games, providing opportunities for all stakeholders to witness achievement of short-term goals, to hit targeted 'milestones' and subsequently to have an opportunity to make achievements highly visible. Such an approach allows for the celebration of these 'quick wins'. The tricky question is, of course, how to create the appropriate milestones and circumstances for authentic and meaningful quick wins. This is where the sharing of the strategic planning exercise comes in, in that the followership can identify 'what success would look like' within, say, the first 3 months, in relation to targets and milestones which they perceive as being appropriate 'wins'.

Effective leaders are able to harness the successes of quick wins, by explaining how they are part of a cumulative route march to achievement of the vision. Quick wins provide early feedback on the appropriateness of both the vision and the strategy. Such early successes are capable of inspiring followership to become fully engaged, irrespective of their initial commitment to the vision. In addition, subsequent to quick wins, cynics' criticisms are put at bay and their power taken away. Indeed, some studies indicate that it is the converted cynics who can become the greatest advocates of the proposed change (Marshall, 2007) and overall build great faith in the collective effort to achieve the vision.

- *Reflect.* Think of a change that you have been involved in that had short-term wins. What was the effect on you? And on others? What did it signal to you about the leadership of the change? How might you use this strategy in the future?

Inspiring 'followership'

Academic abilities – intellectual acuity and technical know-how – are important but not the sole means of inspiring followership. Indeed, the presence of a 'followership' implies the motivation to follow the leader in delivering the required changes in order to realise the vision. Interpersonal skills are absolutely crucial here. Emotional intelligence and resilience are essential to inspiring followership. In general terms, emotional intelligence implies adeptness in relationships, the ability to empathise and to demonstrate motivation, and the possession both of sufficient self-awareness to understand the effect of one's own behaviour on others, and of self-regulation, particularly with respect to controlling one's negative emotions. In the context of leadership, emotional intelligence means managing feelings with respect to the vision and change strategy, and expressing these constructively and appropriately, encouraging people to work together towards the common goals. Many people remark that great leaders make each and every person feel unique and special. This sort of impact is not achieved through written or cascaded communication, but through high visibility and regular engagement from routine day-to-day chat (e.g. 'How's it going today?') through to questioning individuals about their interpretation of the vision and strategy for its achievement.

In addition, to inspire followership requires pacing change so that they remain loyal to the vision. People are much happier following someone who has taken some time to get to know them, know their values, know what motivates them and know the appropriate 'speed' at which to push forwards.

Goleman (1998, pp. 9–10) suggests that:

'Data tracking the talents of stars over several decades reveals that two abilities that mattered relatively little for success in the 1970s have become crucially important in the 1990s: *team building* and *adapting to change*. And entirely new capabilities have begun to appear as traits of star performers, notably *change catalyst* and *leveraging diversity*.' [Emphasis added.]

These four capabilities – team building, adapting to change, acting as a change catalyst and leveraging diversity – are essential for forging alliances and networks to pass on ownership of both the vision and the strategy to those critical to making it happen.

- *Reflect*. How much time do you spend with others who are key stake-holders in your vision for the future? What are you doing in terms of 'oiling the machinery' so that it is working well and will deliver the outputs you require to achieve your vision?

Negotiating and influencing skills

Negotiating and influencing skills are essential for delivering the vision at two levels: first, to bring on board all the personnel and partners who will be responsible for the operational delivery of the change required to realise the vision; and second, to ensure that the local change does not take place within a vacuum, but rather within a larger (i.e. national) process of transformation. Both levels require a high degree of emotional intelligence. The former requires a commitment to spend time communicating in a range of different and appropriate ways with those who will be required to 'make it happen', inspiring them to engage fully not only with the vision but also with the transformational process that will have to take place to bring about the required change. The latter requires, alongside the ability to interpret the likely strategic direction of changes in health and social care, formulating a vision aligned with your reading of what is going on 'out there', and your ability to forge partnerships and influence developments across the wider health service. Networking is thus essential for you to be able not only to understand an increasingly complex environment but also to determine how best to work in partnership across the health services. Networking may require skills or attributes that you feel you do not possess, but these can be learned, if the commitment is there. Greater understanding of the external interface can be gained through a greater involvement in a wide range of networks, thus giving your vision a better grounding for achievement.

- *Reflect*. Think of your vision for the future. To achieve this vision, who will you have to influence? What might you have to negotiate with them about? What will be your bottom line? What might be their bottom line? What new networks may you need to become involved in to make the vision a reality? Can you see any easy 'ins' to these networks?

Role modelling

'Walking the talk' can be costly in terms of time, but pays back in abundance in the long term when it comes to delivering results. Ultimately, such visibility saves time, as it both enhances followership and alerts you to potential saboteurs, potential barriers or blockages, which, with honed negotiating and influencing skills, can be addressed before they derail the change process. A great leader needs to role model integrity, and thus must be guided by a clear set of underpinning values. The NHS Institute for Innovation and Improvement (2005) refers to the fact that:

'there is so much at stake in leading health services. Outstanding leaders bring a sense of integrity to what they do that helps them to deliver to the best of their abilities. Features of this quality include:

- Believing in a set of key values borne out of broad experience of and commitment to the service which stands them in good stead, especially when they are under pressure.
- Insistence on openness and communication, motivated by values about inclusiveness and getting on with the job.
- Acting as a role model for public involvement and the dialogue that all staff, including the front line, need to have with services users.
- Resilience that enables them to push harder, when necessary, in the interests of developing or improving the service.'

The ability to 'walk the talk' is essential if you are to be credible, at the same time as setting both standards and an example for others. Being respectful of others, chairing meetings effectively, good time management and making time for staff are all examples of role modelling which are noted by not only subordinate staff but also by peers and stakeholders more generally.

- *Reflect*. What sort of example do you set for others? What messages are conveyed as a result of your behaviour in different situations. Are you consistent? Do others seek you out for your leadership or managerial advice because of the positive example you set? If not, why not?

Developing leadership

Particularly when you achieve the position of consultant, it is important not only to act as a suitable role model to others, inspiring others to adopt highly professional standards of human interaction and attempting to influence the agenda, but also to provide opportunities for others to hone their leadership skills. This must, ultimately, be to the benefit of the patient and the credibility of the profession. One hand could well be held by a mentor or someone whom you look up to, to help you learn, view the world from alternative perspectives and assist you on your journey of continuous improvement. The other hand should be used to support and guide others, further to your own knowledge, understanding, skills and wisdom. This is what leadership of continuous improvement – of both systems and individuals – is all about.

So, how do you 'upskill', or hone your own skills? There are an increasing number of national programmes aimed at developing both today's and tomorrow's leaders. A number of consultants and prospective consultants have benefited from programmes such as those run by the Leadership Foundation for Higher Education (see http://www.lfhe.ac.uk) and those offered by the NHS Institute for Innovation and Improvement (http://www.institute.nhs.uk). Alternatively, regional or in-house bespoke programmes are increasingly being offered, with leadership development interventions such as mentoring, coaching, action learning sets and leadership development groups proving most beneficial in transforming practice, to the benefit of both staff and patients (for further information email stephanie.marshall@lfhe.ac.uk). I hope this chapter will have served as a stimulus to get more involved and hone those leadership skills!

References

Collins, J. (2001) *Good to Great*. Random House.
Goleman, D. (1998) *Working with Emotional Intelligence*. Bloomsbury.
Goleman, D., Boyatzis, R. & McKee, A. (2002) *The New Leaders*. Little, Brown.
Kanter, R. (2004) *Confidence*. Random House.
Kanter, R., Stein, B. & Jick, T. (1992) *The Challenge of Organisational Change*. Free Press.
Khurana, R. (2002) *Searching for a Corporate Saviour*. Princeton University Press.
Kotter, J. (1996) *Leading Change*. HBS Press.
Kotter, J. & Cohen, D. (2002) *The Heart of Change*. HBS Press.
Marshall, S. (ed.) (2007) *Strategic Leadership of Change in Higher Education: What's New*. Routledge.
Mayo, A. & Nohria, N. (2005) Zeitgeist leadership. *Harvard Business Review*, **83**(10), 45–60.
NHS Institute for Innovation and Improvement (2005) Website of the Board Level Development Team, http://www.executive.modern.nhs.uk.

CHAPTER 17

Management of change

Zoë K. Reed

One of the most important tasks requiring management is securing the implementation of change. That is the focus of this chapter and the approach will be to provide some overall concepts which people have found help them to be effective in these turbulent times.

On one level, the management of change needs no introduction, since it is something we cope with throughout our lives. As we go through the different stages and different educational and economic opportunities, we manage each transition. On a micro-level, our bodies and our social relations are always undergoing minor, and sometimes major, changes and we manage the necessary adjustments. However easy or difficult we find these changes, we manage. The issue is whether we manage them well and whether having the right theories to help guide our thoughts, feelings and behaviours might move us from coping with, to thriving in, change.

'Skills and ability to manage change' is a phrase appearing in most organisations' job descriptions and person specifications these days. Psychiatrists as individuals will be skilled in supporting service users through their personal changes – the clinical change task. This chapter offers an approach which should enable psychiatrists to have a way of thinking which will give them confidence in approaching the managerial and organisational change task.

Why is the management of change necessary?

Society in the UK, as elsewhere in the world, is changing rapidly and will continue to do so. The effects of developments in information and communications technology are well known and support the prediction that constantly adjusting services and provider practices will be a feature of the modern world. This has an impact on all parts of the economy, including the delivery of mental healthcare. The context for that delivery is one where the right to choice is an expectation of service users and being subject to contestability is a fact for service providers. As the public becomes more educated about options and more prepared to voice their needs and wants, the requirement is for services and clinicians to offer flexible and responsive services which are experienced as personalised by each service user.

The other big organisational driver for change is an economic one. All industries have to be constantly aware of the competition, and to check out the relative quality and cost of their products. In the UK, the concepts of *contestability* and *choice* have been introduced into the National Health Service (NHS) as a way of bringing a focus on quality and cost into healthcare. The constant drive to increase the efficiency and cost-effectiveness of services is equally as important as increasing their clinical effectiveness. This is because the need for services will always outstrip available resources and the money for new services is usually locked within existing services.

The final driver for change which is offered here is that of medical advances. Research is continually being undertaken and generates evidence which points to more effective ways to secure the desired outcomes for service users. However, these ways can be at odds with clinical practice as taught during training to become a doctor. Providing evidenced-based care therefore requires good change management skills – to secure changes in both personal practice and in the practice of others.

What change has to be managed?

At its most basic, the change which has to be managed is that of personal behaviour. Individuals have to start to do things differently. Ensuring that the change is sustained in each individual and applied consistently by all individuals is the change management task. To secure this, organisations frequently implement change programmes. These programmes often work on the idea that if you change people's thoughts and feelings, then the *behaviour* change (which is the desired outcome or goal of the programme) is more likely to be sustained and spread throughout the organisation.

An area where there has been much debate about the design of change programmes is that of ensuring equal access, experience and outcomes for all service users, regardless of their ethnicity. The design of change programmes has evolved over the years from ones with the aim of winning 'hearts and minds' (i.e. a focus on thoughts and feelings and emphasising the moral case) to ones which focus on changing behaviours (i.e. emphasising the legal framework and business case).

An effective change programme will therefore include design components which aim to secure spread and sustainability (Fraser *et al*, 2003). This is because, although it is relatively easy to find a few enthusiastic individuals within an organisation to experiment with new ways of working, what is more difficult to achieve is a change programme which is replicable across an organisation and which secures and maintains the desired changes. Key to the success of any design is, first, to be very clear about what the required outcomes are, then to understand the organisational context within which the change has to be achieved, and finally to apply the right concepts to the design of the programme.

What concepts help?

For organisations and individuals to secure the change that is required and to thrive in a context where frequent change is the norm, it is important to work within a theoretical framework which is likely to lead to successful outcomes. Put simply, some ways of thinking can actually be unhelpful and lead to the person asked to lead the change feeling overwhelmed by the task. This is clearly not productive and the key to success is to construct a way of thinking about things that makes the change task seem doable and even enjoyable. The concepts can be grouped into categories in which they are most helpfully applied:

- organisations and systems
- individuals in groups – the leadership task
- individuals.

Theories about organisations and systems

Complexity sciences (Battram, 1998) draw on biological and physical sciences and contain a number of principles and ideas which help designers to shape change programmes. Central to these are the idea that organisations are *complex evolving systems* (Mitleton-Kelly, 2003). This term gives recognition to the fact that organisations are organic and, to quote Mitleton-Kelly, are 'co-evolving within a social ecosystem'. Wheatley describes organisations as:

'A collection of individual agents who have the freedom to act in ways that are not entirely predictable and whose actions are interconnected such that one agent's action changes the context for other agents' (Wheatley, 1999).

This definition can be applied at every level of *nested systems*, which, in the present context, would be each team member within the team, each team within the organisation, each organisation within the health services community, each health services community within the broader public sector.

Thinking about organisations and individuals within them in this way leads to profoundly different designs to change programmes than views of a more traditional nature. Conventional management theories view organisations as machines and staff within them as component parts. From this world-view, designers assume people can be told what to do and that they will do it in a consistent manner. They assume that learning from one area will be automatically replicable in another. They believe that a plan for change can be worked out in advance in detail and that it must be and can be executed as planned.

199

Complexity perspectives provide a more organic and holistic view. Biological metaphors are frequently used to deepen understanding of successful approaches. Two of these are *birds flocking* and *termites building*. Both describe the idea that central command and control is neither necessary nor helpful in orchestrating action. Birds and termites achieve amazing results through the individual agents following a few *simple rules*. Some modern change management programmes focus on seeking to identify the few simple rules – often characterised as values or guiding principles – which will enable all individuals to shape their behaviour for themselves in accordance with organisational goals.

The termite hill *emerges* from the *patterns of behaviour* of the termites following their simple rules. There was no grand plan: the hills simply emerged from the behaviour. The *intrinsic motivation* of the termites coupled with the simple rules ensures that the termites *self-organise* to achieve the desired result. Emergence, intrinsic motivation and self-organisation are key concepts in the complexity sciences. They are the underpinning theory to techniques such as whole-group brainstorming and 'Post It' note exercises. When design is guided by more conventional thinking, there can be a fear of asking a large group of people to generate as many ideas as possible and then to come out with a way forward, because it could feel uncontrollable and potentially non-productive. However, from a complexity perspective there is confidence (and tools and techniques coherent with the theory) that everyone has an intrinsic motivation to be cooperative, that they will self-organise to achieve the objectives and that the solutions will emerge from the process. The aim of such exercises is to involve everybody and to create a *possibility space* (Battram, 1998), in which solutions will emerge. This contrasts with more conventional management methods, where top management create a plan and then seek to persuade staff to follow it through consultation exercises.

Birds are also used to illustrate the need for *attractors* within the system. As a way of getting people to understand that organisations are living entities, not machines, a rock is contrasted with a bird. If you want to get a rock into the corner of a room, with a bit of practice on your aim you will be able to achieve it by throwing. By contrast, if you want to get a bird into the corner of a room you certainly will not achieve it by throwing the bird; instead, your only chance is by placing the attractor (for birds) of bird seed in the corner.

Using words like 'systems' and drawing on biological metaphors has another important message for organisations. It is that life proceeds: things are never static, and flow and movement are an intrinsic part of organisations. This contrasts with more conventional approaches, where there is an assumption that once the change has occurred and the problem has been fixed, the organisation will remain static. Many small changes or adjustments, quickly executed, are a key feature of change programme designs which work in harmony with living systems.

Theories about individuals in groups – the leadership task

Understanding that the management task is about enabling a living system rather than controlling a machine brings a different set of leadership tasks. A metaphor that is frequently used to describe the organisation is a garden, and this can help managers understand that their role is to create the most favourable conditions for emergence and self-organisation. They must tend their gardens with care and continually work on improving the conditions to maximise the chance of healthy development, but what they cannot do is *make* the plants grow! This helps managers and leaders let go of thinking that their role is to figure it all out and then create a plan and force the system to implement it. Instead, the need for a much more nurturing role becomes apparent. A key role for managers and leaders in this world-view is to manage the context and the relationships around their work area to enable the part of the system they are responsible for to thrive and grow. Leaders start something, see what happens and give feedback in a continuous cycle; they watch to see when the required patterns of behaviour emerge and then manage the conditions so that those patterns are reinforced and sustained. Core skills are in the design of the possibility space and close observation in the search for the *tipping point* (Gladwell, 2000), when the whole system starts to move in the required (or desired) direction.

Helpful guidance for managers comes from the idea of *learning organisations,* with the leaders' new work being to act as *designers, stewards* and *teachers* (Senge, 1993): in learning organisations, leaders design the processes and systems within which the vision can be generated and articulated; they are stewards of that vision, with a special sense of responsibility but without being possessive of it; as teachers, they help people achieve more accurate views of reality and hold the creative tension which is generated. This description of leadership contrasts with the more conventional theories of a leader as a hero, leading from the front, or a leader as the most knowledgeable expert on the subject area. It calls for knowledge, skills and attention to process to get the best out of everyone – leadership as guardian of the co-created vision and expert in process rather than expert on content.

Complexity sciences help managers and leaders look for order rather than control; they provide a conceptual framework for inviting participation – every voice is valid – rather than curtailing contribution (for fear that someone will speak out against the plan). They foster a real belief in the intrinsic motivation of people. Even in chaotic circumstances, individuals can make congruent decisions when there are a few simple principles that everyone is accountable for but where the condition within which everyone is operating is one of individual freedom.

In this mind-set, much management time is spent on developing and sustaining a *shared vision*, which will guide and shape the behaviour of the individuals in the team. Creating the conditions for *team learning* becomes an essential leadership task, since the way in which the organisation will move forward and adapt to its shifting context is 'to do something and see what happens – if it's what is wanted then repeat; if not, modify the conditions, do something and see what happens'.

Theories that help individuals thrive in this context

To be effective in complex adaptive systems, people need to have highly developed *emotional intelligence*, which Goleman (1996) describes as:

'The capacity for recognising our own feelings and those of others, for motivating ourselves, and for managing emotions well in ourselves and in our relationships.'

The research evidence is that competent leaders who also exhibit high levels of emotional intelligence lead teams which have the competitive edge. Crucially, if managers are to lead from the perspective that all individuals have intrinsic motivation, then it follows that a high level of emotional intelligence needs to be developed in all members of staff.

Personal mastery and *mental models* (Senge, 1993) are crucial skill areas for continuous development. They complement the development of emotional intelligence and enable individuals to understand what motivates them and to work at clarifying and articulating how they are thinking about people and issues. People's responses to a set of circumstances are based on their particular mental models. Individuals have their own mental models and so crucial to progress in learning organisations is the development of the ability for people to articulate their mental models and suspend them before the group so that others can understand and respond. Individuals in learning organisations need to become skilled in *dialogue* (Battram, 1998) rather than discussion. This approach starts with listening and encourages reflection. Sub-optimal suggested solutions are acceptable, as the focus is on generating many ideas and synthesising the way forward.

Implications for psychiatrists managing change

People who choose to work in the field of mental health are well placed to work within conceptual frameworks which emphasise the humanness of us all. Understanding human strengths and uniqueness is essential to effective clinical practice in the field. This means that psychiatrists, for example, are particularly well placed to assist in the design and implementation of change programmes. This contrasts with doctors who have chosen to specialise in surgery, for example, where it can be argued that the ability to understand the human condition is perhaps less essential to the delivery of quality healthcare.

For psychiatrists to influence and implement change programmes effectively, they have to be active players in the organisational system within which they operate. Each individual's views are valid, within the theoretical framework for change management advocated in this chapter, and so it follows that it is really important for each clinician to be actively engaged in the life of the organisation. Finding opportunities to influence and shape throughout a psychiatrist's career is a good way of proceeding – not leaving it until a role is secured (e.g. as clinical director) which has a specific management component. This is not necessarily easy given the design of university medical training programmes, which favour identification with the medical school rather than the mental health trust where the clinical practice is being carried out. Nevertheless, participation in the life of the mental health trust will ensure that psychiatrists are fully part of the culture of the organisation and understand and enact its values. This is something which service users emphasise as particularly important, since for many of them their psychiatrist is the most important member of the clinical team.

Conclusion

All individuals at work need to develop their emotional intelligence and other skill sets (Box 17.1) to enable them to engage effectively with colleagues, whatever their location in the hierarchy and structure. This is the underlying essential set of competencies required to manage change effectively.

Box 17.1 Tips for successful change leaders

- Develop your emotional intelligence and your humanness
- Undertake continuous professional development in management and change leadership
- Think about your organisation as an organic entity that naturally keeps evolving
- Spend time with the team, building a shared vision
- Believe in people and their capacities and abilities to embrace change
- Develop a way of communicating that allows space for others to have opinions and contribute
- Demonstrate through your behaviour that you positively welcome and value diversity
- Pay attention to *process* as well as *content*
- Make change the norm in the team – doing many little changes quickly
- Catch people doing things right and continue to provide the conditions that have supported that behaviour
- Design processes that involve everyone and enable everyone to participate
- Offer sub-optimal proposals and invite genuine participation in co-creating the best solution
- Go where the energy for change is and support those who wish to achieve improvement – once the tipping point is reached the rest will come through

---

Developing a working knowledge of the other theories highlighted in this chapter should equip all who are asked to lead or implement change with a way of thinking about the context and the task such that they are confident enough to involve those around them in designing the way forward. Taking the first small steps is the key to success, and in a way which involves as many as possible of those who will be required to implement the change. Applying complexity principles to shape the thinking gives the confidence to take those first essential steps. The references and further reading listed below are by way of a sample reading list that will give you all the tools you need to design and implement successful change programmes. Enjoy the management of change!

Acknowledgements

Grateful thanks to Arthur Battram for our early discussions and help in formulating my thinking.

References and further reading

Battram, A. (1998) *Navigating Complexity*. Industrial Society.

Bunker, B. B. & Alban, B. T. (1997) *Large Group Interventions – Engaging the Whole System for Rapid Change*. Jossey-Bass.

Clarkson, P. (1995) *Change in Organisations*. Whurr.

Fraser, W., Conner, M. & Yarrow, D. (eds) (2003) *Thriving in Unpredictable Times*. Kingsham Press.

Gladwell, M. (2000) *The Tipping Point – How Little Things Can Make a Big Difference*. Little, Brown.

Goleman, D. (1996) *Emotional Intelligence*. Bloomsbury.

Mitleton-Kelly, E. (2003) *Complex Systems and Evolutionary Perspectives on Organisations*. Pergamon Elsevier Science.

Senge, P. (1993) *The Fifth Discipline – The Art and Practice of the Learning Organisation*. Century Business.

Senge, P., Kleiner, A., Roberts, C., *et al* (1999) *The Dance of Change – the Challenge of Sustaining Momentum in Learning Organizations*. Nicholas Brealey.

Wheatley, M. (1999) *Leadership and the New Science – Discovering Order in a Chaotic World*. Berrett-Koehler.

CHAPTER 18

Clinical governance

Rosalind Ramsay and Eleanor Cole

The rise of clinical governance

For the first 40 years of the National Health Service (NHS) there was an implicit notion of quality, with the assumption that providing well-trained staff and good facilities and equipment is synonymous with high standards (Halligan & Donaldson, 2001; Palmer, 2002). The arrival of the Thatcher government in 1979 saw the start of the first major reforms to the NHS. These initially focused on funding, management and organisational reform. From 1982, managers became accountable for output measures, at first concentrating on financial and workload concerns. In 1983, the Griffiths report described a lack of clarity in accountability at local level and overturned consensus management, resulting in the appointment of general managers to lead healthcare units (Griffiths, 1983).

More service changes followed with the introduction of the internal market in the early 1990s, but these did not specifically look at how to achieve improvements in quality at a structural level. Quality continued to be seen as inherent in the system, sustained by the ethos and skills of the health professionals working in the NHS. Any quality initiatives tended to be insular activities, not integrated across a whole service.

Quality management ideas developed in the Japanese car industry and taken up by business in the USA were creeping into the US healthcare system in the 1970s, before arriving in Europe. New concepts included total quality management and continuous quality improvement, but these were not widely accepted. However, the rise of consumerism in the postwar generation was starting to challenge the traditional paternalistic role of healthcare professionals in general, and of doctors in particular. Patients wanted more information, choice and involvement in decisions regarding their healthcare. This is illustrated in the rise of the service user movement and with the Major government's introduction of the Patient's Charter in 1992; shorter waiting lists and the right to information and to complain were potential vote winners.

There were also questions about variations in practice as clinicians adopted the principles of evidence-based practice, taking a more rigorous approach to their work. A series of high-profile service failures – an example being paediatric cardiac surgery in Bristol – raised concerns about professional self-regulation and doctors' accountability. These service failures prompted more urgent demands for change and attempts to address quality in a more systematic and explicit way.

The National Health Service and Community Care Act 1990 gave services a statutory duty of quality. Fuller development of this approach came with the first Blair government in the late 1990s. The White Paper *The New NHS* (Department of Health, 1997) stated:

'every part of the NHS, and everyone who works in it, must take responsibility for improving quality ... and it must be the quality of the patient experience as well as the clinical result.'

Clinical governance formalises this focus on the quality of services. The consultation paper *A First Class Service: Quality in the New NHS* (Department of Health, 1998) proposed that clinical governance would be the means by which NHS organisations could discharge their statutory duty to provide high-quality, safe and effective healthcare (Oyebode *et al*, 1999).

Definitions

Clinical governance has been described as:

'the opportunity to understand and learn to develop the fundamental components required to facilitate the delivery of quality care – a no blame, questioning, learning culture, excellent leadership, and an ethos where staff are valued and supported as they form partnerships with patients. These elements have perhaps previously been regarded as too intangible to take seriously or attempt to improve. Clinical governance demands re-examination of traditional roles and boundaries – between health professions, between doctor and patient, and between managers and clinicians – and provides the means to show the public that the NHS will not tolerate less than best practice' (Halligan & Donaldson, 2001).

The commonly used definition of clinical governance is:

'a framework through which NHS organisations are accountable for continuously improving the quality of their services and safeguarding high standards of care by creating an environment in which excellence in clinical care will flourish' (Scally & Donaldson, 1998).

Dame Janet Smith, chair of the Shipman Inquiry (2004), in her fifth report, has written that she did not find this definition particularly easy to understand and that the medical profession has been confused and uncertain as to what clinical governance means in practice. Having decided that it was impossible to define clinical governance, she attempted to describe it as 'a

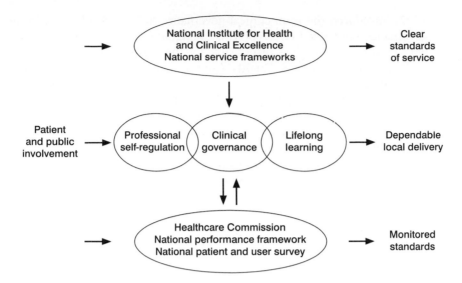

Fig. 18.1 A quality framework. (After Department of Health, 1998.)

system for improving the standard of clinical practice in the NHS and for protecting the public from unacceptable standards of care'. This system is made up of different activities within an integrated framework (Fig. 18.1) that replaces what were previously disparate and fragmented approaches to the improvement of quality of care.

A useful description of clinical governance has been given by Gray (2005), who says it is:

'doing the right thing, at the right time, by the right person – the application of the best evidence to a patient's problems, in the way the patient wishes, by an appropriately trained and resourced individual or team. But that's not all – the individual or team must work within an organisation that is accountable for the actions of its staff, values its staff (appraises and develops them), minimises risks, and learns from good practice, and indeed mistakes.'

Deighan *et al* (2004) have put forward the concept of integrated governance. They see this as a way of allowing governance to move out of its individual silos of clinical governance, corporate governance, research governance, information and financial governance, so that trust boards can more easily agree a common set of objectives and set a high-level direction for the organisation.

Clinical governance in Scotland

With devolution have come some differences in the development of clinical governance and its supporting structures. In Scotland, for example, the White Paper *Designed to Care* (Scottish Executive Health Department,

1997) introduced the term clinical governance to NHS Scotland. Clinical governance was defined as 'corporate accountability for clinical performance', with trust chief executives responsible for the quality of care provided by their organisations. NHS Quality Improvement Scotland (http://www. nhshealthquality.org) was set up in 2003 as the lead organisation to improve the quality of healthcare delivered by NHS Scotland. It works with the Scottish Intercollegiate Guidelines Network (SIGN) (http:// www.sign.ac.uk), which develops national clinical guidelines containing recommendations for effective practice based on current evidence. Quality Improvement Scotland describes clinical governance as the system for making sure that healthcare is safe and effective, that care is patient centred and that the public are involved.

Developing a framework for clinical governance

A First Class Service lists the main components of clinical governance as:

- clear lines of responsibility and accountability for the overall quality of clinical care
- a comprehensive programme of quality improvement activities
- clear policies aimed at reducing risk
- procedures for all professional groups to identify and remedy poor performance.

The New NHS outlined structures that would support the development of clinical governance. These include the National Service Frameworks and the

---

Box 18.1 Commission for Health Improvement (CHI) and clinical governance reviews

The CHI inspected clinical governance arrangements and provided feedback to local NHS organisations to inform development. CHI review teams assessed how well clinical governance was working throughout an organisation by making enquiries at corporate and directorate levels and in clinical teams about the different reviews areas, known as the seven components or 'pillars' of clinical governance:

- clinical audit
- risk management
- research and effectiveness
- use of information
- patient and public involvement
- staffing and staff management
- education and training.

The CHI also described strategic capacity and the patient experience.

National Institute for Clinical Excellence (NICE, since renamed the National Institute for Health and Clinical Excellence but retaining the acronym) to set quality standards, while the Commission for Health Improvement (since renamed the Healthcare Commission) (Box 18.1), the National Performance Framework and the National Survey of Patient and User Experience were to monitor standards.

Further legislation around the quality agenda came with the consultation paper *Supporting Doctors, Protecting Patients* (Department of Health, 1999b), with its proposals for professional regulation, and *An Organisation with a Memory* (Department of Health, 2000) which looked at learning from adverse incidents in the NHS. *An Organisation with a Memory* prompted the creation of the National Patient Safety Agency (NPSA) in 2001 to report on and promote learning from mistakes and problems that affect patient safety.

Another element of the quality strategy is patient and public empowerment. Since 2003, NHS bodies have had a legal duty to involve and consult the public. New developments have included establishing patient advice and liaison services (PALS) and patient and public involvement forums (PPI forums) in trusts as well as the independent complaints advocacy services (ICAS). Another way to empower patients is to provide better information.

Underpinning clinical governance were programmes in information technology, research and development, and education and training (Halligan & Donaldson, 2001).

Standards for Better Health

The *NHS Improvement Plan* (Department of Health, 2004a) has continued the emphasis on the quality of services, with an increased focus on the individual service user, including patient choice, and also public health. At the same time, *National Standards, Local Action* (Department of Health, 2004b) provides the framework for the NHS and local authorities until 2008. Within the framework are the 'Standards for Better Health', which build on the work of the National Service Frameworks and NICE. Standards are to be the main drivers for quality improvement and with fewer national targets there is greater scope for addressing local priorities. The 'Standards for Better Health' have tried to define the level of quality that all NHS organisations – including NHS foundation trusts and private and voluntary sector providers of NHS services – need to meet to assure safe and acceptable services. This is through compliance with the mandatory minimum 'core' standards and promoting service improvement by working towards the goals set in the 'developmental' standards. The standards aim to rationalise the existing standards and guidance into a single framework. They are presented in seven domains:

- safety
- clinical effectiveness and cost-effectiveness

- governance
- patient focus
- accessible and responsive care
- care environment and amenities
- public health.

As we can see, one of these domains covers governance and of the remaining six, five are closely linked to the previous CHI 'pillars' of clinical governance (Box 18.1): safety, clinical effectiveness and cost-effectiveness, patient focus, accessible and responsive care, and care environment and amenities.

Healthcare Commission

The Health and Social Care (Community Health and Standards) Act 2003 replaced the Commission for Health Improvement (CHI) with the Commission for Healthcare Audit and Inspection, generally known as the Healthcare Commission in 2004. The Healthcare Commission (http://www.healthcare commission.org.uk) has the overall function of encouraging improvement in healthcare and public health in England and Wales. It pays particular attention to:

- the availability of and access to healthcare
- the quality and effectiveness of healthcare
- the economy and efficiency of healthcare
- the availability and quality of information provided to the public about healthcare
- the need to safeguard the rights and welfare of children

The Healthcare Commission aims to focus on service users and the public, to work in partnership with others and to be open and accountable for its actions. Its corporate plan for 2004–08, *Inspecting, Informing, Improving* (Healthcare Commission, 2004), made a commitment to reduce the existing system of multiple inspections.

The Healthcare Commission has developed criteria and an assessment process based on 'Standards for Better Health'. This annual health check requires NHS trusts to make public declarations on the extent to which they meet the core standards, supplemented by comments from service users and the local community. The Healthcare Commission will also introduce improvement reviews that focus on particular aspects of the developmental standards, as well as specific populations and conditions.

There has been sharp criticism of 'Standards for Better Health', on the grounds that they are 'inconsistent in depth, scope and specificity', while the seven associated domains (see above) have 'no apparent architecture ... or hierarchy' and do not match any existing conceptual models (Shaw, 2004). It remains to be seen how well the Healthcare Commission can develop its assessment processes. As Shaw commented:

'the Department of Health has misjudged the research, technical expertise and time needed to develop and test a fair and reliable process of external assessment. The burden will fall on the fledgling Healthcare Commission as assessor and on the early guinea pigs who are assessed.'

Implementing clinical governance

Nicholls *et al* (2000) suggest we can understand clinical governance as:

'a whole system cultural change which provides the means of developing the organisational capability to deliver sustainable, accountable, patient focused quality assured healthcare.'

This reflects the view expressed in *The New NHS* (Department of Health, 1997) that 'achieving meaningful and sustainable quality improvements in the NHS requires a fundamental shift in culture'. Nicholls *et al* believe that clinical governance gives us a chance to find ways to move out of the comfort zone of the status quo to a more challenging culture with more active learning. They comment on the central role of the patient, with a real partnership between patient and professional being at the heart of clinical governance (Box 18.2). They also remind us that staff are the key resource for health services.

According to the website of the NHS Clinical Governance Support Team (http://www.cgsupport.nhs.uk), clinical governance requires changes at three levels: by individual professionals, by teams and by organisations.

• Individual healthcare professionals need to embrace change and adopt reflective practice that places patients at the centre of their thinking.

Box 18.2 Involving patients and carers in clinical governance

The NHS Modernisation Agency's *Improvement Leaders' Guide to Involving Patients and Carers* (2005) states that clinical governance reports should clearly describe how teams are developing continuous and effective patient involvement and how this has improved care as a result. One example they give concerns discharge planning from a particular in-patient unit. The service users had reported being confused about who was looking after them and had difficulty remembering contact telephone numbers, particularly at times of crisis. Users and carers received no written information on discharge. The service worked with service users and carers to set up a steering group, which explored the views of service users about discharge planning information. The group adopted an idea from a user to create a 'crisis card', the size of a credit card, that gave contact information about the care coordinator, general practitioner, social services and helplines. The local users helped to design the cards, which are now used for all patients discharged from in-patient care. The service users felt more confident at times of crisis knowing that they could easily make contact with services when needed. There are plans to extend the use of the crisis card to other parts of the service.

- Teams need to become true multidisciplinary groups, where understanding about roles, about sharing information and knowledge and about support for each other become part of everyday practice.
- Organisations need to put in place systems and local arrangements to support such teams and to assure the quality of care provided. Commitment and leadership from the board and throughout the organisation are clearly crucial.

Examining its findings from clinical governance reviews of mental health trusts, the CHI reported a number of common factors among trusts that were performing well and among those that had made less progress (see Table 18.1). Generally, trusts that were making progress in implementing clinical governance had also made good progress in implementing the National Service Framework for Mental Health, developing integrated provision with their social care partners, and in implementing the care programme approach. The CHI also found similar problems and characteristics in organisations that had been subject to investigation.

Table 18.1 Common factors among trusts in clinical governance reviews by the Commission for Health Improvement

Characteristics shared by trusts performing well	Characteristics shared by trusts performing poorly
Lower vacancy rates, particularly in psychiatry, or work to resolve vacancy problems; progress on Improving Working Lives	Serious problems with recruitment generally in psychiatry and in-patient nursing, low morale, cultural and operational divide with social care staff
Good progress with developing National Service Frameworks and the NHS Plan services and the care programme approach	Limited development of new services and implementation of the care programme approach
Leadership cohesive, visible and well regarded by staff and partners	Staff see leadership as remote, weakness in executive/non-executive leadership
Strong relationships between clinicians and managers	Lack of engagement of clinicians in management
Cohesive structures between different parts of the trust	Disconnection between different parts of the trust
Strong structures to support clinical governance in directorates and sectors/localities; understanding of relationship between the board and directorates, sectors and services	Limited structures below corporate level to support implementation and performance management of clinical governance, or structures to support clinical governance components
Well-developed clinical information systems and progress with performance management	Fragmented information systems and little development in performance management
Good progress on organisational and operational integration with primary care	Limited progress with organisational and operational integration with social care
Effective communication systems in place	Poor communication systems in place

Source: Adapted from Commission for Health Improvement (2003).

212

Barriers to clinical governance

A number of barriers to implementing clinical governance have been identified. Palmer (2002) refers to organisational culture, low prioritisation and lack of support. In spite of the rhetoric of a 'no blame' culture, many clinicians and managers feel there is a strong blame culture, with fears, for example, that participation in clinical audit can lead to punishment of poor performers. Historically, clinical audit had a low priority and clinical governance may not be seen as central to an organisation's activity, and this is compounded by a lack of support for clinical governance activity.

Putting clinical governance into practice

Clinical governance was originally seen as being local in its orientation and operation. As a bottom-up mechanism it could inspire and enthuse, and create a no-blame learning environment with excellent leadership, valued staff and an active partnership between staff and service users (Degeling *et al*, 2004). However, government preoccupation with delivery and top-down performance management has undermined its developmental potential. Degeling *et al* (2004) argue that if clinical governance is to work it must reach every level of a healthcare organisation, including clinicians.

Can we redefine clinical governance as an integral part of everyday work and express this in terms that relate to the improvement of patient care? Edwards (2004) comments there are two preconditions for this to be possible. First, the notion of professionalism must include:

- using techniques to improve the safety and effectiveness of care
- standardising care
- taking responsibility for the financial resources required
- being accountable for quality and performance.

Second, policy-makers and leaders must develop objectives and ways of working that will be meaningful to clinicians, supported by performance management and appraisal, and allow them to work more effectively.

Working with individual teams

In taking a bottom-up approach to implementing clinical governance, it is also essential to consider how individuals perceive it and what their understanding is of the concept. Murray *et al* (2004) used the Staff Clinical Governance Scale to explore staff knowledge of, attitudes to and implementation of the seven CHI pillars (see Box 18.1) across three mental health/community trusts. They found considerable goodwill towards clinical governance, although over a quarter of responders had not heard of it. The majority of staff viewed clinical governance as useful, and as clear and welcome,

213

although it was also felt to be complex and tiresome. One directorate which had put some effort into training and communicating about clinical governance had the most positive responses, suggesting the value of having a proactive approach to involving all staff in clinical governance.

Another mental health trust has developed clinical governance portfolios for its teams, to facilitate the recording of all the clinical governance activity a team does (Mynors-Wallis *et al*, 2004). The aim is to increase awareness of clinical governance, ensure that it is central to team activity, encourage clinical governance activity and monitor it. One member of each team acts as the portfolio coordinator. Review of the portfolios allowed the team coordinators to discuss their successes and difficulties in establishing clinical governance at a team level, and to develop an action plan over the following year. The portfolios are linked in with other trust developments rather than being an isolated project. They have also enabled the spread of good practice.

Topic-specific clinical governance: suicide prevention

Degeling *et al* (2004) recommend looking at clinical governance in a condition-specific way, by encouraging staff dealing with a particular type of clinical work to define, describe, assess and manage what they do as a team. We could also look at a particular topic, for example suicide prevention, in this way. What can individual teams do to develop better practice in relation to reducing the risk of suicide among their users?

Suicide is the commonest cause of death in men under the age of 35 and the main cause of premature death in people with a mental illness (Department of Health, 2002). The White Paper *Saving Lives: Our Healthier Nation* (Department of Health, 1999a) has a target to reduce the death rate from suicide and undetermined injury by at least a fifth by 2010. There is no single route to achieving this target, as the factors associated with suicide are many and varied. Developing a coherent suicide prevention strategy needs the collaboration of a range of organisations and individuals. Training in suicide risk assessment and management is required for all teams and individual clinicians.

The National Suicide Prevention Strategy (Department of Health, 2002) proposes six goals and objectives for action. What do these mean in terms of quality of care for practising clinicians? How can we conceive of them in clinical governance terms?

Reduce the risk in high-risk groups

High-risk groups include people who are currently or were recently in contact with mental health services, as well as people who have recently harmed themselves, young men, prisoners and certain occupational groups.

What services are available for individuals in the immediate aftermath of an episode of self-harm? Is there a local implementation plan for the NICE (2004) guideline on self-harm? That guideline covers the first 48 hours after an episode of self-harm and recommends more sophisticated ways of trying to engage with service users and their carers, encouraging the notion of self-management as well recommending those types of psychological intervention for which there is some evidence of effectiveness.

There is continuing concern about the risks in young men, and evidence of their increased risk of suicide has caught the attention of the media. How are clinicians and services trying to engage with this group in their locality? Initiatives include a crisis helpline in some areas (CALM – Campaign Against Living Miserably), supplementing the work of the Samaritans and NHS Direct, and also work with substance misuse services to look at how they can improve the clinical management of alcohol and drug misuse in young men who harm themselves.

The prison service suicide prevention strategy includes a number of plans to improve the screening and management of self-harm in this population, some in collaboration with local mental health services. There are plans to improve the information flow into and across the criminal justice system concerning individuals known to be at risk of suicide.

A particular high-risk time for psychiatric patients has been identified as the week after discharge, and clinicians need to make arrangements for early ('7 day') follow-up for people at high risk, as well as considering access to services at times of crisis.

Promote well-being in the wider population

This is in line with standard 1 of the National Service Framework for Mental Health (Department of Health, 1999c), which aims to promote mental health for all and to combat discrimination against those with a mental illness. The strategy recognises the range of factors that may predispose to self-harm but goes on to take a narrower focus in addressing the needs of particular groups: young people, those bereaved by suicide, older people, Black and minority ethnic people, and women in the perinatal period. The National Service Frameworks for Children and Older People look at these issues further, and the Confidential Enquiries into Maternal Deaths, which report every 3 years, continue to make recommendations.

Reduce the availability and lethality of suicide methods

Some of the recommendations might appear to fall outside a health organisation's remit – including changes in car design and safety measures at identified 'hot spots' (e.g. on the railways and high buildings) – but there may be scope for work with other agencies. For example, in relation to hot spots, London Underground is wanting to work with local services to reduce the risks. There are also questions about hanging, strangulation and asphyxiation. Estates and facilities departments will need to get involved in auditing identified ligature points such as non-collapsible bed and shower rails, while clinical staff can look at the availability of other methods, such as plastic bags. For clinicians there are practice issues around the safe prescribing of antidepressants, including the type of antidepressant prescribed and the amount given in any one prescription. Clinicians can also ask users about unwanted medicines at home and look at their safe disposal.

Improve the reporting of suicidal behaviour in the media

There is guidance available from the Samaritans on suicide reporting in the media. 'Mind Out for Mental Health', the Department of Health's anti-stigma campaign, has tried to influence the ways in which the media report mental health issues, for example by providing workshops and training materials for trainee journalists. There is also scope for individual clinicians (those who have had training and feel confident in handling media contact) to be interviewed to give accurate and non-stigmatising information about mental illness and its effect on individuals and communities.

Promote research on suicide and suicide prevention

There is evidence from epidemiological and clinical studies on risk factors associated with suicide, but no intervention studies in which suicide has been the main outcome, because of the size of the sample that would be needed. The strategy recommends research focusing on high-risk groups, and intervention studies with more common outcomes that can be a proxy for suicide.

Improve the monitoring of progress towards targets

There is already information available through the National Confidential Enquiries into suicide and homicide by people with mental illness, and into maternal deaths; more detailed data may be available in the future to cover, for example, the occupation and ethnicity of individuals if coroners record them.

Clinical governance and service modernisation

Another way to consider and improve the quality of health services is through the use of modernisation tools and related training. The NHS Modernisation Agency had aims shared with clinical governance, namely that of modernising services to improve the experience and outcome for patients. In 2005, the Agency merged with the NHS University and NHS Leadership Centre to form a new body, the NHS Institute for Innovation and Improvement. The NHS Institute is a special health authority in England. It has a number of functions: to identify best practice; to develop the NHS's capability for service transformation; to facilitate local implementation of good practice; and to promote a culture of innovation and lifelong learning for all staff. The Osprey programme is a good example of a modernisation project to improve service quality throughout one healthcare sector.

Clinical systems improvement in south-east London: the Osprey programme (Better care without delay)

'Clinical system improvement' (CSI) is a term used to describe the management of patient flow to improve the efficiency and quality of the patient's experience. The Osprey programme combined with the Improvement Partnership in Hospitals (IPH) to form part of a national pilot project involving a number of strategic health authorities with assistance from the former Modernisation Agency to develop a 'spread programme' for CSI in south-east London. The project's aims were to build foundations and to strengthen the infrastructure for improving patient flow through healthcare systems. CSI engineers and flow redesign capability were the key components of the programme. The CSI engineers supported improvement work across the sector, developing innovative ideas to improve services. This was done by developing capacity for service improvement within the local health economy and through promoting coordination of this work.

Key objectives of the Osprey programme were:

- improving the way information is used
- building CSI skills and expertise locally at consultant and general practitioner level
- communicating and implementing flow management concepts in service design and planning
- linking funding decisions to service redesign.

The Programme design is focused on dissemination of improvement concepts (Box 18.3) and measuring their uptake in health service organisations in south-east London.

Senior clinician involvement is crucial to the successful redesign of services and for sustaining any improvement. A key component of the programme has been the acquisition of skills locally by both consultants and general practitioners. Identified clinicians have taken part in a development programme that included training in service development and improvement methods. The programme provided funding for replacement sessions, which allowed senior clinicians time away from their clinical responsibilities. Individual coaching with a CSI engineer was also available. Clinicians selected a project that dovetailed with the priorities of their organisation.

Box 18.3 Improvement concepts

- Queues are caused by a mismatch between capacity and demand
- Understanding how patients flow through health systems, with their bottlenecks (constraints)
- Understanding how reducing carve-out and implementing pooling stop this
- Understanding the true capacity and demand of the system and how to work towards limiting variation within the system
- Monitoring variation and improvement using statistical process control (SPC)

Both of the authors completed this programme as part of a local service improvement development. Understanding patient flow within the health economy was the overarching theme of the training programme, the contents of which are shown in Box 18.4.

Clinicians completing the training served as an internal resource within their respective organisations; they provided support and expertise to their peers. Participating clinicians were supported in this work by the CSI engineers. Time commitment for the training programme consisted of a term of half-day introductory seminars and workshops. Subsequent monthly half-day learning sets provided an opportunity to test approaches, discuss problems and find solutions as a group.

An example of the work conducted by one of the authors (Box 18.5) was examining bed management, a priority area for most of the participating trusts. Bed management is an area where there is considerable scope for service improvement.

Clinicians can benefit greatly from being involved in service improvement work. The CSI project described is one very important way for clinicians to acquire the necessary skills and make a difference to healthcare quality.

Clinical governance provides a useful framework for service improvement but requires ownership by all clinicians, particularly those in senior positions. Mobilising a whole organisation to improve healthcare delivery remains an ongoing challenge and an exciting and worthwhile goal.

Box 18.4 Content of training programme

- Better understanding of flow
- Principles of demand and capacity
- Construction and interpretation of statistical process control charts
- Process mapping and other diagnostic tools to identify problems with flow
- Understanding and improving the culture of organisations
- Understanding personal styles

Box 18.5 Description of project

Aims
- Establish overview of patient flow through the trust
- Introduce improvements to reduce variation in flow
- Introduce improvements to increase predictability of beds needed for admission on a daily basis
- System to be as efficient as possible

Context
- Capacity exceeding demand for acute in-patient beds
- Numerous interfaces involved in patients' journey through mental health services
- New functional in-patient and community teams bedding down
- Pressures on staff finding beds for patients requiring admission
- Beds mostly being made available in response to bed pressures
- More efficient use of resources required

Outcomes
- No inappropriate admissions
- Reduced length of stay
- No patients in out-of-borough beds ('sleep-overs')
- Reduction of staff stress
- Improvement in patient experience

Performance monitoring
- Top-level analysis trust performance indicators using statistical process control charts to measure effect of any changes
- Total number of admissions to borough acute wards
- Total number of admissions to acute wards mapped to locality number of patients in out-of-borough beds ('sleep-overs')
- Total number of discharges from acute beds
- Length of stay (analysis of two groups, 80% with shortest length of stay and 20% with longest)
- Percentage of patients seen within 7 days of discharge

Other investigations
- Audit of delayed discharges
- Test targeted interventions

References

Commission for Health Improvement (2003) *What CHI Has Found in Mental Health Trusts: Sector Report*. CHI.

Degeling, P. J., Maxwell, S., Iedema, R., *et al* (2004) Making clinical governance work. *BMJ*, **329**, 679–681.

Deighan, M., Cullen, R. & Moore, R. (2004) The development of integrated governance. *Debate*, (3), 1–8. NHS Confederation. http://www.cgsupport.nhs.uk/downloads/Board/integrated_governance_paper.pdf

Department of Health (1997) *The New NHS: Modern, Dependable*. TSO (The Stationery Office).

Department of Health (1998) *A First Class Service: Quality in the New NHS*. Department of Health.

Department of Health (1999*a*) *Saving Lives: Our Healthier Nation*. TSO (The Stationery Office).

Department of Health (1999*b*) *Supporting Doctors, Protecting Patients. A Consultation Paper on Preventing, Recognising and Dealing with Poor Clinical Performance of Doctors in the NHS in England*. Department of Health.

Department of Health (1999*c*) *National Service Framework for Mental Health*. Department of Health.

Department of Health (2000) *An Organisation with a Memory*. TSO (The Stationery Office).

Department of Health (2002) *National Suicide Prevention Strategy for England*. Department of Health.

Department of Health (2004*a*) *The NHS Improvement Plan*. Department of Health.

Department of Health (2004*b*) *National Standards, Local Action. Health and Social Care Standards and Planning Framework 2005/06–2007/08*. Department of Health.

Edwards, N. (2004) Commentary: model could work. *BMJ*, **329**, 681–682.

Gray, C. (2005) What is clinical governance? *BMJ Careers*, **330**, 254.

Griffiths, R. (1983) *NHS Management Inquiry Report*. Department of Health and Social Security.

Halligan, A. & Donaldson, L. (2001) Implementing clinical governance: turning vision into reality. *BMJ*, **322**, 1413–1417.

Healthcare Commission (2004) *Inspecting, Informing, Improving*. Healthcare Commission.

Murray, J., Fell-Rayner, H., Fine, H., *et al* (2004) What do NHS staff think and know about clinical governance? *Clinical Governance: An International Journal*, **9**, 172–180.

Mynors-Wallis, L., Cope, D. & Suliman, S. (2004) Making clinical governance happen at team level: the Dorset experience. *Clinical Governance*, **9**, 162–166.

National Institute for Clinical Excellence (2004) *Self-harm*, Clinical Guideline 16. NICE.

NHS Modernisation Agency (2005) *Improvement Leaders' Guide to Involving Patients and Carers*. NHS Modernisation Agency.

Nicholls, S., Cullen, R., O'Neill, S., *et al* (2000) Clinical governance: its origins and its foundations. *Clinical Performance and Quality Healthcare*, **8**, 172–178.

Oyebode, F., Brown, N. & Parry, E. (1999) Clinical governance: applications to psychiatry. *Psychiatric Bulletin*, **23**, 7–10.

Palmer, C. (2002) Clinical governance: breathing new life into clinical audit. *Advances in Psychiatric Treatment*, **8**, 470–476.

Scally, G. & Donaldson, L. J. (1998) Looking forward: clinical governance and the drive for quality improvement in the new NHS in England. *BMJ*, **317**, 61–65.

Scottish Executive Health Department (1997) *Designed to Care*. Scottish Executive Health Department.

Shaw, C. D. (2004) Standards for Better Health: fit for purpose? *BMJ*, **329**, 1250–1251.

Shipman Inquiry (2004) *Fifth Report – Safeguarding Patients: Lessons from the Past – Proposals for the Future*, Cm 6394. TSO (The Stationery Office).

Useful reading for modernisation improvement concepts and methodologies

Hart, M. K. & Hart, R. K. (2002) *Statistical Process Control for Healthcare*. Duxbury Thompson.

NHS Modernisation Agency. *NHS Modernisation: The Clinicians' Guide to Applying the 10 High Impact Changes*. See http://www.modern.nhs.uk/highimpactchanges

Wheeler. D. J. (1999) *Understanding Variation: The Key to Managing Chaos* (2nd edn). SPC Press.

CHAPTER 19

Complaints

Frank Margison and Alistair Burns

The general response of clinicians when receiving a complaint tends, very often understandably, to be negative. Irritation, fear, anxiety about the possibility of error and worries about disapproval are common. Sometimes the feelings are very personal. Complaints can still occur when staff have gone far beyond the minimum expected, and so the response is influenced by feelings that patients (and their families) are being particularly unreasonable or ungrateful. Knowing more about the benefits of a good complaints system helps keep any initial negative reaction in check.

An effective complaints system is an essential part of good clinical governance. Complaints can give early warning about systemic failures in a trust's procedures, about services where staff have developed unhelpful or hostile attitudes and, occasionally, can identify a clinician whose performance is below standard. This last point fuels the anxiety that clinicians feel, but in practice a complaint is usually just one element of more general problems in performance.

This chapter clarifies different types of complaint, practical issues in managing complaints, legal issues and how to learn from complaints and offers some ways of dealing with reactions to complaints. The development of the complaints system within the National Health Service (NHS) has been complicated and punctuated by reports expressing dissatisfaction with the seriousness and effectiveness of complaints processes.

The history of complaints processes in the NHS

The next section shows how the current complaints system has grown over the past 10 years to meet the need for the NHS to be more open and more responsive. The current system is detailed in every trust's complaints procedure as they all follow national guidance, with some variations for England, Wales, Scotland and Northern Ireland. The changes in the English policy described in more detail below reflect a common process that has affected all four jurisdictions. The current system is intended to be:

- open
- transparent
- subject to challenge at several levels
- part of a learning culture
- focused on clinical and non-clinical failings
- compatible with medico-legal processes through civil actions.

Perhaps the biggest change affecting trusts has been the involvement of the Healthcare Commission, which provides both review and challenge to trusts' own complaints investigations. A common result is a requirement for trusts to make further attempts to find local resolution.

Before 1996, there was a fragmented system whereby complaints in the NHS were dealt with entirely by trusts and there were no enforceable or national standards for the way they were handled. In April that year, a new complaints system came into force for hospital, community and primary care services and which could manage complaints dealing with either administration or clinical treatment, or both. The first stage of any complaint was known as local resolution, whereby local staff and the trust's managers would deal with the complaint and try to resolve it to the satisfaction of the complainant. If complainants continued to be dissatisfied, they could ask the trust to organise an independent review. This request was considered by a non-executive director of the trust, designated the 'convenor'. The convenor could decide to refer the complaint back for further local work towards resolution or decide that no more useful purpose would be served by further investigation. The convenor decided whether a full independent review was needed, with an independent chair from a list of names held by the strategic health authority. The convenor had independent clinical advice from outside the trust. If complainants remained dissatisfied after an independent review, or had been refused one, they could complain to the Health Service Ombudsman.

The overwhelming problem with this system was that it was not perceived as being independent. The convenor was a non-executive director of the trust where the events leading to the complaints had occurred; furthermore, the panel was organised by hospital staff, and the meeting was held on hospital premises. The Department of Health ran an exercise in 1999–2001 (known as 'Evaluation and Listening Exercise') which confirmed the high level of dissatisfaction at all stages. The main reasons, in addition to the perceived lack of independence, were unhelpful attitudes of staff, poor communication between the hospital and complainants, and lack of information and support. It is interesting to note that this public view was also one held by the Ombudsman's office, based on its experience of picking up complaints after the trust had tried to deal with them. The subsequent report, *NHS Complaints Procedure: National Evaluation* (Department of Health, 2001a), made 27 recommendations to improve the system. These included ensuring: a uniform procedure with defined time limits; dissemination of good practice; targets (hardly surprising); clear lines of responsibility;

responsibility specifically for trust boards to ensure training; quarterly reports to the trust board; strengthening of procedures for complaints in primary care; and wide dissemination of reports.

In September 2001, the Department of Health (2001b) issued another document, *Reforming the NHS Complaints Procedure – A Listening Document*, which invited comments both as written responses and within a series of regional events. In April 2003, the Department published *NHS Complaints Reform, Making Things Right*, which gave a new vision of the complaints procedure – open and easy to access, fair and independent, responsive, and providing an opportunity for learning and developing. It said that responsibility for the review would be placed with the new Commission for Health Care Audit and Inspection (CHAI, now renamed the Healthcare Commission).

The need for change was underscored by a number of inquiries, such as the Bristol Inquiry in 2001, the Neale and Ayling inquiries in September 2004, the last part of the Shipman Inquiry in January 2005, and the Haslam and Kerr inquiries in 2005. The inquiries had considered why existing systems did not recognise and act sooner on the difficulties with which they had dealt.

In parallel with the changes to the formal complaints system, the NHS Plan (Department of Health, 2000a) proposed the creation of patient advice and liaison services (PALS), which were put in place in NHS trusts by 2002 (see below for a discussion of their role). Part of their remit was to provide on-the-spot advice and information to patients and they often gave views about resolving complaints. Although they were not initially designed to be directly involved in complaints, they have now taken on part of this role and they have acted as a catalyst for the setting up of a new service – the independent complaints advocacy services (ICAS), which in conjunction with the PALS were to take over the role of the community health councils (CHCs), which were abolished in December 2003. In January 2003, another agency was established, the Commission for Patient and Public Involvement in Health Care (CPPIC), which had the broad remit of making sure NHS services took account of the view of the public; it set up patient and public involvement forums (one for each trust), whose role was to provide direct independent input into the day-to-day management of health services. In July 2004 the CPPIC was abolished but the patients and public involvement forums (PPI forums) continued.

As these changes were occurring in the complaints process, the Chief Medical Officer published a report, *Making Amends – A Consultation Paper* (Donaldson, 2003), that set out proposals for reforming the clinical negligence system, as the existing system was slow, unfair, encouraged defensive practice and was costly. A new NHS-based system was devised, under the remit of the NHS Litigation Authority (NHSLA), which now deals with medical negligence on behalf of NHS trusts.

The Health Ombudsman produced a report on the complaints procedure in 2005. It was felt that the system still had five major weaknesses, which needed to be resolved (Health Service Ombudsman, 2005):

1   The complaints systems are fragmented, not only within the NHS but between the NHS and both the private health system and social care.
2   The complaints system is still not centred on patients' needs.
3   There is a lack of competence among staff to deliver a high-quality service.
4   Leadership, culture and governance are not in place
5   Just remedies are still not being achieved for justifiable complaints.

The Health Service Ombudsman's and subsequent discussion with the Healthcare Commission led to the current process whereby the Healthcare Commission now has the responsibility for complaints that have not been resolved at the local level. The Healthcare Commission can refer back for further local work, uphold a complaint or investigate further with independent advice. The Healthcare Commission has already commented on the weakness of trusts' procedures and has encouraged trusts to make their processes more robust. It is in a position to monitor this process through its referrals back for local resolution. The Healthcare Commission has set timescales which trusts are expected to meet in managing complaints.

The Health Service Ombudsman can still receive a referral if the complainant is not satisfied with the Healthcare Commission's intervention.

The Citizens' Charter Complaints Task Force (Department Of Health, 1995) defined a complaint broadly as 'an expression of dissatisfaction requiring a response'. This definition is somewhat tautological, as it does not clarify what forms of dissatisfaction require a response. It is wise to think that any such expression is potentially a complaint and should be recorded in the trust's complaints system. However, the vast majority of these expressions of dissatisfaction are resolved immediately and do not require any further investigation.

The trust's chief executive is responsible for the overall system and signs the responses to complainants after the investigation has been completed. There are time limits for the different stages of complaint response and trusts are judged against these performance standards. In practice, this means that the chief executive has oversight of the policy and procedures, but the actual investigation is usually carried out by local managers with someone coordinating the process on behalf of the chief executive.

The guidance from the Department of Health states:

'In the majority of cases, complaints are made orally. All complaints, whether oral or written, should receive a positive and full response, with the aim of satisfying the complainant that his/her concerns have been heeded, and offering an apology and explanation as appropriate, referring to any remedial action that is to follow. The trust chief executive will be responsible for ensuring that there is appropriate local policy and procedural guidance in place that is available to all staff' (http://www.dh.gov.uk/en/Publicationsandstatistics/Publications/PublicationsPolicyAndGuidance/Browsable/DH_5133265)

Written and verbal

Written complaints are sometimes seen to be more 'formal', but in fact there should be no real distinction between written and verbal complaints, in the sense that both need a timely and accurate reply. It is good practice to make a written note of any oral expressions of dissatisfaction, so that someone who has difficulty in putting things in writing is not disadvantaged. Once the account has been recorded and signed by the complainant, a written response has to be provided and signed by the chief executive, as described below.

Informal and formal

There is often confusion about formal and informal complaints. 'Informal' usually means that a complaint can be resolved by local agreement and subsequent action, whereas a 'formal' complaint is typically managed centrally, with a manager asked to investigate it by gathering information from everyone involved.

Some patients or relatives may use the term 'formal' to mean that they do not want local resolution but want a written response from the chief executive following an investigation. Complainants are entitled to this level of response, but sometimes when the procedure is explained properly complainants are happy that a local resolution will provide what they want. In either case, the complaint has to be recorded and counted in the trust's figures on complaints, so in that sense all complaints are 'formal'. However, the chief executive has a statutory obligation to respond to written complaints, as well as all oral complaints that are subsequently put into writing with the content agreed by the complainant, and so the term 'formal' is often used to refer to any written complaints or complaints subsequently put in writing on behalf of a patient or relative.

It is important to remember that if a people contact you with what they believe is a complaint, then it is a complaint to them, however unjustified you may think it is. If the complainant raises the same or similar issues repeatedly, despite receiving a full response, there may be underlying reasons for this persistence (how to deal with unreasonable complainants is discussed towards the end of the chapter).

Local resolution

'The purpose of local resolution is to provide an opportunity for the complainant and the organisation (or individual) subject to the complaint, to attempt a rapid and fair resolution of the problem. The process should be open, fair, flexible and conciliatory, and should facilitate communication on all sides.' (http://www.dh.gov.uk/en/Publicationsandstatistics/Publications/PublicationsPolicyAndGuidance/Browsable/DH_5133265)

Clinical and administrative staff need to have the expertise to identify the key issues being raised and to find a resolution wherever possible. In some situations, the issues raised have to be managed more formally. Examples include cases of potential fraud or exploitation of patients, or cases which raise threats to safety.

When the issue looks particularly complex or serious, the complaints manager gets involved more closely. This might be to arrange a fuller investigation or to arrange meetings with senior staff to deal with the issues raised. When the trust's central complaints department is involved, an investigator is usually appointed to pull the evidence together. These processes characterise a complaint that is following 'formal' procedures.

Complainants can seek support from an ICAS or any other agency offering advice, advocacy and/or information, regarding their case.

Customer care and complaints

Customer care refers to the range of skills used by staff to make patients and relatives feel they are being heard and treated with respect. In the context of complaints, customer care training reduces the tension arising when a patient or relative feels aggrieved and let down by the service. The skills required have considerable overlap with good clinical interviewing. They include the ability to listen, clarify, summarise and feed back in the context of someone who may be angry or distressed.

The additional points are about trying to achieve a resolution. In very straightforward situations, this may involve nothing more complex than giving information and explanation (e.g. 'We have an information leaflet to explain how you can change an appointment and I will make sure the consultant knows you need an afternoon time in future'). Some situations need more information but are not complicated to answer (e.g. 'I will check with the doctor and ring you back with the results and let you know whether you need to book an earlier review appointment'). Where a complaint is more complicated or serious and needs investigation, the skill is in conveying to the patient that any concerns have been heard and will be investigated. In all of these situations it is crucial that the staff hearing the complaint 'deliver' on what they have said they will do.

Patient advice and liaison services

The PALS support patients and carers over a whole range of service issues, but they have a particular role in supporting patients who want to complain. They provide:

- confidential advice and support to patients, families and their carers
- information on the NHS and health-related matters

- confidential assistance in resolving problems and concerns quickly
- information on and explanations of NHS complaints procedures
- how to get in touch with someone who can help.

The content of complaints

Events

Where complaints concern a discrete event that can be investigated, they are usually the simplest to deal with. Some merely require the facts to be gathered and an apology given if something went wrong, but the principles of root cause analysis are important in identifying underlying problems that can addressed and rectified (see below).

There should be some agreement between the content of these complaints and incident reports that have already come in from staff involved in the incident. In practice, this is often not the case, as incident systems tend to be focused on the more severe end of the spectrum. This is not an adequate explanation though, as good incident systems should document about 40 times as many minor events as serious incidents (Department of Health, 2000b). So, while it would be reasonable to expect that most complaints could be investigated initially by looking at the log of the incident, sadly this is not often the case.

Complaints can function as a back-up to these incomplete systems so that less serious incidents and near misses can be recorded more effectively. Good clinical governance should see complaints and incident reporting as part of an integrated system. Indeed, current practice encouraged by the Clinical Negligence Scheme for Trusts is for complaints and incidents (as well as health and safety events and claims) all to be reported to the trust board in an integrated way, with explicit statements about 'lessons learned'.

Events can range from quality issues that cause irritation but no serious harm (e.g. no water in the cooler in the waiting room) to serious issues that need to be reported as adverse incidents as well as complaints (e.g. errors in giving the wrong medication through to allegations of being physically assaulted by a member of staff).

Problems with process

Commonly it is a process that goes wrong, rather than a specific event: clinics being cancelled, a letter going to a person who has died, addresses being wrong and so on. From a service design point of view, many complaints systems fail to learn from these. An unhelpful underlying attitude in an organisation may be that 'stuff happens'; a minimal apology is given and people move on, without ever learning what the cause was. Often staff running systems who hold these attitudes feel angry and frustrated themselves but feel powerless to do anything about the poor tools with which they work, such as out-of-date software, or about clinicians who do not update their holiday dates with clinic managers, for example. Whatever the underlying reason, the apparent indifference leads to a more forceful complaint in the end.

These process issues have a surprisingly large effect on how a business is seen, and this certainly applies to the NHS. The corollary is that using complaints about process issues can significantly improve the quality of a service, as they often include crucial details about what is going wrong.

Attitudes

Concerns about staff attitudes are common reasons for complaints. These are often difficult to investigate, as they often arise from one-to-one interviews. Sometimes there is a straight contradiction of facts. For example, the patient may say that the consultant used the words 'You are wasting my time!', which is then denied by the consultant. It is very hard to uphold a complaint in these circumstances.

However, the person investigating is left with a patient who feels he or she has been treated discourteously and who may well feel aggrieved if the complaint is not upheld. The clinician, equally, may feel aggrieved that there is a complaint at all when he or she feels nothing untoward happened. It may be that the patient has grasped some disquiet on the part of the clinician, but reads this as hostility rather than, say, puzzlement or frustration about the behaviour of others in the system. When things go well in the investigation both parties may feel that the underlying problem has been identified and dealt with. Unfortunately, the investigator is often left at an impasse, with two irreconcilable accounts.

Quite different issues arise if the clinician has been the subject of several similar complaints from a range of patients and carers already, all with similar features. There may still be the same problem in getting evidence to uphold this particular instance, but it may be reasonable to raise the pattern with the clinician to reflect upon, perhaps through the appraisal process. A constructive outcome may be agreement to take part in 360° appraisal, which, if done properly, will assist the clinician to see any contribution he or she is making to the complaints.

Absence of service

Complaints often arise about the lack of availability of a service. Again, these complaints raise difficult issues for the investigator, as the trust may not have any remedy to offer, other than raising the concern with commissioners. Sometimes the complaints process may reveal other avenues for help that had not been considered by the clinician.

Complaints requiring further specific action

Some complaints raise concerns that require action beyond the complaints process itself. This means that the complaints process needs to be closely linked to other aspects of clinical governance. Where safety or protection issues are raised, these must follow their own course while the complaint is investigated. The first categories requiring additional action concern protection of children and vulnerable adults.

Child protection

The local child protection procedures need to be activated when a complaint raises concerns about child safety. Every trust should have a lead nurse and a lead doctor responsible for child protection; sometimes a manager is responsible for child protection. These staff can indicate the need for referral to the child protection leads for the area, who will advise on whether, and how, to refer to the formal child protection agency for the area. It is possible to complete some complaints investigations while the child protection concerns are being resolved, but often there will need to be liaison between the two processes.

Vulnerable adults

Complaints sometimes raise the possible exploitation or abuse of vulnerable people. Every trust has to have a process approved by its board for investigating and if necessary remedying such concerns. These have some similarities to child protection processes, in that there will be an area policy adopted by the trust, and a recognised method of investigating these incidents, including links with the police at an early stage.

Health and safety concerns

Sometimes a complaint will raise a health or safety concern that needs urgent attention. These are often matters that affect staff as well as patients. For such situations, trusts have procedures to manage the immediate concerns, but the complaints process must also receive proper attention. A simple example might be a complaint that the floor is slippery and the complainant almost fell. As well as responding to these individual concerns it is obvious that someone needs to check the floor and remedy any problem.

It may not be quite so easy for staff to see that similar worries should be raised when a clinical error is raised, such as receiving the wrong medication. In addition to investigating the error so that an appropriate apology can be given (if indeed the error did occur), it is important that the error is referred to the person responsible for errors of this type; typically this will be the chief pharmacist or someone from the medicines management committee in the trust. He or she may find a systematic error in the way that checks are carried out, or a previously unreported error in dispensing, administration or prescribing.

Criminal proceedings

Rarely, complaints will raise matters that involve breaches of criminal law. Examples might include a complaint that raises the possibility of fraud or theft. Other examples might overlap with the vulnerable adults procedure, such as allegations of sexual assault or rape. In the latter cases, the police *must* be involved; in situations of potential fraud within the NHS the counter-fraud services within the Health Service may need to be involved. The presence of such services may not be known to all staff, and so it is crucial that referral to the counter-fraud service is made at the earliest opportunity.

Disciplinary action

The disciplinary process should always be kept separate from the investigation of a complaint. However, in investigating a complaint it may be that disciplinary action needs to be considered. For example, there may be concerns about serious malpractice raised in interviewing a witness. It is essential that the complaints process links at the earliest opportunity with the investigation processes leading to a potential disciplinary hearing. This protects both the staff and the patient, as there are clear procedures for gathering and considering evidence by an investigating officer. It is essential to keep the processes distinct, as the key aim of a complaints process is to improve services and offer apologies when things have gone wrong. The purpose of a disciplinary proceeding is to hold people to account for their actions. If the complaints process is to be kept open, within a learning environment, it is crucial that staff know when there is a change of the process that may lead to criticism or, sometimes, formal penalties.

Practical issues

How to write a report

Clinicians are often asked to provide a report to form the basis for the reply from the Chief Executive to the complainant.

It is important before you write a report to examine carefully the terms of reference for the investigation. Part of the skill of carrying out an investigation is to have terms of reference (and questions) that can be answered within the timescale and resources allowed. Remember to answer only those questions you were asked, not the questions you think the investigators should be asking.

Your answers should be concise, to the point and written in a style that an intelligent lay person can understand. If you do not know the answer to a question, or if the answer is outside your area of expertise, then you should say so. People get into trouble by pretending they know the answers to something and, even worse, when they think they know more about something than the investigators.

It is always good practice to have a colleague to read over a report you have prepared, and it also good practice to check with your medical defence union about what you are writing (it will sometimes ask for a copy for its files). Even if the investigation is not critical of you in any way, your report may inadvertently implicate others.

How to draft a response

Sometimes, you will be asked to comment on things that others have written. The same principles apply here as do in writing a report.

How to meet users and carers

The current generation of trainees and newly appointed consultants will have been well used to the involvement of people who use the service and their carers. Always take time to explain things in simple, straightforward language, but avoid any tendency to be patronising. Generally, users and carers tend to speak their minds more openly, unshackled by traditional professional constraints, so be prepared for that but try not to take it personally. Remember, because of the privileged position they hold, users and carers can be your best advocates!

How to apologise

Never be reluctant to apologise where appropriate. Be careful, however, not to apologise on behalf of others (e.g. 'I am sorry the junior doctor did not see your mother because he was busy with something else') or for the inadequacy of services (e.g. 'I am sorry, we should have got a social worker to see your brother, but they are grossly under-resourced and didn't respond to our request'). Be clear what you are apologising for. For instance, it is good practice to apologise for any distress caused by an incident but without necessarily apologising for the incident itself (and therefore seeming to take responsibility).

Bereavement

The Health Service Commissioner has investigated a number of complaints about the inadequate management of events around the death of a patient in hospital. Clearly, there needs to be sensitivity in talking with the family and friends of patients who die in hospital, and dying patients. There are health service guidelines on bereavement that provide advice on this.

Guidance from the Department of Health drew attention to some areas of concern that could lead to complaints if they are not addressed:

- keeping accurate records of how to contact the patients and friends of the patient
- keeping relatives and close friends aware of the treatment and prognosis for the patient
- religious and cultural practices of the patient and family
- wishes of the dying patient
- talking to relatives about organ transplant
- advising and counselling bereaved parents
- arranging funerals for patients who have no close relatives or friends
- handing over the belongings of the dead patient
- telling the family as soon as possible if a coroner's post-mortem examination needs to be conducted.

In mental health services for older people these issues form part of day-to-day work. With the introduction of the Mental Capacity Act 2005 (see Chapter 14) and advanced directives incorporated into a legal framework, it will be important for staff to be well trained in these issues, to pre-empt possible complaints.

Patients who have difficulty feeding or swallowing may suffer distress and their relatives may become equally distressed. A process for managing difficult situations such as these needs to be incorporated into a policy and training programme. A particularly sensitive issue is in coming to decisions about the extent of resuscitation attempts, and it is easy for relatives to misunderstand what the clinician is explaining, perhaps confusing the need to share decision-making with the patient and relatives with suggestions of euthanasia. Understandably, relatives can become very upset and it is not uncommon for them to be unable to express their concerns other than through a complaint.

For other mental health services, sadly, it is often in the context of suicide that bereaved relatives are met. The distress of any bereavement is compounded by the nature of the death, and relatives may deal with their feelings by blaming staff. At the same time, staff will be facing an internal investigation, and it is not surprising that staff find it extremely difficult to talk openly and empathically when they are facing a range of distressing feelings themselves.

How to achieve resolution

Local resolution

The purpose of local resolution is to provide an opportunity for the complainant and the organisation, or individual, subject to the complaint to attempt a quick resolution of the problem. The process has to be open and flexible if it is to work effectively.

Staff need to be conciliatory but sometimes they confuse a conciliatory approach with simply appeasing someone. Conciliation involves much more than appeasement (which is ultimately patronising and ineffective). It involves the staff trying actively to see the situation from the other person's point of view. In training sessions staff often feel that this is easy to achieve when in fact they merely imagine how they themselves would react (or would like to react) in the situation. Perhaps the complainant is experiencing fear and remembering past incidents where they felt they were treated unjustly.

Without an active attempt to understand why the other person feels so strongly about the event, it is difficult to respond well. A complaint that on the surface is about something practical – say, having access to a cup of tea on an in-patient ward when the person wants it – may in fact be a patient's expression of feeling completely out of control of life. This feeling may be even more extreme if the practical issue concerns something of personal import. Access to hair and skin products appropriate to particular ethnic groups or dietary needs and preferences commonly form the focus for concerns. In a responsive ward environment, the patients' forum should have already identified and dealt with these concerns, but if the staff are not aware of the deficit, they need to rely on early resolution of complaints as a way of maintaining high-quality services.

Front-line staff have an important role in dealing with local resolution issues – they are often the first point of contact for the complainant and may have support from a PALS or patient advocate to resolve the issue without recourse to the complaints manager. The complaints manager may nevertheless have a useful role in picking up complaints where local resolution is still possible. Complainants can seek support from the ICAS or another agency offering advice, advocacy and information regarding their case.

In cases where the issue looks serious or complex, the complaints manager can intervene to coordinate, in conjunction with appropriate staff, the resolution of the issue. Where this is not successful, the process follows the formal route and an investigating manager is appointed who works with the complaints manager. Even at this point, complaints are commonly resolved when the underlying issue is understood. However, the resolution at this stage will need to be followed up in writing by the chief executive, as there is a statutory obligation to respond to all written complaints, and all oral complaints that are subsequently put into writing and signed by the complainant.

Resolving formal complaints

Once a complaint has been logged as formal, its progress is tracked through the system and tight deadlines need to be built in. However, opportunities for resolution will still arise. Ultimately, the chief executive will write to the complainant with the findings of the complaints investigation and a summary of what will be done in response. This may well include an apology for things which went wrong. Part of the process leading to resolution may be an offer for the complainant to meet with the clinicians involved in the incident. These can be difficult meetings, but often the complaints manager or someone with experience of these meetings (such as a clinical or medical director) will be there as well to help to provide structure. It is helpful in these meetings to summarise the outstanding issues and suggest an agenda for the meeting, ideally with a desired outcome clarified at the outset. Often clinicians are surprised at how limited and reasonable a complainant's desired outcome is.

Learning from incidents

As has been alluded to above, complaints processes are part of what makes a trust a 'learning organisation'. To formalise the learning process, trusts are expected to state explicitly what they have learned, to set objectives for remedying any fault and to use clinical audit to ensure that the lessons are embedded in the service. Complaints often fall into themes that can be considered together and so lessons learned are general and do not usually link back to a single identifiable complaint (although there may be exceptions). Recommendations from complaints and adverse incidents should be 'SMART', that is specific, measurable, achievable, realistic and time-linked. Expressing recommendations using this formula makes them much easier to monitor.

Root cause analysis

Increasingly, the methods of root cause analysis (RCA) are being applied to complaints investigations. These principles, drawn from accident investigation in industry and as applied to adverse incidents, help the investigator to be systematic and look for underlying causes of particular types. The principles are simple and include a systems approach to problem-solving.

Initially, a clear description of 'what', 'when' and 'with whom' is given in the fact-finding stage. Where appropriate, a time line is constructed to help to make sense of complex cases. Then an analysis focusing on root causes is undertaken. A suggested list of factors to account for in the analysis, taken from a toolkit prepared by the National Patient Safety Agency (NPSA; see http://www.npsa.nhs.uk), is given below:

- patient factors
- individual factors
- task factors
- communication factors
- team and social factors
- education and training factors
- equipment and resource factors
- working condition factors
- organisational and management factors.

Dealing with difficult complainants

Complainants may be considered 'difficult' for several reasons: some raise multiple issues, apparently with no clear focus; others come back repeatedly to the same issue even when the whole process has been carried out exhaustively. The Department of Health gives guidance on some of the characteristics of habitual or vexatious complainants. They may:

- complain about every part of the health system regardless of the issue
- seek attention by contacting several agencies and individuals
- always repeat the full complaint even if part has already been ostensibly resolved
- automatically respond to any letter from the trust
- insist that they have not received an adequate response
- focus on a trivial matter
- be abusive or aggressive in their manner.

Although many people managing complaints will recognise this or similar patterns, it is important to try to understand the underlying reason for the persistence and forcefulness of the complainant. However difficult, it is essential that every complaint is given attention, as there have been examples of patients who habitually complain being targeted by people who perpetrate abuse, as they know that 'no one will listen'.

Nevertheless, it can be a difficult task to be rung frequently and abusively, and in some situations trusts have to call a halt to the process, not least to protect their own staff. This is a last resort, and should be seen as applying to as narrow a range as possible. For example, a complainant may say that a particular doctor treated him or her badly, and after full investigation and appeal to the Healthcare Commission the person may repeatedly raise the issue. That complaint may be closed, but it is important that this does not generalise beyond the specific instance so that the complainant cannot raise new issues, for example about food being poor on the ward.

Rarely, the complainant may show similarity to some vexatious litigants, where the preoccupation with their grievance has become all-consuming, and may be a manifestation of illness. Even in these circumstances, it is crucial that the complaints are managed effectively and courteously, as the next stage of the complaints process (referral to the Healthcare Commission) will require the trust to undertake further work if the complainant has not received civil and efficient responses.

Practical steps with vexatious or unreasonably persistent complainants

The Department of Health suggests that the following steps are taken:

'Policy outline - vexatious or unreasonably persistent complainants:
- regardless of the manner in which the complaint is made and pursued, its substance should be considered carefully and on its objective merits
- complaints about matters unrelated to previous complaints should be similarly approached objectively and without any assumption that they are bound to be frivolous, vexatious, or unjustified
- particularly if a complainant is abusive or threatening, it is reasonable to require him or her to communicate only in a particular way - say, in writing and not by telephone - or solely with one or more designated members of staff; but it is not reasonable to refuse to accept or respond to communications about a complaint until it is clear that all practical possibilities of resolution have been exhausted.
- it is good practice to make clear to a complainant regarded as unreasonably persistent or vexatious the ways in which his or her behaviour is unacceptable, and the likely consequences of refusal to amend it, before taking drastic action
- decisions to treat a complainant as unreasonably persistent or vexatious should be taken at an appropriately senior level; and senior management – probably the board or a committee of the board – should monitor such decisions' (http://www.dh.gov.uk/en/Publicationsandstatistics/Publications/Publications PolicyAndGuidance/Browsable/DH_5133265).

Confidentiality

Confidentiality is a crucial part of handling complaints. Complaints managers are usually aware of the need for confidentiality and will work within nationally agreed systems, and refer specific issues to the trust's Caldicott guardian and/or data protection officer when necessary. There are some tricky situations where advice may be needed: the police may be investigating a possible crime, a local politician may make enquiries to chase up a complaint investigation, or there may be matters related to a family court, for example. In all of these situations it is wise to seek assistance, as there are recognised systems to deal with these.

Under the Data Protection Act 1998, all patients have a right of access to their clinical records, unless the contents of those records were to pose a serious threat to their mental stability. Complaints about any aspect of an application to obtain access to health records can be made under the NHS complaints procedure.

Complaints records should be kept separate from health records, subject to the need to record information which is strictly relevant to the patient's health. Such records must be treated with the same degree of confidentiality as normal medical records and would be open to disclosure in legal proceedings.

The Data Protection Act (1998) controls the release and sharing of information about individuals. These procedures apply during the complaints process, but without the consent of the complainant to access information many investigations are very difficult to carry out. Some guidance is given on the sharing of information in the Guidance to Support Implementation of the NHS (Complaints) Regulations (2004).

The Data Protection Act and the Medical Records Act control the release and sharing of information about individuals during the complaints process. When a complaint is made, it is necessary to share patient information with those involved in the investigation.

Acknowledgement

The authors thank Helen Hobday, Corporate Services Manager and complaints lead manager at Manchester Mental Health and Social Care Trust, for her invaluable advice on this chapter.

References

Department of Health (1995) *Citizens' Charter Complaints Task Force: Good Practice Guide*. TSO (The Stationery Office).

Department of Health (2000a) *The NHS Plan. A Plan for Investment. A Plan for Reform*. The Stationery Office.

Department of Health (2000b) *An Organisation with a Memory*. TSO (The Stationery Office).

Department of Health (2001a) *NHS Complaints Procedure: National Evaluation*. Department of Health.

Department of Health (2001b) *Reforming the NHS Complaints Procedure – A Listening Document*. Department of Health.

Department of Health (2003) *NHS Complaints Reform, Making Things Right*. Department of Health.

Donaldson, L. (2003) *Making Amends: A Consultation Paper Setting Out Proposals for Reforming the Approach to Clinical Negligence in the NHS. A Report by the Chief Medical Officer*. Department of Health.

Health Service Ombudsman (2005) *Making Things Better? A Report on Reform of the NHS Complaints Procedure in England* (HC413). The Stationery Office.

Healthcare Commission (2004) *Reforming the NHS Complaints Procedure*. Healthcare Commission.

237

CHAPTER 20

Revalidation, relicensing and continuing professional development

Sheila Mann

Over the past two or three decades, the public has become painfully aware of the sometimes inadequate supervision of doctors' practice. A number of authorities are involved in supervising that practice: the medical schools and similar bodies are responsible for training and checking that doctors have reached the required standard before graduating in medicine; the medical Royal Colleges and equivalent institutions are broadly responsible for setting the standards required for basic specialty and general practice training; and the Postgraduate Medical Education and Training Board has overall responsibility for assessing whether an individual's higher training is acceptable for practice in the UK, wherever training was acquired.

The General Medical Council (GMC) has the duty of regulating medical practice in the UK, including initial undergraduate training, and also of assessing the training and performance of all doctors seeking registration. It sets standards, keeps the Medical Register, and controls the right to practise of those who fall short of expected standards for whatever reason. Few were aware that, providing a doctor paid the annual subscription, kept the Council informed of any change of address and did not fall foul of the Fitness to Practise procedures, there was no overview of an individual doctor's practice. The general public assumed that there would be regular checks, as indeed there are in some countries, for example the USA. Unsurprisingly, the public (in other words patients) demands that this should change.

Revalidation

Over the past 30 years or so, there has been increasing concern about doctors whose practice is not up to the required standard, whatever the cause. Problems caused by the doctor's ill health – often psychiatric illness viewed as stigmatising and little understood by many non-psychiatrists – were considered by the Merrison Committee. As a result the Health Procedures were introduced in 1980. These made it possible for doctors with health problems for which they were not seeking and accepting medical advice, and which could impair their fitness to practise, to be assessed and, if necessary, for restriction on their practice to be put in place.

For most of its life, the GMC appeared to carry out the process of regulating individual medical practitioners by 'exception reporting' – in other words, expecting that those doctors who failed to reach the expected standard would be referred for investigation of their practice. This system relied on reports from colleagues and others acquainted with the individual's practice. It is perhaps not surprising that, all too often, colleagues ignored indications that a doctor's practice gave cause for concern and were extremely reluctant to refer to the GMC – which was seen as an organisation to be avoided at all costs except for maintaining registration. Referrals were very often for 'professional' matters, such as canvassing for patients, advertising, giving false medical certificates and improper relationships with patients – not because of doubt about fitness to practise.

There remained major concerns about those doctors whose practice appeared unsatisfactory but who could not be dealt with under the Health Procedures because there was no identified health problem. A number of 'medical scandals' where doctors continued to practise – with harm to patients – even though their deficiencies and poor practice were known to colleagues and managers – caused further major concerns. The Performance Procedures of the GMC were introduced in 1997 but dealt with only a small number of doctors, many of whom had major deficiencies. There remained dissatisfaction that doctors could still work while their practice was unsafe without any of the then current procedures being involved.

The Merrison Committee's report (Committee of Inquiry into the Regulation of the Medical Profession, 1975) mentioned 'relicensure' but did not recommend it at that time and it was not included in the Medical Act 1978. Pressure grew for a system that would identify poor or deficient performance before major problems had become evident.

In 1998 the GMC suggested proposals for 'revalidation' – similar in principle to the relicensing discussed by the Merrison Committee. The plan was that revalidation would be based on a 'revalidation folder' containing a broad range of information on the doctor's practice, including:

- evidence of satisfactory continuing professional development (CPD)
- compliments
- complaints and the outcomes of investigation
- audit results
- comments from clinical governance visits.

Since 2003, doctors have been under a professional obligation to keep such a folder of information drawn from their medical practice and showing that they are practising in accord with the standards of competence, care and conduct set out in *Good Medical Practice* (General Medical Council, 1995, 2007).

At about the same time as the GMC was proposing to introduce revalidation, the four UK health departments introduced annual appraisal for doctors.

Appraisal

Appraisal can, and does, mean different things to different groups. Educational theorists believe it to be a formative process between an appraiser and an appraisee intended to identify educational and developmental needs which could result in an improvement in performance of the appraisee. In this form of appraisal, appraisees would be encouraged to and should be able to discuss their deficiencies. Another view of appraisal is that it is effectively a performance review which should concentrate on whether the needs of an organisation are being met rather than the personal objectives of the appraisee.

Although appraisal delivered by employers such as the National Health Service (NHS) was originally intended as a formative process, it did not always seem to be so.

The GMC proposed introducing a 'licence to practise' without which a doctor would be unable to practise. Doctors who did not wish to have a licence to practise but who wanted to remain on the Medical Register would be able to do so, but without the associated privileges (such as prescribing).

A crucial part of the original GMC plan was that there would be a 'revalidation folder' which would be reviewed at an annual appraisal and that at intervals – probably every 5 years – the doctor would appear before a revalidation panel. This view appeared to gain considerable acceptance and, for example, the Royal College of Psychiatrists talked about creating a structured folder with clear indications as to what doctors were required to collect for their appraisal/revalidation. The revalidation panel would comprise a majority of doctors but at least one lay member and would include a colleague in a similar field but not in the same organisation as the doctor undergoing revalidation. If the panel was satisfied, the doctor would be 'revalidated' for another 5 years and given a licence to practise. If the panel was not satisfied with the evidence of the doctor's practice, then it could refer the doctor to the GMC to undergo consideration as to whether it was necessary to involve the Fitness to Practise procedures, to issue a licence with conditions, or, indeed, to suspend the doctor. Even with this proposed detailed mechanism, it was accepted that incompetent doctors might not be picked up at a very early stage.

The revalidation/relicensing process as set out initially inevitably attracted much comment and not a little criticism, especially concerning the cost in terms of the financial implications and the medical time involved. The GMC then considered whether revalidation might be based on the evidence of satisfactory workplace appraisals (which were being put in place) and suggested this. However, the appraisal system was not intended for this purpose and there were substantial concerns that it might not be fit for purpose, in other words, to identify a doctor's unsatisfactory practice.

The chairman of the Harold Shipman Inquiry (Smith, 2004) appeared unconvinced that the then current proposals would meet the necessary requirements. The Secretary of State for Health asked the Chief Medical Officer for England to undertake a review and report to him on further measures which are necessary to:

- strengthen procedures for assuring the safety of patients in situations where a doctor's performance or conduct poses a risk to patient safety or the effective functioning of services;
- ensure the operation of an effective system of revalidation;
- modify the role, structure and functions of the General Medical Council.

The Chief Medical Officer published his proposals in 2006 in 'Good Doctors, Safer Patients' (Department of Health, 2006), and definite proposals have been put forward in a White Paper Trust, Assurance and Safety – The Regulation of Health Professionals in the 21st Century (Secretary of State for Health, 2007). These are now being widely considered by all involved with or concerned about, present arrangements.

While this makes it difficult to be precise about what the procedure of revalidation will entail and how organisations and doctors should prepare, it is worth pointing out that healthcare regulation as a whole has become an important concern, and regulation of the various health professions is being revised and improved. The same is true of social services provision. The GMC would emphasise that it is necessary to make regulation more meaningful, in other words, not to have a situation where a doctor obtains full registration and then this is never questioned unless there is a major concern leading to referral to the Council or other interested body.

Nevertheless, there is no doubt that some form of revalidation will be agreed. There are clear indications to some of the information that is likely to be needed from doctors who are wishing to retain a licence to practise.

Doctors work in a wide variety of environments with greater or lesser degrees of contact with colleagues, availability of advice and supervision. The GMC has suggested that working environments should be considered either 'approved' or 'not approved' and that this should be a key to the revalidation progress. It has suggested that approved working environments would:

- have an effective system of clinical governance or equivalent systems if outside the NHS
- have an effective annual appraisal system based on Good Medical Practice
- be independently regulated or quality assured
- have effective complaints handling procedures which meet relevant external standards.

Such approved working environments would include organisations both within and without the NHS. For doctors working primarily in GMC approved working environments, it was suggested that evidence of suitability for revalidation would come from confirmation of their participation in appraisal, and certification from an appropriate named person within the doctor's employing or contracting authority that there were no significant unresolved concerns about their fitness to practise. It is anticipated that this would simplify the process of revalidation for many doctors.

There is at present no agreed process but a considerable amount of work has been done, including the setting up of a UK revalidation steering group. It appears possible that a process will first be established in primary care.

Good medical practice and revalidation

It seems likely that relicensure will be required for all practising doctors. A licence will probably include satisfactory appraisal. This will probably be based on a revised system of NHS appraisal based on generic standards of practice by the GMC and any known concerns will be valid for 5 years. All doctors will have to participate in 360° appraisal.

For those on the specialist or GP register of specialists, recertification will be necessary to practise, and this will, in addition to a licence to practise, require the doctor to have reached specific, relevant standards set up by the appropriate medical Royal College or specialist body. The White Paper suggests that to demonstrate that they have met the standards, doctors may draw evidence from a range of sources and activities, including employer appraisal, clinical audit, simulator tests, patients' feedback, CPD or observation of practice. Information from these processes would be passed to the GMC, which would, if revalidation was successful, issue or renew the licence to practise, including (if appropriate) specialist or GP registration.

For doctors within the NHS, it will be necessary to undergo a formal appraisal looking at practice in the light of GMC standards (General Medical Council, 2007). These standards include the duties of a doctor registered with the GMC. First, patients must be able to trust doctors with their lives and well-being. Second, to justify that trust, doctors have a duty to maintain a good standard of practice and care and to show respect for human life. In particular doctors must:

- make the care of the patient their first concern
- treat every patient politely and considerately
- respect the patient's dignity and privacy
- listen to patients and respect their views
- give patients information in a way they can understand
- respect the rights of patients to be fully involved in decisions about their care
- keep their professional knowledge and skills up to date

- recognise the limits of their professional confidence
- be honest and trustworthy
- respect and protect confidential information
- make sure that their personal beliefs do not prejudice their patient's care
- act quickly to protect patients from risk if they have good reason to believe that they or a colleague may not be fit to practise
- avoid abusing their position as a doctor
- work with colleagues in the ways that best serve patients' interests
- never discriminate unfairly against their patients or colleagues
- always be prepared to justify their actions to patients or colleagues.

Good clinical care

The GMC identifies good clinical care as including:

- adequate assessment of a patient's condition, based on history and clinical signs, and, where appropriate, examination
- providing or arranging investigations or treatment where necessary
- taking suitable and prompt action when necessary
- referring the patient to another practitioner when indicated
- recognising and working within the limits of professional competence
- being willing to consult colleagues
- being competent when making diagnoses and when giving or arranging treatment
- keeping clear, accurate and contemporaneous patient records which report the clinical findings, decisions made, information given to the patient and any drugs or other treatment prescribed
- keeping colleagues well informed when sharing the care of patients
- paying due regard to the efficacy and the use of resources
- prescribing only the treatment, drugs or appliances to serve the patients' needs
- in an emergency offering anyone at risk the treatment that a doctor could reasonably be expected to provide.

Maintaining good practice

A workplace appraisal should identify whether the doctor achieves a satisfactory standard. This is best fulfilled by ensuring that the individual is aware of and meets the standards set for their specialty. The Royal College of Psychiatrists has issued a series of booklets to aid those in the profession, commencing with *Good Psychiatric Practice* in 2000 (updated in 2004). It would involve maintaining CPD, for which the College has an exemplary framework. This is aimed at continuing an individual's lifelong learning.

The College recommends that participants in CPD should form a peer group, normally of three to six psychiatrists, who should meet at least twice a year and who can review and validate the other members' CPD plans. To do this, each will require a job plan, and be able to identify objectives which are realistic and appropriate to the particular participant. This in many ways relates closely to the educationalist's vision of appraisals. One of the duties of the peer group is to identify an individual's needs which he or she may not be aware of, and to enable the group to assess the success remedying these.

A satisfactory appraisal includes the production of a CPD plan. In addition, there will need to be information and accurate figures concerning the doctor's practice and, if possible, outcome figures. At the time of writing, employer organisations (including many trusts) have very disparate levels of accuracy in the statistics they collect. When such figures are suspect, it is essential that managers endeavour, as soon as possible, to change this. Revalidation/relicensing is almost certain to require hard, accurate evidence.

Teaching and training

It seems likely that there will be a need for evidence of the teaching commitments of individual doctors, for example with evidence of educational supervision being carried out. It is possible that other evidence, such as feedback forms from lectures, training sessions and so forth, will be included.

Relationships with patients

There has been considerable discussion about the validity of patient surveys, especially with regard to their accuracy in reflecting the doctor's practice. It seems almost certain that the GMC will expect that patient questionnaires are used wherever possible to obtain direct feedback.

Working with colleagues

The GMC recommends that there should be information from colleague questionnaires. The Royal College of Psychiatrists has been working on 360° appraisal for colleagues. This is now available for use in some psychiatric specialties and has been very successful.

Probity

Probity is likely to be ensured though a signed statement. However, for doctors working in an approved environment it is likely that some questions may have been raised if probity is in question.

Health

Again, it seems likely that the GMC will accept a statement that the doctor is suffering from no health problems likely to affect care of the patients.

Registration and revalidation

The GMC has revised the ways in which it assesses, formally, doctors' practice. This includes revalidation, which would be dealt with by the Registration Section of the General Medical Council. Before the reforms, the Registration Committee, comprised of members of the Council, would make decisions on all aspects of registration, including those which would relate to relicensing and revalidation. However, the GMC has now split its functions so that Council members take no part in assessing a doctor's fitness to practise, whether it be through Fitness To Practise procedures or because of issues over registration.

The Council has appointed associates, who are selected through widespread advertisement and on the basis of their attributes and ability to make appropriate independent decisions, by the NHS Appointments Committee. Members of this pool of Associates are likely to sit on registration panels to assess whether there is need to restrict registration of doctors passing through the revalidation process as well as other registration processes.

Registration decision panels, as the name implies, adjudicate in cases where there is a question of the doctor's appropriate registration status. This can be in either a *meeting*, where the parties are not present and which is not in public, or in certain circumstances a *hearing*, which is in public, unless a case is made for it to be in private, and the doctor can be represented legally.

Registration appeals panels provide an appeal mechanism for a doctor who disputes the decision on registration; they are held in private unless the doctor asks for it to be in public.

The actual procedures are set out in detail on the GMC website (http://www.gmc-uk.org). It is suggested that medical managers should acquaint themselves with this website, which gives a broad and detailed insight into medical registration in the UK and which includes information on possible changes, often with a request for comment. The GMC has produced a considerable number of documents over the past few years on licensing and revalidation. These can all be found on the GMC's website – of particular interest are the draft document *Licensing and Revalidation: Formal Guidance for Doctors* (General Medical Council, 2004) and *Developing Medical Regulation: A Vision for the Future* (General Medical Council, 2005), which is the response of the Council to the call for ideas by the Chief Medical Officer in England. However, relicensure and revalidation are still the subjects of further discussion; the final agreement may be very different to the present expectations.

Acknowledgements

The views expressed in this chapter are the responsibility of the author.

I am most grateful to my Secretary, Pauline Gardner, and to colleagues at the GMC for their assistance.

References

Committee of Inquiry into the Regulation of the Medical Profession (1975) *Report of the Committee of Inquiry into the Regulation of the Medical Profession* (The Merrison Committee report) (Cmnd 6018). The Stationery Office.

Department of Health (2006) *Good Doctors, Safer Patients. Proposals to Strengthen the System to Assure and Improve the Performance of Doctors and to Protect the Safety of Patients*. Department of Health.

General Medical Council (1995) *Good Medical Practice*. GMC.

General Medical Council (2004) *Licensing and Revalidation: Formal Guidance for Doctors (Draft)*. GMC. http://www.gmc-uk.org/doctors/licensing/archive/l_and_r_formal_guidance_for_docs.pdf

General Medical Council (2005) *Developing Medical Regulation: A Vision for the Future* (GMC). http://www.gmc-uk.org/doctors/licensing/archive/developing_medical_regulation_200504.pdf

General Medical Council (2007) *Good Medical Practice*. GMC.

Royal College of Psychiatrists (2000) *Good Psychiatric Practice 2000* (Council Report CR83). Royal College of Psychiatrists.

Royal College of Psychiatrists (2004) *Good Psychiatric Practice* (2nd edn) (Council Report CR125). Royal College of Psychiatrists.

Secretary of State for Health (2007) *Trust, Assurance and Safety – The Regulation of Health Professionals in the 21st Century* (Cm 7013). The Stationery Office.

Smith, J. (2004) *The Shipman Inquiry. Fifth Report: Lessons from the Past – Proposals for the Future* (Cmnd 6394). The Stationery Office.

CHAPTER 21

Confidentiality and management in healthcare organisations

Gwen Adshead and Roy McClelland

Leadership in organisations involves the management of boundaries between different people in different types of relationship. Many of the ethical dilemmas about confidentiality that arise for managers involve tensions between two different kinds of professional space (e.g. should what I learn in this space be told in another?) or tensions between conflicting professional obligations. In this chapter, we review some of these dilemmas and suggest ways of thinking about them.

Confidentiality: ethics

The principle of confidentiality has a lengthy history in medical practice. Respect for this principle is usually grounded in terms of the beneficial consequences of doing so. Keeping patient information confidential benefits the patient by promoting trust between doctor and patient, which is in the patient's interest because it promotes the type of frank discussion that is essential to any therapeutic encounter. If the patient does not feel able to trust the doctor with information, this may mean that the doctor's clinical opinion is compromised in a way that may do harm to the patient.

However, respect for confidentiality is grounded in something of arguably more meaning than just the good consequences. For most of us, when we give away personal information, we are giving away something of ourselves. Theoretically, we make ourselves vulnerable when we give away our secrets to a doctor, especially in psychiatry, when we may be disclosing information that is shameful or traumatic. So the principle of confidentiality is as much about protection of the vulnerable as it is about the consequences of keeping confidences. The tradition of confidentiality probably arose in order to stop doctors gossiping as much as to promote clinical dialogue.

The idea that patients entrust doctors with something precious when they disclose information about themselves finds support from the requirement that we get consent from patients before we share their information with others; that is, it is not ours to do with as we please. Getting consent for disclosure is an act of respect for the autonomy of the patient, without which we do the patient a wrong, not just a harm. In fact, it would be better to conceptualise the whole discussion of confidentiality as really being about the process of getting consent (and refusal) to disclose information.

It makes sense that vulnerability is a key issue in confidentiality, because preventing harm to the vulnerable is the commonest justification for disclosing clinical information. The most obvious examples relate to the requirements of the Children Act 1989, under which doctors are expected to disclose clinical information about their patients in the interests of children, as a matter of good practice. It is children's vulnerability to exploitation that justifies the breaching of the principle of confidentiality.

Confidentiality: law and policy

The common law in England assumes a duty of confidence held by doctors to their patients. Most of the legal advice on confidentiality is based on cases that make up this common law duty and not on specific statutes. Breach of medical confidence is both a legal wrong in its own right and may be evidence of clinical negligence.

The Human Rights Act 1998 allows individuals to pursue in UK courts claims under the European Convention on Human Rights for established torts, such as breach of confidence, or to bring an action against a public authority on the basis of the Convention's right to privacy under article 8. The Human Rights Act also underpins other legislation concerned with confidentiality. For example, public authorities are required to construe the legislation under which they operate in accordance with the Convention and to ensure that their actions and those of their staff are consistent with it.

The Data Protection Act 1998 gives effect in UK law to European Community Directive 95/46/EC and introduces eight data protection principles that set out standards of information processing or handling. The term 'processing' includes the collection, use and disclosure of personal data. The 1998 Act is now a central plank in the statutory framework underpinning confidentiality in clinical information management.

The first data protection principle states that:

personal data shall be processed fairly, lawfully and shall not be processed unless at least one of the conditions in Schedule 2 is met and in the case of sensitive personal data at least one of the conditions in Schedule 3 is also met.

Schedule 2 requires that processing (use) is necessary for the exercise of functions of a public nature and in the public interest by any person. Schedule 3 requires that processing is with the consent of the data subject, or that:

the processing is necessary for medical purposes and is undertaken by a health professional (or a person owing a duty of confidentiality equivalent to that owed by a health professional).

The term 'medical purposes' includes preventive medicine, medical diagnosis, medical research, the provision of care and treatment, and the management of healthcare services.

If processing takes place without consent, 'data controllers' (doctors frequently) must be able to show that it will not be possible to achieve their purposes with a reasonable degree of ease without the processing of 'personal' data. The Data Commissioner takes the view that when considering the issue of necessity, data controllers must consider objectively whether such purposes can be achieved only by the processing of personal data and the processing is proportional to the aim pursued.

There is an obligation on doctors who are data controllers to provide certain information to data subjects when collecting their personal data. This information is often referred to as 'fair processing information'. We should ensure that our patients are told the purpose or purposes for which their clinical information is typically used. For example, patients are likely to expect that basic information will be recorded as to the diagnosis and treatment. They may, however, by surprised to find that other information has been recorded, such as the circumstances in which an injury was acquired.

Patients require information as to specific disclosures. Given the sensitivity of medical information, patients should be informed of any non-routine disclosures of their information. Patients must be given information as to whether any secondary uses or disclosures are optional. Where patients have a choice, this should be brought to their attention. The Commissioner points out that patients who will have their personal data processed for additional purposes will need to be provided with this further information in order to satisfy 'the fair processing' requirements.

While the Data Protection Act does not provide any guidance on the meaning of the term 'lawful', the principle means that the data controller must comply with all relevant rules of law, whether derived from statute or common law. Indeed, it is the Commissioner's assumption that the processing of health data by a health professional is subject to a duty of confidence even though explicit consent for processing is not a requirement of Schedules 2 and 3 – based essentially on case law.

Conflicts of interest

The key message from the foregoing is that data protection legislation assumes that patients own their information and, generally speaking, have a claim to control it. All trusts must have data protection policies and staff to manage those policies. As there is a potential conflict between the need to use patient information for good clinical care and patients' expectations that their information will not be shared with others, each trust is expected to have an official whose task it is to monitor good practice.

Other sources of conflict in relation to patient information are the extent of its use for the public good and the limitations of consent. There has been considerable debate about the extent to which personal patient information can be used without consent for research and audit purposes, with the current emphasis being on patient consent and privacy trumping the public interest. Section 60 of the Health and Social Care Act 2001 creates a power for the Secretary of State to make orders requiring the disclosure of patient data that would otherwise be prevented by a duty of confidence. This is intended essentially as a temporary measure until anonymisation measures or appropriate recording of consent can be put in place for some secondary uses. A major stimulus is the requirements of registries, particularly cancer registries. An independent statutory Patient Information Advisory Group oversees all applications for exemptions from the duty of confidence to use identifiable patient information.

The first regulations to be made under section 60 of the 2001 Act were the Health Service (Control of Patient Information) Regulations 2002, which support the use of identifiable patient information without consent in respect of communicable diseases and other risks to the public. In contrast to the privilege approach taken with ordinary patient information, in cases where there is a presumed risk to the public, the policy of the National Health Service (NHS) appears to suggest that healthcare professionals should disclose information in the public good. We turn now to discuss disclosure of patient information in more detail.

Disclosure

The default position is that no patient information can be disclosed to third parties without the patient's express consent. The Data Protection Act sets out in a general way how patients should be informed that their information is being disclosed and in what circumstances. Essentially, if patients are asked for their consent to disclose and they agree, there can be no breach of confidentiality.

The key issue, then, is in what circumstances can doctors disclose patient information to third parties, either in the absence of consent (i.e. without consulting the patient) or in the face of the patient's refusal to allow disclosure.

Absence of consent

Doctors are required to disclose patient information under the terms of some specific legislation, for example that pertaining to notifiable diseases and road accidents. The ethical argument here is that disclosure of this information will help to prevent harm to the community. In these circumstances, consent is irrelevant: the patient may be informed that the information is being given (although this is not required, the Data Protection Act makes it good practice) but is not given the choice. The breach of confidentiality is justified with reference to the public good.

The Children Act 1989 and the Crime and Disorder Act 1998 allow doctors to disclose under appropriate circumstances but do not require them to do so; that is, they provide justification rather than obligation.

Doctors may also be required by a court to disclose information about patients. Again, this breach of patient autonomy is justified by the public interest in ensuring that the justice process is fair.

Refusal of consent

A more complex issue arises when the doctor perceives the patient to present a risk to others because of his or her condition and asks consent to disclose this to appropriate third parties. If the patient consents, then there is no breach of confidence and all is well. More commonly, however, the doctor may find that the patient refuses to consent to the disclosure. The commonest examples are individuals with sexually transmitted diseases, who may be putting current sexual partners at risk but refuse to allow the doctor to share the information with anyone. Box 21.1 presents an example.

When this issue came before the General Medical Council (GMC) (especially when HIV was first identified as a cause of AIDS), it advised that doctors could breach confidentiality in these circumstances, as the prevention of harm to unsuspecting others justified the breach of patient confidentiality. Although overriding a competent patient's consent or refusal is a major insult to autonomy, the GMC (1997) clearly takes the view that the prevention of harm to others justified this.

When this advice was given, it was not suggested that it was mandatory for doctors to disclose such information, only that they would not be guilty of

---

Box 21.1 Refusal of consent: a case example

On an in-patient ward, Helen accuses Jim, another patient, of rape; Jim denies it. Jim is HIV-positive. Helen refuses to let staff tell her husband about her rape allegation, which is the subject of a criminal investigation. Jim refuses to let staff tell Helen about his HIV status. This situation persists for a number of weeks. Eventually, Brian, who is a member of staff, decides to tell Helen's husband what is going on, about both the rape allegation and Jim's HIV status. Brian is disciplined under local management procedures. He claims that it was his professional duty to prevent harm to Helen's husband. Helen's husband sues the trust for failing to protect his wife. We do not know the outcome for Jim and Helen.

professional misconduct if they did. Since then, however, preventing patients harming other people has come to be seen as a medical duty, especially in mental health. The issue is sensitive for doctors, first because it makes them into agents of public order, which many do not like, and second, and perhaps more importantly, because they lose their beneficent status with the patient. The patient's interests are no longer the doctor's first concern; in fact, the patient then knows that the doctor thinks that another person's interests are more important than the patient's claim to privacy. Further, disclosure of patient information may have negative 'personal consequences' for the patient (General Medical Council, 2004). By disclosing such information, despite a refusal, the doctor appears to give a message that he or she is not concerned about the consequences for the patient.

Because these issues are sensitive and complex to discuss with patients, many healthcare professionals avoid having the discussion with the patient altogether. Fearing that the patient may refuse consent to disclose, they instead debate disclosure of information in the absence of consent. It seems that many healthcare professionals would rather deceive patients than have a painful discussion with them. Perhaps some doctors are fearful of conflict with patients, which in turn suggests a lack of communication skills. It is also true that doctors (especially psychiatrists) cannot guarantee that significant negative consequences for patients will not arise as a result of disclosure of their personal information.

The ethical dilemma for doctor managers is between conflicting duties: the duty to the patient, the duty to the public interest and the duty they have to the organisation. A healthcare organisation may expect a manager to be committed to the aims of an organisation, and to protect its welfare, so it can continue to provide care. But it may be that protecting the organisation means overriding ethical obligations to patients, and this often takes the form of disclosure of clinical information.

Different types of disclosure

Disclosure to fellow professionals

Health service managers will probably have most to do with policies and procedures relating to the ordinary management of patient information within an organisation, where the main tension is the 'Caldicott' one, of balancing privacy against the need of health services for good quality information (Department of Health, 1997).

There are two main ethical dilemmas faced by managers of mental health services in the context of disclosure to fellow professionals. First, many service users may not fully understand that their information is being used for audit and governance purposes. Second, doctor managers may come across information in their work that they know is relevant to their clinical ethical duties, but they are bound by professional duties to the organisation. The Bristol Royal Infirmary Inquiry (Secretary of State for Health, 2001) criticised a doctor manager who did not disclose and use clinical information that came to his attention, apparently because it could have caused managerial difficulties for him (*Roylance v The General Medical Council*, 1998). The GMC (2006) appears to take the view that the medical ethical role trumps other ethical duties; the doctor cannot serve two masters equally.

Doctor managers may also come across the problem that different professionals may have different understandings of their ethical duties and different perspectives about what counts ethically. The best example arises in child health services, where social workers have a mandatory duty to disclose information that may prevent harm to children, whereas doctors have an interpretable duty of 'good practice' in disclosure. The manager may have to listen to both arguments and be able to understand both perspectives as meaningful. In addition, doctor managers may be uncomfortably aware that they are expected to take decisions that make their employing trust look good and to do nothing that would make the trust look 'bad'. Indeed, trusts expect their doctor managers to put the interests of the trust first, in direct contradiction of the GMC's advice. A kind of solution is to have agreed protocols between all relevant professionals working in multidisciplinary teams to cover different situations.

Disclosure to carers

A significant feature of most accounts of bioethics is that they assume a two-person relationship, namely between the patient and the doctor. Further, these accounts assume that the patient is fully autonomous and capable of acting so within a medical relationship. In mental health, these assumptions fall short of the reality of service users' lives. All mental (and many physical) disorders compromise autonomy in various ways and for varying periods of time. Many service users live with the disability of mental illness in ways that mean that they live within a network of dependent relationships, so that the concept of autonomy becomes more complex. Agich (1993), writing about decision-making in old age, has described this as 'interstitial autonomy'; it could also be thought of as 'relational autonomy', where a kind of autonomy emerges from the different relationships around the patient, as in adolescence (Sutton, 1997). However, doctors do have to acknowledge and respect autonomous decisions of patients and therefore will have to decide what constitutes an autonomous decision.

What this means is that relationships between professionals and carers are also more complex, in terms of disclosure of information. Providing information to carers is often a way to provide good care for patients; but it is more than that. Sometimes a person's mental well-being will depend on the well-being of the carer, so that working with carers indirectly provides help for the patient. Alternatively, there are cases where the carers have a negative effect upon the patient, and where disclosure to the carer is not beneficial to the patient, even if there is policy and legal justification for it. Doctor managers may find that the demands of policies and trust procedures do not do justice to the ethical complexities of these relationships.

Disclosure to public bodies: managing risk

A key feature of dilemmas about confidentiality is that they arise at the boundary between different domains in a patient's life and thus different domains for professional action. General practitioners may wonder whether to tell an employer about a patient's drinking habits; a psychiatrist may wonder whether to tell hostel staff that a resident is using cannabis. Clinicians can find themselves sitting on the disclosure 'fence', surveying the various foreseeable possible outcomes and wondering uneasily what outcomes they have *not* foreseen. They may find themselves thinking about their duties (ethical, legal, professional, personal) and becoming uncomfortably aware that they have duties to more than one person or organisation and that these duties conflict. They know, above all, that they will have to come down from the fence and make a decision.

Nowhere is this dilemma more pointed than in relation to disclosure of personal information in order to prevent serious harm to others. Since the early 1990s, there has been a growing perception that people who are mentally ill pose a risk of serious harm to the public, despite evidence to the contrary. Several national policies now exist that commit healthcare professionals to disclosing personal patient information to third parties if they have reason to think this will prevent serious harm to others (Department of Health, 2003; Home Office and National Probation Service, 2003). The question of consent is not even mentioned.

Disclosure of confidential information to third parties (i.e. parties outside the NHS) may be justifiable on the basis of the benefits it brings and the harms averted by disclosure. Where failure to disclose information may expose others to risk of death or serious harm and there is a high probability that disclosure of information would lead to a reduction in that risk, then disclosure is justified. Here, three key decisions need to be made, about whether:

- failure to disclose would result in harm
- that harm is serious
- that serious harm is likely to occur.

The problem is that are all these decisions involve probability and data that can be interpreted different ways. They are decisions about risk, which naturally entails a degree of anxiety on the part of the decision-maker. The more anxious decision-makers are, the more likely they will be to include some forms of information and exclude others; and the information may or may not be relevant.

The disclosure of information about potential risk to others often has highly significant negative consequences for patients (such as deprivation of liberty), so respect for justice means that we need the best possible evidence to justify disclosure. However, decisions about risk are often made by anxious people, who have very particular perspectives on the situation. Risk assessment is not a simple algorithmic process: it is a human process, and because of that, it is likely to be influenced by conscious and unconscious factors, both individual and group.

Managers of teams, or of organisations, will have to contain the anxieties of their teams or groups when dealing with risky situations. Managers in particular hold institutional or group memories, especially if they have been in post for some time; memories of previous disasters may hugely affect risk assessment decisions and therefore decisions about disclosure. A manager in a trust which has not experienced a homicide inquiry may have a different perspective on risk from one who has, so their decisions will be different, with different consequences for the patient.

Managers dealing with decisions about disclosure in relation to risk will find themselves having to deal with policy and procedural advice (including legal precedent) from multiple sources, much of which is likely to conflict. Department of Health policy, the Data Protection Act and the GMC guidance make it clear that patients have to be asked for their consent for disclosure of personal information and need to be advised if their information is being passed on to others, even if there are no personal consequences for the patient. However, if the patient is referred for multi-agency public protection arrangements (MAPPA) (and even this decision obviously involves disclosure), then trusts (and trust employees) are required to cooperate with the MAPPA process (Home Office and National Probation Service, 2003). The MAPPA guidance makes no mention of patient consent or even of patients being informed. There is Department of Health policy that states that NHS employees are permitted to disclose patient information that will assist in the 'detection, prevention and punishment ' of serious crime; again, no mention is made of consent (Department of Health, 2003). Finally, the National Patient Safety Agency has set up a database of patients with histories that suggest they may be a risk to others, which can be accessed by professionals, day or night. Patient information will be entered into this database without consent, based on the perception of clinicians that this is appropriate.

Case law is somewhat clearer. In *W. v. Egdell* [1980], the Court of Appeal found that doctors could disclose clinical information in the public interest if the breach of confidentiality would be justified by the prevention of future harm. In *Palmer v. West Tees HA* [1999] the court found that although the harm was foreseeable (which amounts to risk assessment in the court, with the benefit of hindsight!), there was no duty of care where there was no identifiable victim. The inference here is that it would be a duty of care to an identifiable victim, because then a relationship of proximity would be established. In *T. v. MHRT* [2002], disclosure of patient information was justified on the basis that it *might* relieve an ex-victim's distress.

Overall, the pattern seems to be that patients with a history of both mental disorder and violence can expect little confidential information to be preserved. Information about them can be passed to anyone who might be distressed without it or to whom they are suspected of posing a risk. Information can be passed on to law enforcement bodies without their consent at any time, especially if healthcare professionals perceive there to be a risk of serious harm. There is currently no obligation on professionals to seek their consent, or even their refusal; nor is there any obligation on them to inform such patients that they have done so. There is also no obligation on those professionals to demonstrate that the quality of their information is sufficiently valid to justify this breach of ethics.

Article 8 of the Human Rights Act gives every individual the right to a private life, which includes control over medical information. *Campbell v. MGN Limited* [2004] emphasised the importance of each person having control over their own life, including information about themselves. However, any action under that Act would probably be countered with reference to the right of national law enforcement agencies to use reasonable measures to manage risk to the public. Essentially, each person has the right to control personal information unless someone else sees them as a risk to others, in which case all bets are off.

Decisions to disclose identifiable patient information outside the NHS are matters of judgement – judgements that may be finely balanced. Managers will often be the ones who have the final say in such judgements, which need to take into account the various legal responsibilities at stake, including the duty of confidence to the individual and the public interest in the NHS maintaining confidence. Consideration will need to be given as to whether the harm that could result from disclosure (e.g. the possible damage to the relationship of trust or the likelihood of non-compliance with a programme of healthcare intervention in the future) is likely to be outweighed by the benefit. The potential benefit would need to be soundly grounded on the expectation that disclosure would have the desired effect. All this will go to ensuring that the decision to disclose is a reasonable one.

We should note that many of these situations will require good communication and support to be available for patients whose confidentiality is to be breached. Whether a breach of confidence is justifiable in the public interest will depend to some extent on the scope of disclosure. When deciding whether to disclose, the manager should also consider the extent of the information to disclose and to whom it is appropriate to disclose it. The Royal College of Psychiatrists (2000) advocates disclosing the minimum amount of information to the smallest number of people. We would also recommend that consent be sought from the patient, and that there be an attempt to involve the patient in the risk management process, as a kind of therapeutic joint enterprise.

Ultimately, a court would take careful account of the opinion and guidance of professional organisations as to whether a decision concerning disclosure was one which fell within the reasonable practice of a responsible body of medical practitioners *(Bolam v. Friern Barnett,* 1957). We are, however, facing a moving target and the College's Advisory Group on Confidentiality aims at providing an ongoing source of advice to the College and its members.

Conclusion

Managers in mental health services find themselves on the boundaries between different groups of people. They are always having to manage and negotiate human relationships at work from at least four perspectives: their own, that of their employers, that of those they manage, and the patient's. As in any small group, there are likely to be tensions between different group members and these are often most clearly expressed around ethical dilemmas.

The 'good enough' manager will try to bear all these perspectives in mind and conduct discussions which facilitate the expression of everyone's views. It may not be possible to find a solution that everyone likes, and if that is the case the process of arriving at that conclusion is the 'good enough' part. There is evidence to suggest that decisions that involve many voices, especially dissenting ones, are the best decisions and quality of reasoning is essential for ethical decisions in management (Suworiecki, 2004).

References and further reading

Agich, G. (1993) *Autonomy and Dependency*. Oxford University Press.

Department of Health (1997) *The Caldicott Committee Report on the Review of Patient-Identifiable Information*. Department of Health.

Department of Health (2000) *NHS Trusts and Primary Care Trusts (Sexually Transmitted Diseases) Directions 2000*. Department of Health.

Department of Health (2003) *Confidentiality: A Code of Practice for NHS Staff*. Department of Health.

Fulford, W. K. & Williams, R. (2003) Values-based child and adolescent mental health services? *Current Opinion in Psychiatry,* **16**, 369–376.

General Medical Council (1997) *Guidance on Serious Communicable Disease*. GMC.

General Medical Council (2004) *Confidentiality: Protecting and Providing Information*. GMC.

General Medical Council (2006) *Management for Doctors*. GMC.

Home Office and National Probation Service (2003)*The MAPPA (Multi-Agency Public Protection Arrangements) Guidance* (Probation Circular no. 54/2004). National Probation Directorate.

Information Commissioner (2002) *Use and Disclosure of Health Data: Guidance on the Application of the Data Protection Act 1998*. Information Commissioner.

Royal College of Psychiatrists (2000) *Good Psychiatric Practice: Confidentiality* (CR85). Royal College of Psychiatrists.

Secretary of State for Health (2001) *The Report of the Public Inquiry into children's heart surgery at the Bristol Royal Infirmary 1984–1995: Learning from Bristol* (CM 5207). TSO (The Stationery Office).

Sutton, A. (1997) Authority, autonomy, responsibility and authorisation. *Journal of Medical Ethics*, **23**, 26–31.

Suworiecki, J. (2004) *The Wisdom of Crowds*. Doubleday.

Bolam v. Friern Barnett General Hospital Management Committee [1957] 2 All ER 118.

Campbell v. MGN Limited [2004] UKHL 22.

Palmer v. West Tees HA [1999] Lloyds Rep Med 351.

Roylance v. The General Medical Council [1998] Privy Council Appeal no. 49.

T. v. MHRT [2002] QBD Feb 22.

W. v. Egdell [1990] 1 All ER 835.

CHAPTER 22

Service users' expectations

Diana Rose

It is now a central plank of government policy that the National Health Service (NHS) should be 'patient driven', that there should be a high level of patient and public involvement in health services and that there should be a rapid expansion of choice. This represents a cultural shift and a rebalancing of power relations between patients and doctors. The Department of Health recognises that this is not easy, as doctors may not wish to hand over power to patients (Department of Health & Farrell, 2004).

In this context, there is a crucial dilemma for psychiatrists. This culture shift is supposed to be transferable to all medical disciplines and the mental health user movement has long struggled to bring this about in the psychiatric domain. It has to be said that there have been some successes here. The dilemma is that psychiatrists have the power to take all choice and control away from psychiatric patients, by use of the Mental Health Act 1983. The Bill that was to lead to a new Mental Health Act made the grounds for compulsory treatment wider. Many psychiatrists were opposed to this but it shows that government policy is pulling in two directions at once – more choice and involvement on the one hand and more control and coercion on the other.

In this chapter I look at the mental health user movement, what it has achieved and what it has still to achieve. I then look at research which has tried to determine what users want and do not want in terms of services. Much of this research has been user led.

The user movement

Campbell (1996) shows how there have been protests by psychiatric patients since the days of Bedlam. In the mid-19th century, John Perceval set up the Alleged Lunatics' Friend Society to protest about the conditions in Victorian institutions. In the 1970s there were two small and very radical groups, called the Mental Patients' Union (MPU) and the Campaign Against Psychiatric Oppression (CAPO). Both these groups were influenced by the ideas of R. D. Laing (1959) and Thomas Szasz (1972). They were anti-psychiatry and part of the radical culture of the time.

A more recent phenomenon that led to the rise of more user groups was the closure of the old asylums and the reprovision of care to the community. A dozen user groups grew up across the UK to make sure that reprovision was working properly. These were mixed groups, comprising users, carers and professionals. Later a 'user group' was taken to mean a group wholly made up of users or one where users held the majority in decision-making.

In the 1980s there were national user groups operating in the UK. The best known was Survivors Speak Out, which campaigned for less use of medication, more information, more dignity for service users in hospitals and less stigma in society as a whole. The group drew up a Patients' Charter.

It is often said that the user movement is the child of consumerism – the market economies of Thatcher and Major, who took the view that people should stand on their on two feet and not rely on the 'nanny state'. Certainly the user movement grew exponentially at this time. In 1985 there were around 15 user groups but some 20 years later there were over 700 (Wallcraft *et al*, 2003). The rise of local user groups saw the demise of the national radical ones and a much more practical approach, which we can call 'user involvement'. Where groups have funding, it often comes from statutory bodies and there is an expectation that the group will have some influence on the body. Whether this is real or window dressing is a moot point (Rose *et al*, 2002).

According to Wallcraft *et al* (2003), the commonest activities of user groups are self-help and mutual aid, followed by consultation with planners, policy-makers and mental health professionals. That users commonly consult with planners and policy-makers is a novelty worth commenting on as it is not an easy process. Professionals may want to hear the authentic voice of experience but as soon as it becomes too authentic they pull back and relabel the person as ill. For today's user movement, what users expect from professionals, including psychiatrists, is to be listened to and have their views taken seriously.

Consultation often takes the form of sitting on committees and this can be intimidating for service users. Use of jargon and acronyms makes proceedings incomprehensible and there always is the suspicion that decisions have already been made behind closed doors (or, indeed, in the canteen). Nevertheless, the fact that it has become possible for service users to occupy such high-status positions is a major advance. There is also some involvement at government level, although this is not without its problems.

There are now active groups of patients in many medical specialties, but, as far as I know, the mental health service user movement was the first and remains the most sceptical. This brings us back to the dilemma facing doctors described at the beginning of this chapter. For many service users in the field of mental health, it is lack of power that prevents them having more influence. Power relations between psychiatrists and their patients are the most imbalanced in health services as a whole. From here comes the concept of 'empowerment', meaning that users themselves or in negotiation with their doctors need to take back control over their lives.

Research on what users expect from psychiatry

It is apparent that not all users are part of the movement described above. In fact, they are a small minority. In 2001, two reports were published that aimed to find out what 'ordinary' users want and do not want from services. These two reports came from user-led research teams based in large charities in London. The first was the Strategies for Living (S4L) team based at the Mental Health Foundation (Faulkner & Layzell, 2001). The second was the User-Focused Monitoring (UFM) team based at the Sainsbury Centre for Mental Health (Rose, 2001). Both these projects were user-controlled. Questionnaires or topic guides were devised by a group of users. They then used them to interview their peers. These service users were not experienced researchers. The coordinators of the projects taught them basic research skills, especially questionnaire construction and interviewing skills. These coordinators were also service users but in this case researchers as well. The difference between these two investigations was that S4L was largely qualitative, while UFM was largely quantitative. Below I describe the issues that were most important to 'ordinary' service users.

Information and choice

The single most important finding is that users want more information and choice about a range of issues that affect their lives. One of these is medication, which I discuss below. But users also want information about opportunities for work or leisure in their localities. They want information about welfare benefits, which most are obliged to rely on, partly because of stigmatisation by employers, which prevents them from securing jobs.

When in hospital and detained under the Mental Health Act, they want more information about their rights. The first UFM team conducted site visits to four acute units and observed that there was scant information about the Mental Health Act or the Mental Health Commission on notice boards. Some of those interviewed said they had not, or could not remember having had, information leaflets about their section. Some users did not know whether they were voluntary or not, as practice in the units (e.g. over the right to leave) was applied universally. It did not seem to matter whether restricted leave was via section 17 of the Mental Health Act or not – everybody was subject to restricted leave. This mirrors the findings of the McArthur study, which showed that there was a discrepancy between actual coercion and perceived coercion (Lidz *et al*, 1995).

Medication

Users wanted more information and choice about medication, especially about dosage and side-effects. Those who received their medication from hospital pharmacies were the most frustrated in this respect, as they did not even receive an information sheet. Observation of hospital notice boards during UFM site visits revealed a lack of information leaflets about medication, what it was for, the intended effects and the side-effects. Further, the S4L study found that users were ambivalent about taking medication. Many did take it but with misgivings about whether they really needed it or fear that withdrawal would be difficult. The UFM study found that when a doctor negotiated medication with users, they were happier overall with their mental healthcare. The most important aspects of this negotiation that were reported were what the medication was for and its side-effects. Thirty per cent of people in the UFM study said they were overmedicated.

Medication has been an issue for activists for many years and some psychiatrists have said that this is unimportant as activists are 'unrepresentative'. It is interesting, then, that the people in these two studies expressed the same concerns about medication that activists do and have done for a long time. The implication for psychiatrists is that they should provide full information about medication and negotiate with their patients about dosage and side-effects. Psychiatrists need to take account of a person's life circumstances. For example, it is counterproductive to ask people to take highly sedative medication if they are in work and need to be alert for the working day. Psychiatrists should think carefully about dosage. Patients want the minimum effective dose and to avoid unwanted effects. It is alarming that nearly a third of the participants in the UFM research felt overmedicated.

Self-help

The S4L study found that the users interviewed often used self-help measures to cope with their mental distress. They might do this alongside psychiatrists or on their own. The study by Wallcraft *et al* (2003) found that self-help and mutual aid were the activities most important to user groups, large and small. For example, MDF – the Bipolar Organisation (formerly the Manic Depression Fellowship) runs a network of self-help groups covering the whole country. Self-help activities can be individual as well as collective. Again, MDF – the Bipolar Organisation has developed a strategy for 'self-management'. People with bipolar disorder are helped to manage their condition with more autonomy than is usual. A video has been produced and people with bipolar disorder are trained to help others like themselves to become skilled in managing their own distress. A similar strategy is being developed by Rethink, a UK charity for people with severe mental illness and their carers.

Another self-help network is the 'hearing voices' initiative, which began with the work of Romme & Escher (1993) in the Netherlands. People meet in organised groups where they discuss their voices and are encouraged to come to terms with them. It is interesting that all these organisations aim to help people with severe mental health problems rather than those at the milder end of the spectrum. Professionals may think such groups would not be able to do this.

Other respondents to the S4L survey wanted to use complementary therapies and wished to see these available in National Health Service facilities. The implications of this emphasis on self-help and alternative therapies for psychiatrists are that patients should be given some autonomy and that their rights to pursue their own strategies for living should be respected.

The care programme approach

The UFM project found that most of the users interviewed were not aware of the care programme approach (CPA), did not know who their keyworker was and did not know they had a care plan. Still less were they involved in drawing up their care plan or getting involved in setting up their review. Not a single person knew they could take an advocate to the review. The original UFM work was done in the late 1990s, but current UFM work is finding the same thing, as are professionally led and collaborative studies.

When presented at a workshop for rehabilitation workers who came from the more 'progressive' end of the profession, these findings did not come as a surprise. The participants said that patients were not interested. When asked how long it had taken for them to learn about CPA and then how long they had spent explaining it to their clients, the typical response was a 2- to 3-day course for the professionals. But some of them had not explained CPA at all to their clients and the typical time spent on this discussion was 10 minutes. Such a discrepancy indicates an unhealthy and continuing power imbalance between professionals and their clients.

Involvement in individual care was covered by both the UFM and the S4L projects. Users did not feel involved in their care. However, the UFM work found that on the rare occasions when users were involved in their own care – drawing up care plans, arranging review meetings – they were more satisfied overall with their treatment.

Care coordinators generally see service users more frequently than do psychiatrists. Sometimes users see their psychiatrist only at CPA meetings and maybe once in between for follow-up. So this is an important occasion and the meeting should be taken very seriously, and should involve the service user as much as possible. He or she should not have to sign a care plan drawn up in advance of the meeting but should be asked about needs and preferences for care.

In-patient treatment

The UFM project sometimes conducts site visits to hospitals and interviews people about their experience of in-patient care. As with the questionnaires for community care, the questions for the site visits and interviews were drawn up by a group of service users. These service users had experienced in-patient care. Some of the questions they constructed were very basic indeed but they came from the experience of people who had been in hospital themselves. For example, they asked whether people could get a drink when they wanted one and whether there was privacy in terms of sleeping areas. They also asked whether rights under the Mental Health Act had been respected and I have touched on this already in terms of information.

During site visits, the team would observe the ward and also interview anyone who was prepared to be interviewed. The basic questions described above were discovered to be relevant. Kitchens were often locked and drinks provided at set times. Where there were water coolers, they were usually empty and there were no cups. This is important, as one side-effect of many medications is a very dry mouth. In terms of privacy, many wards had dormitories with only thin and torn curtains between the beds. Women often felt unsafe, as male patients could wander into female dormitories. Staff were criticised as being inaccessible, staying in the office unless an incident occurred.

Perhaps the single most important thing that in-patients experience is crushing boredom. There is little to do, especially in the evenings and at weekends. Some units had gyms but patients could not use them as there was no one to staff them. A further feature of acute wards was the lack of access to fresh air. Even where a psychiatrist had given permission for someone to have escorted leave, the staff would say they did not have the capacity to provide someone to do the escorting. This sometimes meant that patients had to remain on stuffy wards for days on end with no access to fresh air.

These points are relevant for psychiatrists. Although trainees may spend more time on the wards, a large number of consultants generally come on the ward only once or twice a week, for ward rounds. They may be unaware, therefore, of what it is like to be on a ward in a routine way. They may not know that basic rights and dignity are not being respected, that patients have nothing to occupy themselves with or that their agreement to escorted leave is not being carried out. In any event, patients often find ward rounds intimidating, especially in teaching hospitals, where students may be there. In this context, service users may be reluctant to raise issues that preoccupy them, such as those described above.

Advanced directives and joint crisis plans

Many users would like to have an advanced directive. This is a document, prepared when users are well, which sets out the treatment they would like if a situation arises where they are unable to articulate their desires. However, advanced directives have no legal force in the UK and are trumped by the Mental Health Act.

Henderson *et al* (2004)) have studied an alternative to advanced directives which they term 'joint crisis plans' (JCPs). JCPs are negotiated between users and the team that cares for them, with a facilitator helping in the negotiation. They determine what users would like should they lose the capacity at a subsequent date to articulate their wishes. JCPs may lay down medications which the user does and does not want, as well as practical issues like whom to contact in a crisis and how to make sure that a property is secure, pets are fed and so on. The JCP is held by the user and copied to important parties. Henderson *et al* found that JCPs significantly reduced the number of involuntary admissions. They also found that users were more satisfied and more engaged with their care if they have a JCP.

Conclusion

From the above discussion we can summarise what it is that users would like to see their psychiatrist providing. They would like more information and choice – about medication, financial matters and leisure opportunities. They also would like more information if detained under the Mental Health Act. They would like to negotiate with their doctor instead of being treated like passive subjects. They would like this negotiation especially in respect of medication and CPA. They would like their psychiatrist to know more about what routinely goes on in their ward. The important elements are rights, dignity and safety, relations with staff and the issue of escorted leave – the fact that it is sanctioned by the doctor but not carried out by the nursing staff. Finally, many users would like to have advanced directives. Further research will tell us about the efficacy and acceptability of JCPs. My argument is that resolution of all these issues would be facilitated if there were a rebalancing of power relations between psychiatrists and their patients.

References

Campbell, P. (1996) The history of the user movement in the United Kingdom. In *Mental Health Matters: A Reader* (eds T. Heller, J. Reynolds, R. Gomm, *et al*), pp. 218–225. Open University Press.

Department of Health and Farrell, C. (2004) *Patient and Public Involvement in Health*. Department of Health.

Faulkner, A. & Layzell, A. (2001) *Strategies for Living*. Mental Health Foundation.

Henderson, C., Flood, C., Leese, M., *et al* (2004) Effect of joint crisis plans on use of compulsory treatment in psychiatry: single blind randomised controlled trial. *BMJ*, **329**, 122–123.

Laing, R. D. (1959) *The Divided Self*. Tavistock.

Lidz, C. W., Hodge, S. K., Gardner, W., *et al* (1995) Perceived coercion in hospital admission: pressures and process. *Archives of General Psychiatry*, **52**, 1034–1039.

Romme, M. & Escher, S. (1993) *Accepting Voices*. MIND.

Rose, D. (2001) *Users' Voices: The Perspectives of Mental Health Service Users on Community and Hospital Care*. Sainsbury Centre for Mental Health.

Rose, D., Fleischmann, P., Tonkiss, F., *et al* (2002) *Change Management in Organisations in a Mental Health Context. Report to the National Co-ordinating Centre Service Delivery and Organisation Branch*. NCCSDO.

Szasz, T. (1972) *The Myth of Mental Illness*. Granada.

Wallcraft, J., Read, J. & Sweeney, A. (2003) *On Our Own Terms*. Sainsbury Centre for Mental Health.

CHAPTER 23

Measurement of needs

Koravangattu Valsraj and Graham Thornicroft

Defining needs

The US psychologist Abraham Maslow established a seminal hierarchy of need, when he attempted to formulate a theory of human motivation (Maslow, 1954). In Maslow's model, fundamental physiological needs (such as the need for food) underpin the higher needs for safety, love, self-esteem and self-actualisation. He proposed that people are motivated by the requirement to meet these needs, and that higher needs can be met only after the lower and more fundamental needs have been met. This approach can be illustrated by the example of a homeless man, who is not concerned about his lack of friends while he is cold and hungry. However, once these physiological needs have been met, he may express more interest in having the company of other people (Slade & McCrone, 2001).

Since the work of Maslow, several approaches have been developed for defining need with respect to healthcare. The sociologist Bradshaw (1972) proposed a 'needs taxonomy', in which there were three types of need:

1   'felt' or 'expressed' need, which is mentioned by the user
2   normative need, which is assessed by the expert
3   'comparative' need, which arises from comparison with other groups or individuals.

Such an approach emphasises that need is a subjective concept and that the judgement of whether a need is present or not will, in part, depend on whose viewpoint is taken. Other, somewhat more philosophical approaches to needs have also been proposed (Mallman & Marcus, 1980; Liss, 1990). In the Medical Research Council's Needs for Care Assessment, for example, a need is defined as being present when a person's level of functioning falls below, or threatens to fall below, some specified level and when there is some remediable, or potentially remediable, cause (Brewin et al, 1987).

Slade (1994) has discussed the issue with respect to differences in perception between the users of mental health services and the involved professionals, and he has argued that, once differences have been identified, then negotiation between staff and user can take place to agree a care plan.

Despite the current consensus to base services upon assessed needs, there is at present no consensus on how needs should be defined (Holloway, 1994) or who should define them (Slade, 1994). Individual needs, for example, may be defined at the levels of impairment or disability, or in terms of interventions.

Moreover, the fact that a need is defined does not mean that it can be met. Some needs may remain unmet because other problems take priority, because an effective method is not available locally, or because the person in need refuses treatment. Thus, a need may exist, as defined by a professional, even if the intervention is refused by a patient. Further, a needs assessment is not intended to endorse the status quo. It is important to define need in terms of the care, agent or setting required, not those already in place. At the same time, a proper needs assessment process should not lead to the imposition of expert solutions upon patients. A professionally defined need may remain unmet and have to be replaced by one acceptable to the patient.

Stevens *et al* (2001) distinguish need from demand and supply:

- need = what people would benefit from
- demand = what people ask for
- supply = what is provided.

Further, a distinction can be made between provision and utilitisation. Thus:

- A *demand* for care exists when an individual expresses a wish to receive it. Some demands are expressed in an unsophisticated form (e.g. 'Something needs to be done'). The user should be involved in a negotiation as to what interventions should be provided for what problems. This will include an explanation of the options. The process should not be purely directed by experts or professionals.
- *Provision* includes interventions, agents and settings, whether or not they are used. Care coordination entails providing such a pattern of service after initial assessment and then updating the assessment regularly to assess outcomes and to modify the care if needs remain unmet. Over-provision is provision without need. Under-provision is need without provision (unmet need).
- *Utilisation* occurs when an individual actually receives care, for example an in-patient admission.

Just as need may not be expressed as demand, and demand is not necessarily followed by provision, provision is not always followed by utilisation; and there can be demand, provision and utilisation without real underlying need for the particular service used.

Since need has now been defined as the ability to benefit, it is also worth distinguishing need from *efficacy*, *effectiveness* and *outcome* (Stevens *et al*, 2001):

- need is a population's *ability to benefit*
- efficacy is an intervention's/care setting's *potential to benefit in ideal (experimental) conditions*
- effectiveness is an intervention's/care setting's *potential to benefit in everyday conditions*
- outcome is the *achieved benefit* in the local setting.

Another approach to defining need has been proposed by health economists. Their contributions include, first, the proposal that need refers both to the capacity to benefit from an intervention and the amount of expenditure required to reduce the capacity to benefit to zero; it is therefore a product of benefit and cost-effectiveness (Culyer & Wagstaff, 1992). Second is the proposal that diagnosis-related groups are notably irrelevant for mental health services (McCrone & Strathdee, 1994). Third, empirical data should guide operational needs definitions (Beecham *et al*, 1993).

In the particular case of mental health services, needs have been described in terms of the gaps between the service needs of patients and of populations and the services actually provided. Lehtinen *et al* (1990) interpret needs as reflecting an inadequate level of service for the severity of the problem: patients with severe disorders who receive primary rather than specialised psychiatric care would therefore be rated as having unmet need. Similarly, for Shapiro *et al* (1985) unmet needs are defined as the combination of definite morbidity and lack of mental health service utilisation. A third view is that unmet needs represent insufficient provision of particular treatment interventions, and this approach is embodied in the three individual needs assessment instruments described in the next section.

Measuring individual needs

In an ideal planning framework, a comprehensive needs assessment would be undertaken on all patients and the aggregated data would be used to plan the services. In practice, this is seldom possible, but systematic assessment, review and evaluation over months and years of contact should allow teams to work with their users to develop services more appropriate to their needs (Brewin *et al*, 1987).

Individual needs assessments for homeless people who are mentally ill, for example, exemplify these issues. In a study by Herman *et al* (1993), homeless people were asked if they needed 'help with nerves and emotional problems' and were independently rated by the interviewer. A quarter (24%) of the interviewees reported no need for mental health services when the interviewer rated them as having a need. By contrast, Mavis *et al* (1993) reported a study of homeless people who had sought help for substance misuse, who were asked about specific areas of need. Two sub-groups were identified: 78% were the 'economic homeless', with substantial employment and financial problems, and 22% were the 'multi-problem homeless', with significantly greater problems also in physical health, alcohol/drug use, mental health, family and social life. Over 800 clients were interviewed and the study showed the explanatory use of distinguishing the two sub-groups of homeless people.

The issue of how best to make an assessment has taxed both researchers and clinicians, not least because their requirements differ. An ideal assessment tool for use in a routine clinic setting would be one which is brief, easily learned, takes little time to administer, does not require the use of personnel additional to the usual clinical team, is valid and reliable in different settings and across genders and cultures, and, above all, can be used as an integral part of routine clinical work, rather than as a time-consuming extra. In addition, it should be sensitive to change, its inter-rater and test–retest reliability should be high, and it should logically inform clinical management (Thornicroft & Bebbington, 1996). The decision regarding which tool to use will depend on whether the approach is to focus on particular diagnostic or care groups, and on the balance to be struck between economy of time and inclusiveness of the ratings. Ratings should include a range of areas of clinical and social functioning. Three such tools are discussed below.

The Medical Research Council's Needs for Care Assessment

The Needs for Care Assessment (NCA) (Brewin *et al*, 1987) was designed to identify areas of remediable need. As mentioned above, need is defined as being present when:

1   a patient's functioning (social disablement) falls below or threatens to fall below some minimum specified level
2   this is due to a remediable, or potentially remediable, cause.

A need is defined as being met when it has attracted an item of care which is at least partly effective, and when no other item of care of greater potential effectiveness exists. A need is said to be unmet when it has attracted only a partially effective or no item of care, and when other items of care of greater potential effectiveness do exist.

The NCA has proved itself to be a robust research instrument, and there is a substantial body of research describing its use (Brewin *et al*, 1988; Van Haaster *et al*, 1994; Lesage *et al*, 1996). However, it is probably too complex and time-consuming for routine clinical use, and difficulties have arisen when it has been used with long-term in-patients (Pryce *et al*, 1993) and homeless people with a mental illness (Hogg & Marshall, 1992).

The Cardinal Needs Schedule

The Cardinal Needs Schedule (CNS) (Lockwood & Marshall, 2001) is a modification of the NCA. It identifies 'cardinal' problems which satisfy three criteria:

270

1   the 'cooperation criterion' (the patient is willing to accept help for the problem)
2   the 'co-stress criterion' (the problem causes considerable anxiety, frustration or inconvenience to people caring for the patient)
3   the 'severity criterion' (the problem endangers the health or safety of the patient, or the safety of other people).

The instrument involves the use of the Manchester Scale for mental state assessment and the REHAB scale, as well as a specially designed additional information questionnaire. A computerised version known as AUTONEED is also available. Again, given the detail of this instrument, it is probably more suited to experienced researchers.

The Camberwell Assessment of Need

The Camberwell Assessment of Need (CAN) is an individual needs assessment instrument for use with adults with severe mental illness. Four broad principles governed the development of the CAN (Phelan *et al*, 1995; Slade *et al*, 1999a):

1   Everyone has needs, and although people with mental health problems have some specific needs, the majority of their needs are similar to those of people who do not have a mental illness, such as having somewhere to live, something to do and enough money.
2   The majority of people with a severe mental illness have multiple needs, and it is vital that all of them are identified by those caring for them. Therefore, a priority of the CAN is to identify, rather than describe in detail, serious needs. Specialist assessments can be conducted in specific areas if required, once the need has been identified.
3   Needs assessment should be both an integral part of routine clinical practice and a component of service evaluation, so the CAN should be usable by a wide range of staff.
4   Need is a subjective concept and so there will frequently be differing but equally valid perceptions about the presence or absence of a specific need. The CAN therefore records the views of staff and patients separately.

The specific criteria that were established for the CAN are that it:

- has adequate psychometric properties
- can be completed within 30 minutes
- can be used by a wide range of professionals
- is suitable for both routine clinical practice and research
- can be learnt and used without formal training
- incorporates the views of service users, staff and carers about needs (Hancock *et al*, 2003)
- measures both met and unmet need

- measures the level of help received from friends or relatives as well as from statutory services.

There are three versions of CAN: Research, Clinical, and the Short Appraisal Schedule (CANSAS). All versions assess need in the same 22 domains of health and social needs:

1   accommodation
2   food
3   looking after the home
4   self-care
5   daytime activities
6   physical health
7   psychotic symptoms
8   information about condition and treatment
9   psychological distress
10 safety to self
11 safety to others
12 alcohol
13 drugs
14 company
15 intimate relationships
16 sexual expression
17 child care
18 education
19 telephone
20 transport
21 money
22 benefits.

Camberwell Assessment of Need Short Appraisal Schedule

The Camberwell Assessment of Need Short Appraisal (CANSAS) (Slade *et al*, 1999*a,b*) is a short (single-page) summary of the needs of a mental health service patient. It can be used in clinical settings since it is short enough to be routinely used for review purposes. It can also be used as an outcome measure in research studies, especially when a number of assessment schedules are being used.

CANSAS records the views of the patient, carers and staff about the needs of the service user. Questions are asked about each domain, to identify:

- whether a need or problem is present in that domain
- if so, whether that need is met or unmet.

On the basis of the interviewee's responses, a *need rating* is made:

- 0 = no serious problem (no need)
- 1 = no/moderate problem due to help given (met need)
- 2 = serious problem (unmet need)
- 9 = not known.

CANSAS may be used for at least three purposes:

1   CANSAS data can be used at the level of the individual patient, by providing a baseline measure of level of need and then charting changes over time for that patient, for example. Another approach would be to use the CANSAS routinely in initial assessments of new service patients, to identify the range of domains in which they are likely to require further assessment and (possibly) help or treatment.

2   CANSAS data can be used for auditing and developing an individual service.

3   CANSAS can be used as an outcome measure for research purposes, such as the impact on needs of two different types of mental health services, or the reasons why staff's and service users' perceptions differ.

Other versions of the CAN

The CAN has now been translated into 16 languages and further information is available at the website of the Health Services and Population Research Department of the Institute of Psychiatry (http://www.iop.kcl.ac.uk/departments/?locator=4). In addition, standardised translations have been made into Danish, Dutch, German, Italian and Spanish in the European version of the scale (CAN-EU) (McCrone et al, 2000; Thornicroft et al, 2006). Further specialised versions of the CAN have been published for older adults (CANE) (Reynolds et al, 2000; Reynolds & Orrell, 2001; Orrell, 2003), people with intellectual disabilities (CANDID) (Xenitidis & Bouras, 2001; Xenitidis et al, 2000, 2003) and forensic patients (CANFOR) (Thomas et al, 2003, 2004; Harty et al, 2004). A version for mothers who are mentally ill is in press (Howard et al, 2008). Specific applications of needs assessment in relation to other client/user groups – carers, children, ethnic groups, primary care settings, drug and alcohol misuse, eating disorders and services in rural areas – have been discussed by Thornicroft (2001).

Comparing staff and service user ratings of need

There is now growing evidence that needs rated by service users, especially unmet needs, may be more informative that those rated by staff. The comparison of these two perspectives on needs are discussed here in relation to three illustrative studies, from England, Scandinavia and Italy.

The first example comes from the PRiSM Psychosis Study (Leese et al, 1998; Thornicroft et al, 1998). This staff–user CAN comparative project was nested within a larger, prospective, non-randomised controlled trial of two different types of community mental health team in south London. The needs of an epidemiologically representative sample of 137 patients from a catchment area psychiatric service in south London who had an ICD–10 diagnosis of a functional psychotic disorder were assessed cross-sectionally by patients and staff, using the CAN.

Staff rated patients as having, on average, 6.1 needs, whereas patients gave themselves an average rating of 6.7 needs ($t = 2.58$, d.f. $= 136$, $P = 0.011$). This difference was accounted for by the staff rating of 1.2 unmet needs and the patient rating of 1.8 unmet needs ($t = 3.58$, d.f. $= 136$, $P < 0.001$). There was no difference in the ratings of total number of met needs. There was no difference in ratings in relation to any patient socio-demographic characteristics. There was moderate or better agreement on the presence of a need for 13 of the 22 CAN domains (Slade et al, 1998), but while staff and patients agreed moderately about met needs, they agreed less often on unmet needs. The domains more often rated by staff were specific psychotic symptoms and safety to others. The items more often rated by the service users were: information about condition and treatment, company, welfare benefits, sexual expression, and public transport. For example, there was most disagreement between staff and users on four key items: information (about diagnosis, treatment and prognosis), telephone, public transport and welfare benefits. Staff rated a mean of 0.90 needs for these four domains, while service users rated 1.57 (difference 0.67, 95% confidence interval 0.47–0.85).

The study therefore found that although staff and users rated about the same number of needs as each other, and although there was agreement for many of the domains of the CAN, the most disagreement occurred not about clinical issues but primarily in relation to practical aspects of the everyday lives of the services users.

The second illustration of staff–user comparative assessments of need is the Nordic Multi-Centre Study (Hansson et al, 2001), which undertook a comparison of keyworker and patient assessments of needs for people with schizophrenia living in the community. In this study, ten centres in five Scandinavian countries (Denmark, Sweden, Finland, Iceland and Norway) participated, within a larger study of case management. The CAN was used by 300 matched pairs of staff and service users to rate needs. The authors found moderate or good agreement in 17 of the 22 domains, more than in the London study. On the other hand, there was more disagreement on whether the right type of help was being given than in the earlier project.

Domains that were more often rated by staff were specific psychotic symptoms, psychological distress, and self-care and presentation. Items that were more often rated by service users were on the domain information about condition and treatment. Overall, there was relatively poor agreement for the domains information about condition and treatment, welfare benefits and telephone.

The authors also compared responses on whether the right type of help was being offered for the needs identified. Here there was close agreement for only 5 of the 22 domains. Staff and users were least likely to agree that interventions in the following areas were the correct form of treatment or care: physical health, psychological distress, basic education, self-care and presentation, and intimate relationships.

The third example of staff–user differences is the South Verona OUTPRO study, described in detail by Lasalvia *et al* (2000). Patients resident within a local catchment area of 75 000 were identified from a case register of all those in contact with specialist mental health services. Within a larger study which implemented outcome measures in routine clinical practice, 247 staff–patient pairs used the Italian version of the CAN. While this group had somewhat less disability than the sample in the Nordic study of those in contact with case managers, the usual pattern of met needs exceeding unmet needs was found for those receiving care. The needs more often rated by staff were: physical health, psychological distress, self-care and presentation, and specific psychotic symptoms. Users more frequently rated needs in the domains of information about condition and treatment, welfare benefits, safety to self, food and meals, intimate relationships, telephone, basic education, and money.

The Verona group went further than the other researchers and identified predictors of high levels of need. High staff-rated levels of need were associated with: higher level of disability, unemployment, and more service contacts. High user-rated levels of need were associated with higher disability only. Disagreement on the total number of needs was most strongly associated with a lower level of global clinical and social functioning. These results once again demonstrate the clinical/social difference in orientation typified in the studies discussed above.

Measuring population needs for services

Measuring the population's ability to benefit from healthcare generates two very specific information requirements (Wing, 1992):

1   Top-down sources of information are required, such as the local prevalence and incidence of disease, ranged by severity. Prevalence, the number of cases per unit population at a point in time, or over a period, is usually the appropriate measure for chronic disease; and incidence, the number of new cases per unit time, is usually appropriate for measuring acute disease.

2   The type of information required concerns the efficacy of the care and care settings available or potentially available to cope with it.

In practice, several more detailed types of information are needed to assist judgements on how far mental health services meet need at the population level, especially resource costs and the number and characteristics of patients treated. Another potential approach is the measurement of diagnosis-related groups (Mitchell *et al*, 1987), which suggests that diagnosis is of little help in attempting to measure prospectively the resources required by individual in-patients.

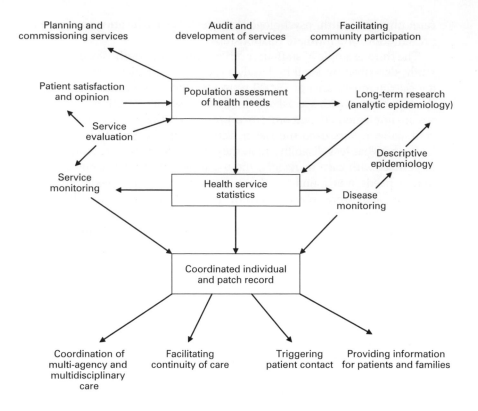

Fig. 23.1 Uses of mental health information systems (Fryers & Greatorex, 1992).

The relationship between individual-based needs assessment (bottom-up) and population-based information (top-down) is illustrated in Fig. 23.1. Bottom-up approaches, that is the aggregation of individual-level data to give information about patient populations, are somewhat less common (Bebbington *et al*, 1996).

Traditionally, service-level needs have been approximated from service utilisation data, especially hospital bed use. This is often inaccurate because: in-patient care is a small and diminishing part of mental healthcare; in many respects in-patient care actually represents an alternative model of care to that practised (i.e. community-based care) for certain patients; the chronicity and episodic nature of mental illness means that episodes are often part of a longer sequence and differ greatly in length and intensity; and there is a greater diversity of health professional contacts (i.e. psychiatrists, psychologists, community psychiatric nurses, and occupational therapists).

In terms of the needs for general adult mental health services for a defined population, Table 23.1 presents data from multiple sources and suggests that:

Table 23.1 Estimated need for and actual provision of general adult mental health services (in-patient and residential care): places per 250 000 population, estimated for England, 1992–96 (for population aged 15–64 years only)

Category of service	Johnson et al (1997)[a]	Strathdee & Thornicroft (1992)[a]	PRiSM (1996)[b]	Actual level of provision per 250 000		
				Outer London	Inner London	Range in London
Medium-secure unit	1–10	1–10	5–30	8	27	0–58
Intensive-care unit/local secure unit	5–15	5–10	5–20	8	16	0–41
Acute ward	50–150	50–150	50–175	73[c]	110[c]	48–165
24-hour nurse-staffed units/hostel wards, staff awake at night	25–75	40–150 for these 2 categories together	12–50	55	35	0–164
24-hour non-nurse-staffed hostels, night staff sleep-in	40–110		50–300	99	162	28–330
Day-staffed hostels	25–75	30–120	15–60	17	43	14–292 for these 2 categories together
Lower-support accommodation	n/a	48–100	30–120	55	95	

[a] All estimates given assume that each category of service exists in the given appropriate range of volume. The Wing (1992) estimates include old age assessment places, and the Strathdee & Thornicroft (1992) figures apply only to general adult services for those aged 16–65.

[b] Johnson et al (1997) estimated need levels based upon: London actual values, and an expected fourfold variation of need from least to most deprived parts of England, for most categories of service, with a far greater variation in medium-secure beds, and the NHS Executive's 1996 guidance for an average of 25 places in 24-hour nurse-staffed accommodation per 250 000.

[c] Includes respite beds and supported self-contained flats. As not all agencies gave information on these categories, these estimates as conservative.

Sources: Glover (1996); Ramsay et al (1997); Thornicroft & Strathdee (2001).

- the emphasis should be upon the number of places available rather than upon the number of beds
- a range of provisions should exist
- the number of places needed in each category depends upon the extent of provision in the other categories
- the overall requirement for services will correlate closely with the degree of socio-economic deprivation experienced by that particular population, as shown in Table 23.1.

Conclusion

The assessments of needs for care and needs for services have been relatively recently developed. As yet, the issue of how service users participate in defining need is largely unexplored territory (Beeforth & Wood, 2001; Thornicroft & Slade, 2002). Just as formidable is the question 'What are the consequences of conducting proper needs assessment?' (Goldman, 1999). In assessing need, we are likely to confront previously inconspicuous layers of psychiatric morbidity and disability. This leads to two further questions: How shall we prioritise services? And is the pursuit of quality of life a reasonable proxy where staff are not able to provide a complete cure for mental disorders (Slade *et al*, 2004)?

Finally, it is sometimes helpful to step back from the detail of how to measure needs for healthcare and to ask *why* we should measure needs. In our view, an approach to health services that is fundamentally based upon need is in essence a moral choice. It is a view that attaches importance to the relief of suffering, whatever the circumstances of the person who is unwell, and which claims that a civilised society will offer services in proportion to the needs of those who may benefit from them. This sentiment has been more poetically expressed by Isabel Allende (1985), when she wrote:

'They also forced me to eat. They divided up the servings with the strictest sense of justice, each according to her need.'

References

Allende, I. (1985) *The House of the Spirits*. Black Swan Books.

Bebbington, P., Brewin, C. R., Marsden, L., *et al* (1996) Measuring the need for psychiatric treatment in the general population: the community version of the MRC Needs for Care Assessment. *Psychological Medicine*, **26**, 229–236.

Beecham, J., Knapp, M. & Fenyo, A. (1993) Costs, needs and outcomes in community mental healthcare. In *Costing Community Care* (eds A. Betten & J. Beecham). Aldgate.

Beeforth, M. & Wood, H. (2001) Needs from a user perspective. In *Measuring Mental Health Needs* (ed. G. Thornicroft), pp. 190–199. Gaskell.

Bradshaw, J. (1972) A taxonomy of social need. In *Problems and Progress in Medical Care: Essays on Current Research: 7th Series* (ed. G. McLachlan). Oxford University Press.

Brewin, C. (2001) Measuring individual needs for care and services. In *Measuring Mental Health Needs* (2nd edn) (ed. G. Thornicroft), pp. 273–290. Gaskell.

Brewin, C. R., Wing, J. K., Mangen, S. P., *et al* (1987) Principles and practice of measuring needs in the long-term mentally ill: the MRC Needs for Care Assessment. *Psychological Medicine*, **17**, 971–982.

Brewin, C., Wing, J., Mangen, S., *et al* (1988) Needs for care among the long-term mentally ill: a report from the Camberwell High Contact Survey. *Psychological Medicine*, **18**, 457–468.

Culyer, A. & Wagstaff, A. (1992) *Need, Equity and Equality in Health and Healthcare*. Centre for Health Economics, Health Economics Consortium, University of York.

Fryers, T. & Greatorex, N. (1992) Case registers of service use and at risk groups. In *Measuring Mental Health Needs* (eds G. Thornicroft, C. Brewin & J. K. Wing), pp. 81–98. Gaskell.

Glover, G. (1996) Health service indictors for mental health. In *Commissioning Mental Health Services* (eds G. Thornicroft & G. Strathdee), pp. 311–318. HMSO.

Goldman, H. H. (1999) The obligation of mental health services to the least well off. *Psychiatric Services*, **50**, 659–663.

Hancock, G. A., Reynolds, T., Woods, B., *et al* (2003) The needs of older people with mental health problems according to the user, the carer, and the staff. *International Journal of Geriatric Psychiatry*, **18**, 803–811.

Hansson, L., Vinding, H. R., Mackeprang, T., *et al* (2001) Comparison of key worker and patient assessment of needs in schizophrenic patients living in the community: a Nordic multicentre study. *Acta Psychiatrica Scandinavica*, **103**, 45–51.

Harty, M., Shaw, J., Thomas, S., *et al* (2004) The security, clinical and social needs of patients in high security psychiatric hospitals in England. *Journal of Forensic Psychiatry and Psychology*, **15**, 208–221.

Herman, D., Struening, E. & Barrow, S. (1993) Self-assessed need for mental health services among homeless adults. *Hospital and Community Psychiatry*, **44**, 1181–1182.

Hogg, L. I. & Marshall, M. (1992) Can we measure need in the homeless mentally ill? Using the MRC Needs for Care Assessment in hostels for the homeless. *Psychological Medicine*, **22**, 1027–1034.

Holloway, F. (1994) Need in community psychiatry: a consensus is required. *Psychiatric Bulletin*, **18**, 321–323.

Howard, L., Slae, M., O'Keane, V., *et al* (2008) *The Camberwell Assessment of Need for Pregnant Women and Mothers with Severe Mental Illness*. RCPsych Publications. In press.

Johnson, S., Ramsay, R., Thornicroft, G., *et al* (1997) *London's Mental Health*. King's Fund.

Lasalvia, A., Ruggeri, M., Mazzi, M. A., *et al* (2000) The perception of needs for care in staff and patients in community-based mental health services. The South-Verona Outcome Project 3. *Acta Psychiatrica Scandinavica*, **102**, 366–375.

Leese, M., Johnson, S., Slade, M., *et al* (1998) The user perspective on needs and satisfaction with mental health services: the PRiSM Psychosis Study (8). *British Journal of Psychiatry*, **173**, 409–415.

Lehtinen, V., Joukamaa, M., Jyrkinen, E., *et al* (1990) Need for mental health services of the adult population in Finland. Results from the Mini Finland Health Survey. *Acta Psychiatrica Scandinavica*, **81**, 426–431.

Lesage, A. D., Fournier, L., Cyr, M., *et al* (1996) The reliability of the community version of the MRC Needs for Care Assessment. *Psychological Medicine*, **26**, 237–243.

Liss, P. (1990) *Healthcare Need: Meaning and Measurement*. Studies in Arts and Science.

Lockwood A. & Marshall, M. (2001) The Cardinal Needs Schedule – a standardised research instrument for measuring individual needs. In *Measuring Mental Health Needs* (2nd edn) (ed. G. Thornicroft), pp. 261–272. Gaskell.

Mallman, C. A. & Marcus, S. (1980) Logical clarifications in the study of needs. In *Human Needs* (ed. K. Lederer). Oelgeschlager, Gunn & Hain.

Maslow, A. (1954) *Motivation and Personality*. Harper & Row.

Mavis, B., Humphreys, K. & Stöffelmayr, B. (1993) Treatment needs and outcomes of two subtypes of homeless persons who abuse substances. *Hospital and Community Psychiatry*, **44**, 1185–1187.

McCrone, P. & Strathdee, G. (1994) Needs not diagnosis: towards a more rational approach to community mental health resourcing in Great Britain. *International Journal of Social Psychiatry*, **40**, 79–86.

McCrone, P., Leese, M., Thornicroft, G., *et al* (2000) Reliability of the Camberwell Assessment of Need – European Version. EPSILON Study 6. European psychiatric services: inputs linked to outcome domains and needs. *British Journal of Psychiatry*, **177** (suppl. 39), S34–S40.

Mitchell, J., Dickey, B. & Liptzin, B. (1987) Bringing psychiatric patients into the medicare prospective payments system: alternatives to DRGs. *American Journal of Psychiatry*, **144**, 610–615.

Orrell, M. (2003) *Camberwell Assessment of Need for the Elderly (CANE)*. Gaskell.

Phelan, M., Slade, M., Thornicroft, G., *et al* (1995) The Camberwell Assessment of Need: the validity and reliability of an instrument to assess the needs of people with severe mental illness. *British Journal of Psychiatry*, **167**, 589–595.

Pryce, I. G., Griffiths, R. D., Gentry, R. M., *et al* (1993) How important is the assessment of social skills in current long-stay in-patients? An evaluation of clinical response to needs for assessment, treatment and care in long-stay psychiatric in-patient population. *British Journal of Psychiatry*, **162**, 498–502.

Ramsay, R., Thornicroft, G., Johnson, S., *et al* (1997) Levels of in-patient and residential provision throughout London. In *London's Mental Health* (eds S. Johnson *et al*), pp. 193–219. King's Fund.

Reynolds, T. & Orrell, M. (2001) Needs assessment in mental healthcare for older people. In *Measuring Mental Health Needs* (2nd edn) (ed. G. Thornicroft), pp. 393–406. Gaskell.

Reynolds, T., Thornicroft, G., Abas, M., *et al* (2000) Camberwell Assessment of Need for the Elderly (CANE). Development, validity and reliability. *British Journal of Psychiatry*, **176**, 444–452.

Shapiro, S., Skinner, E. A., Kramer, M., *et al* (1985) Measuring need for mental health services in a general population. *Medical Care*, **23**, 1033–1043.

Slade, M. (1994) Needs assessment: who needs to assess? *British Journal of Psychiatry*, **165**, 287–292.

Slade, M. & McCrone, P. (2001) The Camberwell Assessment of Need (CAN). In *Measuring Mental Health Needs* (2nd edn) (ed. G. Thornicroft), pp. 291–303. Gaskell.

Slade, M., Phelan, M. & Thornicroft, G. (1998) A comparison of needs assessed by staff and an epidemiologically representative sample of patients with psychosis. *Psychological Medicine*, **28**, 543–550.

Slade, M., Thornicroft, G., Phelan, M., *et al* (1999a) *Camberwell Assessment of Need (CAN)*. Gaskell.

Slade, M., Beck, A., Bindman, J., *et al* (1999b) Routine clinical outcome measures for patients with severe mental illness: CANSAS and HoNOS. *British Journal of Psychiatry*, **174**, 404–408.

Slade, M., Leese, M., Ruggeri, M., *et al* (2004) Does meeting needs improve quality of life? *Psychotherapy and Psychosomatics*, **73**, 183–189.

Stevens, A., Raftery, J. & Mendelsohn, R. (2001) The commissioner's information requirements on mental health needs and commissioning for mental health services. In *Measuring Mental Health Needs* (2nd edn) (ed. G. Thornicroft), pp. 59–83. Gaskell.

Strathdee, G. & Thornicroft, G. (1992) Community sectors for needs-led mental health services. In *Measuring Mental Health Needs* (ed. G. Thornicroft), pp. 140–162. Gaskell.

Thomas, S., Harty, M.-A., Parrott, J., *et al* (eds) (2003) *CANFOR: Camberwell Assessment of Need – Forensic Version. A Needs Assessment for Forensic Mental Health Service Users.* Gaskell.

Thomas, S., Leese, M., Dolan, M., *et al* (2004) The individual needs of patients in high secure psychiatric hospitals in England. *Journal of Forensic Psychiatry and Psychology*, **15**, 222–243.

Thornicroft, G. (2001) *Measuring Mental Health Needs* (2nd edn). Gaskell.

Thornicroft, G. & Bebbington, P. (1996) Quantitative methods in the evaluation of community mental health services. In *Modern Community Psychiatry* (ed. W. Breakey), pp. 120–138. Cambridge University Press.

Thornicroft, G. & Slade, M. (2002) Comparing needs assessed by staff and by service users: paternalism or partnership in mental health? *Epidemiologia e Psichiatria Sociale*, **11**, 186–191.

Thornicroft, G. & Strathdee, G. (2001) Local catchment areas for needs-led mental health services. In *Measuring Mental Health Needs* (2nd edn) (ed. G. Thornicroft), pp. 171–189. Gaskell.

Thornicroft, G., Strathdee, G., Phelan, M., *et al* (1998) Rationale and design. PRiSM Psychosis Study 1. *British Journal of Psychiatry*, **173**, 363–370.

Thornicroft, G., Becker, T., Knapp, M., *et al* (2006) *International Outcome Measures in Mental Health. Quality of Life, Needs, Service Satisfaction, Costs and Impact on Carers*. Gaskell.

van Haaster, I., Lesage, A., Cyr, M., *et al* (1994) Problems and needs for care of patients suffering from severe mental illness. *Social Psychiatry and Psychiatric Epidemiology*, **29**, 141–148.

Wing, J. (1992) *Epidemiologically Based Needs Assessment. Report 6. Mental Illness*. NHS Management Executive.

Xenitidis, K. & Bouras, N. (2001) Measurement of needs in people with learning disabilities and mental health problems. In *Measuring Mental Health Needs* (2nd edn) (ed. G. Thornicroft), pp. 379–392. Gaskell.

Xenitidis, K., Thornicroft, G., Leese, M., *et al* (2000) Reliability and validity of the CANDID – a needs assessment instrument for adults with learning disabilities and mental health problems. *British Journal of Psychiatry*, **176**, 473–478.

Xenitidis, K., Slade, M., Thornicroft, G., *et al* (2003) *Camberwell Assessment of Need for Adults with Developmental and Intellectual Disabilities (CANDID). A Comprehensive Needs Assessment Tool for People with Learning Disabilities and Mental Health Problems*. Gaskell.

CHAPTER 24

Managing the psychiatrist's performance

David Roy

'Patients in the United Kingdom rightly have great confidence in their health professionals. When we need care, we entrust ourselves to doctors, nurses and a range of other skilled and dedicated professionals ...

... Professional regulation must create a framework that maintains the justified confidence of patients in those who care for them as the bedrock of safe and effective clinical practice and the foundation for effective relationships between patients and health professionals.

The danger is that in addressing the issue at all we risk highlighting too much the poor practice or unacceptable behaviour of a very small number of health professionals. It is all too easy to focus on the incompetent or malicious practice of individuals and seek to build a system from that starting point, instead of recognising that excellent health professionals far outnumber the few who let patients down substantially. For every time that Harold Shipman and Beverley Allitt are mentioned, we must recall the hundreds of thousands of extraordinary individuals who dedicate themselves impeccably to their patients every day' (Hewitt, 2007: p. 1).

A somewhat bleaker but perhaps more realistic assessment of medical practice is essayed by Richard Smith in his preface to *Problem Doctors: A Conspiracy of Silence* (Lens & van der Wal, 1997):

'We shouldn't be surprised by problem doctors. Why wouldn't they exist? Think how surprised we would be by a community of 130 000 people where nobody committed terrible crimes, went mad, abused drugs, slacked on the job, became corrupt, lost confidence and competence, or exploited their position. Such a community cannot be imagined, and yet doctors behave as if they are surprised by the existence of problem doctors.'

Donaldson (1994) describes the problems arising over a number of years in a large hospital within the National Health Service (NHS), including poor attitude, disruptive and irresponsible behaviour, lack of commitment to duties, badly exercised clinical skills and inadequate medical knowledge, dishonesty, sexual overtones in dealings with patients or staff, disorganised practice and poor communication with colleagues. He drew two conclusions:

1 Dealing with such problems requires experience, objectivity and a willingness to tolerate unpleasantness and criticism.
2 Existing procedures for hospital doctors within the NHS are (were) inadequate to deal with serious problems.

Since that time, the procedures have changed. There is a new framework for dealing with doctor's performance, as set out in the document *Maintaining High Professional Standards in the Modern NHS* (Department of Health, 2005a). Also, the climate is somewhat altered, with further initiatives regularly being announced by the Department of Health. This is to be welcomed. There has been a change in the public perception of medical performance regulation and, since the report of the Shipman Inquiry (2004), the way in which doctor's performance is accounted for and monitored is changing at a rapid pace. All doctors, including doctors in training, will be included in the programme of revalidation (on which, see Chapter 20).

It is important for those trying to deal with less-well-performing doctors always to start from the premise that most clinical staff who work in the NHS do so because they want to deliver high-quality services. All doctors have areas of performance which are sometimes less good than they would wish and all doctors should be open to the notion of continuously striving to improve their own performance and the performance of their teams.

Key categories for a poorly performing doctor can be outlined as follows (Department of Health, 1999):

• clinical performance and professional conduct
• personal misconduct
• failure to fulfil contractual requirements
• clinical performance serious enough to warrant referral to the General Medical Council (GMC).

In this chapter I outline how a psychiatrist's performance should be assessed and validated and the link to appraisal and revalidation. Through these and related processes, occasionally a problem doctor emerges, and I outline some of the tools available to manage performance. Finally, if all else fails, the more formal processes are available to take action, and these are also described below.

The way in which doctors judge their own performance, or the way in which their performance is judged by others, can be simply put in three basic questions:

1 *What does* the doctor do? This includes the outline of the job plan, the contractual arrangements, case-loads, hours worked, and so on.
2 *What should* the doctor do? This includes the standards of clinical practice against which an individual's practice can be measured, ethical and moral standards, clinical effectiveness and evidence base and so on.
3 *How well* does the doctor do it? This includes the actual practice of the individual doctor and the team, including outcomes, relationships

within the team and with colleagues, relationships with patients, carers and referrers, feedback on effectiveness of teaching and research, and so on.

What should the psychiatrist do?

What the psychiatrist should do is set out by various professional standards. The first editions of *Good Medical Practice* and *Maintaining Good Medical Practice* were published by the General Medical Council in 1996 and 1999, following a period of consultation with the profession; they outline the professional, ethical and moral parameters within which all doctors should practise and conduct themselves. The latest, combined edition of the two appeared in 2006. The Royal College of Psychiatrists has published *Good Psychiatric Practice* (2001, revised 2004), which provides all practising psychiatrists with the core attributes of a psychiatrist (Box 24.1) and clearly links these to the basic tenets of *Good Medical Practice*. More importantly, *Good Psychiatric Practice* includes explicit indications of what constitutes unacceptable practice. It is now possible to refer to a set of standards when psychiatrists are asked to describe 'what I do' and 'how well do I do it'.

Box 24.1   The core attributes of a psychiatrist

- Clinical competence
- Being a good communicator and listener
- Being fully sensitive to gender, ethnicity and culture
- Commitment to equality, antidiscriminatory practice and working with diversity
- Having a basic understanding of group dynamics
- Being able to contribute to creating an atmosphere within a team where individual opinions are valued and team members have a sense of ownership of decisions
- Ability to be decisive
- Ability to appraise staff
- Basic understanding of the principles of operational management
- Understanding and acknowledgement of the role and status of the vulnerable patient
- Bringing empathy, encouragement and hope to patients and their carers
- A critical self-awareness of emotional responses to clinical situations
- Being aware of the power inherent in the role of doctors and its potentially destructive influence on relationships with colleagues in other disciplines, with patients and with carers, and respecting boundaries
- Acknowledging situations where there is a potential for bullying or harassment, either through one's own actions or those of others

---

What does the psychiatrist do?

Appraisal

Consultants within the NHS – and doctors working outside of managed organisations, doctors in training and staff and associate specialists (SAS) – are being asked to account for their performance in a more structured way than ever before, and one means by which this can be achieved is through the annual appraisal process. Advance Letter (MD) 6/2000 states: 'Appraisal must follow a standardised format if it is to be applied and satisfy the GMC's requirements for revalidation' (Department of Health, 2000). The paperwork claims to provide a framework that is 'formal, supportive and consistent'. Many doctors find the new process more demanding of time, both in working through the documentation and in providing data in a way that has not been expected or required previously (perhaps made more difficult where clinical information systems are poorly developed, currently a particular issue for mental health services generally compared with some other branches of medicine).

The principles of good appraisal are well established, and the formality of the approach and the direct link to the revalidation process will surely change the way in which doctors review and assess their own performance through the year. The NHS appraisal document spells out the reflective questions doctors should ask of themselves, extending 'what do I do, what should I do and how well do I do it?' to 'how good a consultant/leader/doctor in training … am I, how well do I perform, how up to date am I, how well do I work in a team, what resources and support do I need, how well am I meeting my service objectives and what are my development needs?'

NHS appraisal for doctors does not include 'how well do I engage with the patient and carers?' in any detail but this issue must be central to all good mental health services.

In its Council report *Good Psychiatric Practice: CDP*, the Royal College of Psychiatrists (2001) describes appraisal and performance review as:

'two overlapping yet distinct processes whereby doctors relate to their employers. Appraisal is the process in which the potential and development needs of the employees are identified in conjunction with peers or employers, while performance review brings the work, achievements and aspirations of individual practitioners into a relationship with the aims, objectives and working practices of the organisation. Revalidation describes an external process of professional self-regulation ensuring the individual practitioners continue to meet at least the minimum standards set by the profession.'

Pragmatically, most organisations run the two processes of appraisal and performance review as one, although good job planning (see below) will be more linked to organisational aims and objectives than appraisal.

A good appraisal should provide the opportunity for doctors to take stock of their professional performance through the year and link that performance to an active and forward-looking development plan. Although appraisals could be considered to be 'data heavy', in the most successful appraisals the doctor brings a range of evidence to the table, including detailed indicators and narratives of what they do, and as many indirect indicators of how well they do it as they have managed to collate through the year.

An additional key development within the appraisal process is the use of more formal 360° appraisal 'tools', whereby doctors ask colleagues, referrers, patients and others to comment confidentially on perceptions of the doctor's strengths and weaknesses; these are compiled in a confidential report that outlines themes and sometimes key areas for improvement.

A long-term challenge for appraisal within the NHS is that the process currently provides the key source evidence for the relicensing (revalidation) decisions of the GMC. It is perhaps inevitable that if the only means by which consultants in particular provide the revalidation process with evidence is through the appraisal process, appraisal will focus in the main on 'performance review' rather than personal development. Personal development requires trust and confidentiality within the appraisal process, to encourage doctors to be open and reflective about both their weaknesses and their strengths, so that a cycle of continuous improvement can be initiated. This process will inevitably play a poor second to 'performance review', which will contain the hard data for revalidation ('is this doctor good enough?'). The doctor will then want to use the appraisal process to show that he or she is indeed good enough and not that there are areas of performance which could be improved in a constructive way. The process for doctors in training and SAS grades will inevitably be part of ongoing personal/educational supervision and the appraisal process should be a natural adjunct to this.

Alongside and contributing to the appraisal process is the requirement for all psychiatrists to have a 'personal development plan' (PDP). This is partly achieved by a process of peer review, whereby groups of psychiatrists (should) come together to review the activities and objectives of their programmes of continuing professional development (CPD) (trainees in all grades will do this through their training programmes and SAS doctors either through supervision or through peer groups). The result of this cycle is individual psychiatrists preparing a peer-agreed summary of CPD activities. As psychiatrists (particularly at consultant level) develop confidence in the peer review process and different styles emerge of enabling these review groups to work, it may well be that this development and support network becomes a key and integral part of the psychiatrist's working life.

What is less clear is how this peer-reviewed personal development plan (form E in the current College documentation) links to the personal development plan (form 4 of the Department of Health's appraisal documentation). The College's form E, concentrating on CPD, informs the development of an agreed 'appraisal PDP', which should be a mix of CPD and other objectives (which may include service developments, more specific career choices and other activities) which consultants undertake through their often varied careers. This process should help to redress the balance that leans heavily towards performance review within the annual cycle of appraisal and to ensure that the personal development of each consultant is planned and incorporated within the process.

A new development, still to be clarified (Department of Health, 2007), is the role of the College in assessing psychiatrists with specialist qualifications for 'recertification'.

Trusts will have a key role to play in ensuring that sufficient information is available for consultants to draw together the data that will enable appropriate monitoring of performance. It is difficult to see how appraisers and eventually revalidation teams will be able to make much sense of raw data provided by individual consultants unless there are comparative data also provided for other similar teams or services. The trust should be able, with the consultant, to provide some narrative which will outline what the data actually means and how they reflect on individual practice. Table 24.1 gives a practical overview of the type of information which psychiatrists should provide for appraisal, and the link in the future to the 'external revalidation' process (relicensing and recertification).

Job planning

Job planning is also a two-way process. It is central to effective appraisal and performance management and review. The job plan helps psychiatrists at consultant grade to be explicit about what they do and when they do it, and helps to clarify the expectations of the service of the individual doctor as well. The relationship between the 'job plan' and the notional weekly timetable needs to be reviewed and the structure and expectation of services provided by NHS psychiatrists should become more realistic as a result.

Trusts have traditionally invested little time and effort in the appointment and induction process for new consultants (and SAS grades) and this critical phase can ensure that performance meets service need. Anecdotally, it is common for services to bring in a new consultant 'thrown in at the deep end', leaving only the job description and timetable as a blueprint for that consultant's performance in the early years. In addition, it seems equally common that services are often disappointed (after the first few years of a new consultant appointment) that the consultant has not achieved the expectations that the service harboured. A challenge to services is that consultants are often not given clear objectives which explicitly spell out the service expectation of their first few years, given feedback of their performance against these expectations, and given the mentoring and support required to achieve these objectives.

The reasons why this might occur are complex and numerous, but include service reluctance to engage in the feedback process for new consultants (this is often left to a hard-pressed and under-resourced medical manager).

New Ways of Working (Department of Health, 2005*b*) provides a strategic framework for psychiatrists (and the services in which they work) to re-evaluate what psychiatrists do, and whether there is a better (locally appropriate) way of working that meets both the long-term career aspirations and needs of the psychiatrist and the delivery of better care to patients and their carers.

How well does the psychiatrist do it?

'Every consultant being appraised should prepare an appraisal folder. This is a systematically recorded set of all documents: information, evidence and data which will help inform the appraisal process.' (Department of Health, 2001)

This document goes on to state that:

'the appraisal process will not result in the generation of significant amounts of new evidence or information, rather it will capture the information that already exists. What goes into the folder will, for the most part, be available from clinical governance activity, the job planning process and other existing sources. One result of the appraisal process will be to identify gaps to be filled or where perhaps data needs to be better collated or presented. This is likely to be more apparent in the early years after appraisal is launched.'

However, if the revalidation process requires a level of data collection that is not in place in the early years for appraisal, there is considerable room for concern and confusion for psychiatrists.

The development of positive measures of performance will be key in the coming years. Most consultants work as members of one or more clinical teams, and it is often the performance of the team against which consultants measure their own performance. Team performance varies over time, often for reasons well beyond the control of the individual consultant, and extrapolating these measures of performance as direct indicators of the doctor's is tricky. More useful measures will be gained by looking at absolute figures directly relating to the work of the doctor, for example prescribing practices within a team. Few services are currently configured to provide consultants with accurate data to support these important aspects of performance review, although the development of well-designed clinical information systems will go some way to doing so.

Doctors will also routinely present 'indirect' data of 'how well they do' of varying relevance to answering the actual question, such as complaints from patients, serious untoward incidents and related investigations (some excellent doctors work within a service that generates significant complaints, because of the nature of either the service itself or the patient group, and some poorly performing doctors are rarely complained about by patients even though colleagues and members of the team are well aware of their deficiencies).

Giving and receiving feedback

Doctors have traditionally not been trained in giving and receiving feedback about performance. This is changing, and as part of the appraisal process psychiatrists are increasingly seeking effective means of receiving high-quality feedback from peers, managers, referrers, members of the clinical team, doctors in training and patients and carers. A number of simple and brief 360° appraisal tools are available. The Royal College of Psychiatrists has developed a comprehensive 360° appraisal package specific to psychiatrists that is now available for widespread use.

Dealing with poorly performing doctors

How to approach poor performance in a colleague

Medical and non-medical managers alike have traditionally shied away from proactively dealing with doctors where questions about performance are raised. Raising a 'cause for concern' at an early stage can go some way to resolving the problem, although some doctors will respond poorly to perceived criticism even at an early and 'reflective' stage. The culture of medical practice still militates against doctors, and particularly those at consultant level, accepting feedback as something other than negative and unjustified criticism or interference in their 'autonomous practice'.

The profile of a poorly performing doctor

McManus & Vincent (1997) describe principal characteristics of the poorly performing doctor broadly as follows:

- medical and technical errors of judgement
- personality factors of various kinds
- inability to work in a team
- poor communication and lack of social skills
- mental health problems.

Some further characteristics of poorly performing doctors (not in any order) are listed below:

- being out of touch
- poor recognition of the roles of the multidisciplinary team
- poor time-keeping
- bullying
- little understanding of the workings of the NHS
- intolerant of risk management processes
- resistant to peer review
- no previous participation in any form of supervision

- denial of problems identified by others
- defensive and offensive when challenged
- feels that quality improvement is what other members of the team need to do
- reflective and open practice is resisted
- believes that users and carers have a high regard for their practice despite evidence to the contrary
- indecisive and at the same time controlling
- often described as arrogant by members of the team
- always offers only concrete solutions to problems (e.g. more resources, more doctors).

Checklist for managers in improving doctors' performance

Clearly thought out employment structures provide a framework for improving performance, and equip the medical manager with the skills and support to undertake the task at hand when individual performance occasionally falls below an acceptable standard. Such structures will include the following:

- *Clear lines of accountability within services.* Trusts should outline clearly to whom doctors are accountable, both professionally and managerially.
- *Clear job plans.* Newly appointed doctors often have to rely on rather flimsy outlines of what is expected of them (see 'Job planning', above). Services should ensure that all newly appointed doctors have a full induction; this is often well laid out for doctors in training, but less so for new consultants; it could be anticipated that consultants (and career-grade non-consultant staff) who are clear about the service and its expectations of them will find it easier to perform their job well.
- *Recruitment and retention.* Having full recruitment into medical posts can be critical in ensuring doctors are then able to perform to the highest standard. Services which rely on locum cover or on consultants extending their remit well beyond what they could safely do place both the service and the medical staff at risk. Even hard-pressed clinical services where recruitment is a particular problem should think very carefully before recruiting or continuing to tolerate a poorly performing doctor. Doctors should be appointed only after careful scrutiny of appropriate references, and it is advisable for employing organisations always to ensure that they have had a reference from the most recent employer; if not, they must be fully satisfied as to the reason why. *New Ways of Working* gives employers an opportunity to review the profile of consultant posts that are hard to fill and possibly to come up with 'better jobs'. However, if the local pool from which psychiatrists are being recruited is small, even the best jobs may not attract recruits.

- *Professional roles*. As indicated above, a professional's role should be outlined in a proper period of induction. It is often difficult for organisations to ensure that doctors are fully cognisant of policy, procedure and practice developments. It is useful as part of 'in-house' education and training programmes to keep doctors up to date with the trust's clinical priorities, and to get them actively participating in setting the agenda for policy and practice.

- *Advice and training*. Medical managers, consultants and tutors should have access to sound advice and training on the principles of dealing with performance problems.

- *Collaboration*. Consultants who work in isolation are often most vulnerable. Trusts should increasingly encourage clinical teams to work more closely together, as this will provide a way in which consultants associated with those teams can receive support. The same applies to medical managers, who need to share expertise and receive high-quality support from other managers, as well as to able to access support at a more personal level from medical managers within the organisation or from other trusts.

- *Mentoring and coaching*. Mentoring (particularly but not exclusively for new consultants) and coaching for more experienced consultants and those taking on medical management roles will help maximise their personal effectiveness.

- *Leadership*. There are a range of initiatives in developing the leadership role of doctors. The concept of co-leadership and the leadership role of the doctor alongside team leader or other senior clinicians provides for interesting models and training opportunities.

- *Peer review*. The Royal College of Psychiatrists expects all consultants to participate in formal, regular peer review processes. The College has laid out clear standards for participation in CPD. While many doctors may find the detail of the process daunting, the basic principle of meeting with a small group of professional colleagues three or four times a year to agree the outline of individual CPD needs and plans is both simple and compelling.

- *Appraisal*. The appraisal process is usually an annual cycle, and on rare occasions it may be the first opportunity an appraiser has to bring a concern about performance to the attention of a consultant. However, it is both unwise and unhelpful to deal with significant performance concerns only through this process, and if a service is aware of performance concerns these should have been brought to the attention of the doctor well in advance of an appraisal meeting. However, conversely, it is equally inappropriate to be engaged in the management of poor performance and not have this formally recorded within the appraisal process.

- *Human resources and disciplinary policies*. All medical managers are advised to refer closely to all relevant human resources policies when considering any issues relating to the performance or conduct of doctors. Copies of relevant policies should be made available to any doctor under investigation, and the terms and parameters of the investigation should be clearly laid out (see 'Suspension (exclusion) of doctors', below).

The process of dealing with poor performance

The National Clinical Assessment Service (NCAS), now part of the National Patient Safety Authority, provides advice and assessment where serious performance concerns are expressed about a doctor.

The disciplinary procedures for doctors are set out in the document *Maintaining High Professional Standards in the Modern NHS* (Department of Health, 2005a); these replaced an older set of procedures, dating from 1990. The steps in the new disciplinary procedure are described below.

Identification of the problem

This is possibly the most complex and important element of the process. Although staff are often quick to bring a performance problem to the attention of managers or senior colleagues, it often proves difficult to translate this into a clear outline of the nature and severity of the problem. Staff are often anxious about their concerns being made known to the consultant, fearing that this might lead to bullying or harassment, and certainly a potential change in the functioning of the clinical team. However, without a clear and open concern being expressed it is difficult to proceed with even an informal investigation to ascertain the facts. It is often unhelpful to proceed with fact-finding without the knowledge of the consultant, as it can contribute to more entrenched positions being taken up.

The 'whistle-blowing' policies of the Public Interest Disclosure Act 1998 came about because of the reluctance of staff to raise concerns about more senior colleagues. They allow complainants to remain anonymous, which, as outlined above, can make it difficult to move effectively to an open investigative phase without problem. Those policies should certainly protect any employee from being targeted or victimised for having 'blown the whistle'.

Service-wide data on performance may be available which show up deficits in the work of an individual consultant, but, on occasion, the only way forward is to initiate a formal collection of particular service-wide data. This information may confirm a suspected performance deficit. Looking for evidence of poor decision-making, for example, by going on a 'fishing expedition' through a consultant's case-load without explicit agreement, or without or at least making it known to the consultant that a serious performance problem is being investigated, often leads to early souring of relationships and difficulty in the re-establishment of working relationships. It can also be challenged if a formal disciplinary process ensues (and any decision to dismiss based on such a process would most likely fall foul of any employment tribunal).

Recording of the facts

If performance problems concerning a consultant are raised through any channel, expert advice should be sought from the trust's director of human resources. Given the difficulties that can arise at a later date, the chief executive should also be informed. The cause for concern should be recorded; if it is given verbally, attempts should be made to have a written account prepared by the person making the complaint or bringing the problem to the attention of the organisation. Careful records should be kept that note the times and dates of correspondence and communications, as these could be called for at a later date, from a number of different sources.

Cause for concern

It is often the case that less than optimal performance in an individual occurs in a number of different modalities at different times, which can make it difficult for the medical manager to deal with as a single issue in a focused way. An example of this would be a consultant who has difficulties with the multidisciplinary team, from whom a number of complaints are then received. Each complaint is about a different issue and there is little relationship between them, or necessarily with the problem encountered in team working. The complaints are dealt with individually, and then the consultant handles a clinical case in a way which gives cause for concern. Each of the problems is, in itself, enough for a single discussion, but if the consultant is unwilling to engage in a reflective discussion about these multiple but essentially unrelated issues, the system makes it difficult to proceed to a more formal intervention until further evidence or another incident has occurred. In addition, poor performance in consultants who have proceeded through higher training and been established within the NHS for some time is often combined with problems in personal and professional relationships, and this causes added problems for the manager responsible for responding to and dealing with poor performance. However, a series of complaints indicating poor team working can be dealt together, but it is essential that there is good communication between managers to enable this to happen.

It is helpful for services to identify what they consider to be less than optimal performance earlier rather than later and this can be done by bringing any concerns to the attention of the consultant informally. This can then be linked to the appraisal process in terms of personal development plans and any special measures that may be agreed to help the consultant deal with these difficulties. It is a measure of how anxious medical managers are at bringing these issues to the attention of a colleague that, often, a serious investigation is launched into the performance of an individual who is hearing this concern for the first time.

Equal opportunities

Most doctors will at some time be directly involved in the employment and management of other doctors and must have received training in equal opportunities employment procedures. This is thrown into clear relief in all issues relating to performance, for which a (basic) knowledge of the legislation is required, with particular reference to the Sex Discrimination Act, the Race Relations Act, the Disability Discrimination Act, the Employment Equality Regulations and the Race Relations Amendment Act. As a result of such legislation, a number of possible actions on the part of employers are now identified as clearly unlawful. A core standard against which to measure all actions in relation to either employment or poor performance is that all aspects of the process are *fair* and that the medical management and employer can justify those actions.

Conclusion

The assessment of medical performance and the management of poor performance are complex and time-consuming. In this chapter I have outlined some broad principles and related them to practical issues. Progress has been made in setting standards for psychiatric medical practice, as with the introduction of the new medical disciplinary framework. On those rare occasions where there is a link between poor performance and issues of medical discipline, it remains to be seen whether the new processes actually help medical managers and organisations (and the poorly performing doctor) to address the issues and move appropriately to improve performance and to protect patients.

At the time of going to press the ground is moving under the profession with regard to revalidation and professional regulation and the roles of the GMC and the Royal Colleges, but we can hope that common sense will prevail and medical managers will be able to work with colleagues in a collaborative way to improve performance and, in a small number of cases, given the necessary tools, take the action required to protect patients and the public.

References

Bewley, B. & Bewley, T. (1990) Doctors as an example: smoking and drinking. *Health Trends*, **22**, 45.

Department of Health (1999) *Supporting Doctors, Protecting Patients*. Department of Health.

Department of Health (2000) *Consultants Contract: Annual Appraisal for Consultants* (AL(MD)6/2000). Department of Health.

Department of Health (2001) *Appraisal for Consultants Working in the NHS: Guidance*. Department of Health.

Department of Health (2005*a*) *Maintaining High Professional Standards in the Modern NHS*. Department of Health.

Department of Health (2005*b*) *New Ways of Working for Psychiatrists: Enhancing Effective, Person-Centred Services Through New Ways of Working in Multidisciplinary and Multiagency Contexts. Final Report 'but not the end of the story…'*. Department of Health.

Department of Health (2007) *Trust, Assurance and Safety: The Regulation of Health Professionals in the 21st Century* (Cm 7013). The Stationery Office.

Donaldson, L. J. (1994) Doctors with problems in an NHS workforce. *BMJ*, **308**, 1277–1282.

General Medical Council (1996) *Good Medical Practice*. General Medical Council.

General Medical Council (1999) *Maintaining Good Medical Practice*. General Medical Council.

General Medical Council (2006) *Good Medical Practice*. General Medical Council.

Ghodse, H. (2000) Who heals the healers? In *Doctors and Their Health* (eds H. Ghodse, S. Mann & P. Johnson), pp. 10–14. Reed.

Hewitt, P. (2007) Foreword. In *Trust, Assurance and Safety – The Regulation of Health Professionals in the 21st Century* (Cm 7013). The Stationery Office.

HM Government (2005) *The Kerr/Haslam Inquiry* (vols I & II) (Cm 6640). The Stationery Office.

Lens, P. & van der Wal, G. (1997) *Problem Doctors: A Conspiracy of Silence*. IOS Publishing.

McManus, C. & Vincent, C. A. (1997) Can future poor performance be identified during selection? In *Problem Doctors: A Conspiracy of Silence* (eds P. Lens & G. van der Wal), pp. 7–13. IOS Publishing.

Roy, D. & Secker Walker, J. (1995) Deal with colleagues with problems. In *How To Do It, Vol. 1: Management, Employment and Counselling* (3rd edn) (ed. D. Reece), pp. 66–75. BMJ Publishing.

Royal College of Psychiatrists (2001) *Good Psychiatric Practice: CDP* (CR90). Royal College of Psychiatrists.

Royal College of Psychiatrists (2004) *Good Psychiatric Practice*. Royal College of Psychiatrists.

Shipman Inquiry (2004) *Fifth Report – Safeguarding Patients: Lessons from the Past – Proposals for the Future*, Cm 6394. HMSO.

Chatterjee v. *City and Hackney Community Services NHS Trust* [1998] 49 BMLR 55.

CHAPTER 25

Clinical audit

Adrian James

Clinical audit is a central component of clinical governance and is the principal tool for ensuring that healthcare is delivered to the required standard and continuously improves. It has been defined as:

'a quality improvement process that seeks to improve patient care and outcomes through systematic review of care against explicit criteria and the implementation of change. Aspects of the structure, processes, and outcomes of care are selected and systematically evaluated against explicit criteria. Where indicated, changes are implemented at an individual, team, or service level and further monitoring is used to confirm improvement in healthcare delivery' (National Institute for Clinical Excellence, 2002: p. 1).

Participation in clinical audit by hospital doctors was made mandatory with the publication of a *First Class Service* (Department of Health, 1998) and is a requirement set out in *Good Psychiatric Practice* (Royal College of Psychiatrists, 2004). Done well, it can lead to significant and sustained improvement in outcomes for users, but at its worst it can be a demoralising waste of time that diverts precious clinical time away from patients. This chapter provides a framework to ensure that clinical audit is a worthwhile component of the quality improvement toolkit.

History

Clinicians have for millennia audited outcomes and it is reported that King Hammurabi of Babylon in 1750 BC instigated audit for clinicians with regard to outcome, with hazardous outcomes for those not performing well (Clinical Governance Support Team, 2005). Medical audit became part of mainstream practice in the National Health Service (NHS) after the publication of *Working for Patients* (Department of Health, 1989) and, in recognition of the multidisciplinary nature of healthcare delivery, became clinical audit in the 1990s (Department of Health, 1997).

Clinical audit can be considered the first pillar of clinical governance to be erected and was a key component of the Commission for Healthcare

Improvement's clinical governance reviews. With the publication of *Standards for Better Health* (Department of Health, 2004), there may appear to be evidence that the pillar is crumbling, as the seven pillars of clinical governance were replaced by seven domains (safety, clinical effectiveness and cost-effectiveness, governance, patient focus, accessible and responsive care, care environment and amenities, and public health) (see Chapter 18). However, closer examination reveals that, far from losing its importance, clinical audit has reached its rightful place, embedded within the other components of quality improvement, and is seen as a methodology to be applied across all aspects of governance. Instead of one pillar, it can be considered the cement that binds the rest of the governance structure together. The Healthcare Commission (http://www.healthcarecommission. org.uk) has assumed responsibility for clinical audit as the independent inspection body for both the NHS and independent healthcare. It is also responsible for the National Clinical Audit programme in England.

Clinical audit in practice

Clinical audit is a cyclical activity that starts with the establishment of clear standards in healthcare, investigates these standards to see whether they are delivered in practice, investigates the performance gap, initiates change in practice and then re-audits to ensure that real change happens. The audit cycle is illustrated in Fig. 25.1.

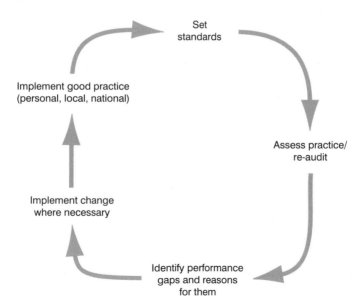

Fig. 25.1 The audit cycle.

Several stages must be completed to carry out successful audit. These include:

- *preparation* – topic selection, identification of relevant individuals to carry out the audit, identification of technical support, and ensuring that those involved are appropriately trained
- *selection of criteria* – identification of the process or outcome of care to be audited, ensuring that criteria are explicit, measurable and related to important aspects of care
- *measuring performance* – finding relevant sources of data, such as patient registers, collecting relevant data
- *making improvements* – feedback of results to relevant individuals, dissemination in a variety of ways and agreement with key stakeholders (including users) as to what needs to be done to improve care
- *sustaining improvement* – continued monitoring and evaluation of improvement, setting up structures to ensure that improvements in care are integrated into clinical governance programmes.

Organisation and resources

In order to progress clinical audit in a systematic way, healthcare organisations will need to have either a free-standing clinical audit committee or clinical audit as a major component within another committee, such as that dealing with clinical effectiveness. The committee, in order to maintain the clinical focus, will need to be led by a senior clinician, and to have representation from across the organisation and across grades, to be truly multidisciplinary and to be supported by a clinical audit infrastructure. Suggested members are listed in Box 25.1.

Box 25.1 Suggested membership of a clinical audit committee

- Chair (senior clinician)
- User or carer representative
- Clinical audit leads from localities, directorates, services
- Representation from all disciplines
- Clinical audit manager
- Clinical audit facilitator(s)
- Information management and technology representative
- Training and development representative
- Social care representative
- Clinical effectiveness representative

It is essential to have good links with users and carers. This can be most easily achieved by having a representative on the committee, but experience has shown that this is often not found by users to be of significant benefit, and attendance at local user forums by a member of the clinical audit committee can be a more effective means of engagement. It is essential to have good links with information management and technology and training departments, and with the other areas of governance. Clinical audit must be seen as a methodology to be used by the other areas of governance and intrinsic to their workings.

A clinical audit programme will require both clinical leadership and effective management of clinical audit resources. It is usual to have a clinical audit manager, who may manage other areas of governance, with facilitators and audit clerks working as part of a combined department. Other models can include facilitators being embedded in directorates. This has the advantage of a closer link-up with the clinical interface but can result in isolation for the facilitators.

Each audit will need an identified lead, working with an audit project team which includes technical support, stakeholders who are involved in bringing about change and a range of people who fully understand the process of clinical care. The clinical audit department will need to arrange an ongoing programme of training, with set-piece training days that individuals from across health organisations can come to, but also for specific teams.

It is essential that the clinical audit department has a budget. Each service and locality will need its own clinical audit lead.

Key tasks for the clinical audit committee include ensuring that audit is effectively supported, prioritising audit that meets appropriate criteria, performance monitoring and feedback through such mechanisms as the Healthcare Commission standards, which are part of the performance monitoring of trusts, and production of a strategy, annual report and work plan, with clear actions and timescales.

Programme

The National Institute for Clinical Excellence (2002) proposed an effective framework for prioritising audits (see Box 25.2). Suggested audit topics are listed in Box 25.3. Audit topics are inevitably dictated to some degree by the state of maturity of the audit environment within the organisation. While audit infrastructure is evolving, the selection of bottom-up, straightforward audit by motivated staff can be prudent. As confidence, support and sophistication develop and the benefits of audit are plain for all to see, more ambitious topics can be taken on. Audit can be undertaken at various levels: individual practice, team, service, trust-wide, regional or national (e.g. the audit of violence and aggression sponsored by the Healthcare Commission and coordinated by the Royal College of Psychiatrists' Research Unit).

Box 25.2   Criteria for prioritisation of clinical audit topics

- Topic has been identified by service users as an area of concern or where change is necessary
- There is evidence of a serious quality problem
- There is potential for involvement in a national audit project
- It is linked to organisational priorities
- There is good evidence to inform standards (e.g. national clinical guidelines)
- The topic is concerned with risk to staff or users
- The topic addresses a high-cost activity
- The topic is linked to a national priority or guidance

Box 25.3   Some suggested clinical audit topics in psychiatry

- Note-keeping
- Documentation for the care programme approach
- Customer care (e.g. information for patients)
- Timeliness of interventions
- Critical incident or sentinel event audit (e.g. following suicide)
- Emergency re-admissions
- Mental Health Act documentation (e.g. consent to treatment)
- Guidelines from the National Institute for Health and Clinical Excellence (e.g. on the treatment of schizophrenia)

A key aspect to all audits is the setting of standards for each topic, as audit should not be seen as merely a monitoring exercise. Care should be delivered according to the evidence of effective practice. Geddes (2005) suggests five stages in applying evidence-based practice:

1   Ask a structured, answerable clinical question.
2   Find the evidence.
3   Critically appraise the evidence.
4   Apply the evidence to the clinical problem.
5   Assess and improve the process.

Some sources of this sort of evidence are suggested in Box 25.4.

Making a difference

Clinical audit is a pointless and even damaging enterprise unless real improvements in patient care result. Much depends upon creating the right environment in terms of structure and culture, to allow audit to

---

Box 25.4   Sources of evidence in mental health practice

- Royal College of Psychiatrists (http://www.rcpsych.ac.uk)
- Cochrane Library – through the National electronic Library for Health (http://www.nelh.nhs.uk)
- *Evidence-Based Mental Health* (http://ebmh.bmj.com)
- *Clinical Evidence* (compendium) (http://www.clinicalevidence.com)
- Mental Health Specialist Library (http://www.library.nhs.uk/mentalhealth)
- National Service Frameworks (http://www.dh.gov.uk/en/Policyandguidance/Healthandsocialcaretopics/DH_4070951)
- National Institute for Health and Clinical Excellence (http://www.nice.org.uk)

---

flourish. Good project design lies at the heart of all quality improvement and this starts with effective strategy, setting appropriate priorities and topic selection (see Box 25.5). A culture must be created where practice is critically examined and professionals feel able to say that they are getting it wrong. At the heart of all good audits lies user and carer involvement, alongside the involvement of those whose practice is likely to change as a result of audit, so that all key stakeholders buy into not only the audit itself but also its outcomes. Many methodologically sound audits flounder because not enough effort is put into communicating findings and achieving change in clinical practice. If action points just entail shouting at the system or mere assertion that certain practices must change, then little effective is likely to happen. Effective education and training must underpin practice advancement.

Box 25.5   Top tips for effective audit

- Good project design
- Preparation
- Involving stakeholders in the audit and outcomes
- Topic selection
- Use of clinical audit facilitators
- A venue to present audits to a wider stakeholder group
- Action points from audits discussed at wider clinical governance meetings and regularly updated
- User involvement
- Information technology representation on audit committee
- End-of-year audit of audits to follow up action points

Standards for Better Health

Standards for Better Health (Department of Health, 2004) provides reporting guidance for quality issues across the NHS. These standards were heralded as a breakthrough in being clear, broad and overarching, while allowing local determination of what works best. The seven traditional pillars of governance were replaced by seven domains (see 'History', above, and Chapter 18). Within each domain, there are core standards (24 in total), which pull together existing standards and are described in the document as being 'not optional', along with ten developmental standards, which suggest improvements needed for the future. *Standards for Better Health* draws together in one place the standards reflecting the complex range of existing standards, guidance and guidelines that already existed for the NHS.

At first glance, clinical audit could appear to have been downgraded in importance with the publication of the document, as there is no separate clinical audit domain. In fact, however, audit runs through each domain as a key tool or methodology to use in assessing performance. It is seen as a resource used to ensure the implementation of safe, clinically effective and cost-effective, patient-focused, accessible and responsive care within an appropriate environment.

Although found within each domain, reference to clinical audit is most explicit within the second domain, of clinical effectiveness and cost-effectiveness. There is specific reference, as a core standard, to clinicians participating in regular clinical audit and reviews of clinical services. Clinical audit methodology is implicit in the developmental standards, such as the requirement to conform to nationally agreed best practice, such as guidance from the National Institute for Health and Clinical Excellence. Under the third domain, of governance, one developmental standard states that healthcare organisations must work together to implement a cycle of continuous quality improvement and, again, clinical audit is a key part of this. Time will tell whether these new arrangements lead to a downgrading of clinical audit, or whether it will achieve its rightful place at the heart of all aspects of clinical governance activity.

Ethics and confidentiality

Ethical consideration should apply to all medical practice. However, audit is often excluded from the remit of research ethics committees. In order to avoid the minefield of ethical consideration, there is an ongoing temptation to label research as audit (Warlow, 2004).

Research investigates what should be done, whereas audit investigates whether it is being done. The reason for distinguishing between the two should not be to avoid appropriate ethical scrutiny. Ethical consideration is necessary when the involved parties have different interests or values and

---

Box 25.6 Circumstances of audit that requires external ethical scrutiny

- Degree of conflict arising from competing interests of the investigator, clinician or other responsible party is great
- Burden on the patient is great (time, effort and discomfort)
- Risks are moderate to high
- Potential benefit to the patient is likely to be small
- Potential benefit for society is likely to be small
- Low likelihood of audit succeeding in its stated aim

---

there is the potential for conflict between the burden and risk imposed on patients or others (including society) and the likely benefits (Wade, 2005). If an audit will involve minimal change in practice and only minor risks and limited burdens, then it would rarely require specific ethical consideration. However, if an audit potentially puts patients at significant risk, if there is potential for great change in practice, or if there is a significant burden, and particularly where benefits are likely to be small, then external ethical review becomes vital and should be obtained from a properly constituted independent ethics committee. Box 25.6 shows the circumstances in which clinical audit is likely to require external ethical scrutiny.

A further issue is that of confidentiality. If changes do occur, then findings need wide dissemination. Identifiable patient data must be anonymised or patient consent obtained. Individual practitioners must be also be anonymised unless they have agreed to be identifiable to a wider audience. However, even if the clinicians are anonymised, it is still important that they are given feedback on the results of audit.

Future developments

The future for clinical audit depends much upon the future of the quality domains in *Standards for Better Health*. Clinical audit is likely to become the key to all quality improvement processes. Much will depend upon mental health services' abilities to develop robust standards and indicators, and to improve information management and technology, in order to provide an effective tool in the quest for quality and in providing a framework to bring about change. Quality improvement is at the heart of audit activity. As methodology and analysis become more sophisticated, the possibility has been raised that routinely collected hospital data and audit findings could be used to anticipate or predict future individual or service poor performance, so that wider interventions can be implemented before major harm is done (Harley *et al*, 2005). This is a fine aspiration but much needs to be done to develop robust systems to enable it to happen.

References

Clinical Governance Support Team (2005) *A Practical Handbook for Clinical Audit*. Clinical Governance Support Team. See www.cgsupport.nhs.uk

Department of Health (1989) *Working for Patients*. TSO (The Stationery Office).

Department of Health (1997) *The New NHS. Modern, Dependable*. TSO (The Stationery Office).

Department of Health (1998) *A First Class Service. Quality in the New NHS*. Department of Health.

Department of Health (2004) *Standards for Better Health*. TSO (The Stationery Office).

Geddes, J. (2005) Evidence-based practice. In *Clinical Governance in Mental Health and Learning Disability Services. A Practical Guide* (eds A. James, A. Worrall & T. Kendall), pp. 149–158. Gaskell.

Harley, M., Mohammed, M., Hussain, S., *et al* (2005) Was Rodney Ledward a statistical outlier? Retrospective analysis using routine hospital data to identify gynaecologists' performance. *BMJ*, **330**, 929–933.

National Institute for Clinical Excellence (2002) *Principles for Best Practice in Clinical Audit*. Radcliffe Medical Press.

Royal College of Psychiatrists (2004) *Good Psychiatric Practice* (Council Report CR125). Royal College of Psychiatrists.

Wade, D. T. (2005) Ethics, audit and research: all shades of grey. *BMJ*, **300**, 468–472.

Warlow, C. (2004) Clinical Research under the cosh again. This time it is ethics committees. *BMJ*, **329**, 241–242.

CHAPTER 26

Quality improvement tools for healthcare

Paul Walley, Simon Baugh and Kate Silvester

A number of recent improvement programmes, such as the Emergency Services Collaborative and Improvement Partnership for Hospitals, have used quality methodologies specially adapted for healthcare. The tools have produced good results and have shown their effectiveness where they have been implemented correctly and used appropriately. Most healthcare organisations have at least a small team involved in quality or process improvement using these tools, but general use of the methods has not yet spread across organisations or between organisations to any great extent. This is partly because of a lack of understanding of the advantages of such approaches. In this chapter, we introduce the main tools and techniques that we see as the most useful for clinicians. Our objective is that all staff should see that external quality improvement methods, rather than being some management fad or political initiative, do actually have a sustainable, positive contribution to make in the development of health services.

Establishing the direction for improvement work

UK collaborative programmes have shown that most UK healthcare systems face similar issues in relation to process and quality improvement. There are some common principles, therefore, that we can adopt to tackle the underlying causes of poor performance.

Harnessing the patient's perspective

Because clinicians and other healthcare staff care about the welfare of their patients, it is difficult for some to accept that current, local approaches to the specification and design of healthcare systems are insufficiently focused on patient needs. The idea of increased 'patient focus' is seen as a piece of management jargon rather than a meaningful attempt to help improve healthcare. In fact, there are a number of ways in which existing methods of specification of health services fall short of the most desirable outcome.

First, clinical protocols tend to focus on the technical aspects of a treatment episode; also, any one protocol can be delivered in many different ways. This restricts the ability of the organisation to deliver the service effectively and it does not factor the patient's service experience into the specification. Second, patient demand for services can be misunderstood. Existing methods of recording clinical activity do not accurately reflect types of demand that are being placed on the system. In most cases, activity measures reflect all attempts to access services, including patients who make multiple (failed) attempts to receive services from different forms of provider within the system (e.g. general practitioner, accident and emergency department, NHS Direct), and they do not reflect the patient's desired first choice or the level of rework caused by quality problems. Third, system design should not simply be about clinical effectiveness at the lowest unit cost. Aspects of patient-focused quality can be used to move organisations away from ineffective, high-utilisation, low-accessibility service design towards ones that have been genuinely designed around aspects of performance that are consistent with patient needs.

Looking at the end-to-end patient journey

In the well-known management book about 'lean thinking', Womack & Jones (1996) explain how the retailer Tesco made large-scale improvements to its procurement and logistics systems. Using a study of one typical product (a pack of cola cans), the company discovered that its supply chain was organised as a series of optimised factories, each doing its bit as efficiently as it could. This meant that these 'factories' were actually incompatible with each other, because each one would refuse to operate 'sub-optimally' (i.e. with low utilisation) from its own perspective. The net effect was work that could have taken less than 2 days to complete if the process was 'seamless' actually took more than 300 days, as a consequence of the mismatches in the system. Almost as worrying, performance measures used to assess the process did not highlight this issue.

Healthcare improvement collaborative work has revealed similar character-istics in patient journeys. How typical is it to see yet another review of radiology, pathology, surgery and so on, with a view to making it 'more efficient'? In a high proportion of cases, these reviews make the department busier but the system less effective. There is still a need to move further away from departmental working and towards a 'process-based' view of healthcare. Organisations like the Institute for Healthcare Improvement (IHI) have been selling this message for a long time, but its significance is not always fully appreciated.

An immediate consequence of the lack of process perspective is the lack of knowledge about the existing intended and actual systems that have been designed or implemented. Experience during our research has shown that processes are routinely re-invented, and any form of standard procedure frequently does not exist. Two patients requiring the same treatment at the same time can conceivably experience two completely different processes. This creates chaos and waste in the system.

Using difference metrics and measurement approaches

A lot of performance reporting within the National Health Service (NHS) is focused on the achievement of targets and the annual reporting mechanisms for auditing purposes, and so on. These systems often lead to a poor choice of measures and the results are presented badly. For example, many hospitals report bed occupancy as a measure of the effective use of beds. This has a number of flaws. For one thing, occupancy is a surrogate measure for utilisation and we know that many occupied beds are not being used effectively. System utilisation is also a meaningless figure. Any of the following will lead to a reported increase in utilisation:

- delays to patient discharge (e.g. batching discharge, by doing rounds only twice per week)
- in-hospital waiting for the results of tests
- delays in the consultant seeing a patient admitted in emergency
- an increase in the hospital-acquired infection rate.

We would not want any of the above to happen, even though they would cause an apparent increase in resource utilisation.

Conventional management performance measurement systems share another characteristic with clinical audit processes. They use comparative statistics that do not necessarily factor in complex system changes over time. Simple two-point comparisons are inappropriate for quality improvement, as they do not take this time factor properly into account.

The effect of change needs to be measured and understood

The theoretical underpinning for this aspect of quality improvement comes from systems theory. Complex processes, such as hospital treatment, can be viewed as systems with feedback loops and amplifying effects. There is often a disconnection between the symptoms of a problem and the root causes. Systems theorists see that many attempts to improve processes fail because the interaction between different parts of the same system is not accounted for, and hence the diagnosis and remedies for the situation are flawed. 'Symptomatic relief' often makes the situation worse, not better. Improvements intended to provide long-term solutions are not sustained as the system responds to a change over time, rather than instantaneously and permanently. A classic case in point was the action by many hospitals to manage a perceived 'winter crisis' for emergency admissions by temporarily increasing the number of beds, without balancing the rest of the system. The consequence was that ward rounds slowed down owing to the extra discharge workload, reducing the discharge rate and increasing the length of stay, making the beds crisis worse.

Taking the patient's perspective

Patients' needs can never really be understood until people involved in service improvement fully appreciate all that goes on in a patient journey through the system. Process mapping has been used for many years, but the conventional methods of charting the patient journey merely identify the sequence of existing events, without consideration of the actual patient service experience. Furthermore, existing methods do not always provide mechanisms for improving the process. Two key concepts can be added to enhance the analysis to improve quality and reduce waste: asking what it is the patient should see, and looking at the value-adding steps.

What should the patient see?

'Blueprinting' as a concept has been used in the service sector extensively. According to the original idea of Shostack (1987), some parts of the process are not seen by the customer and some parts should not been seen. As a general principle, the greater the customer interference in a process, the higher the risks of quality failure. However, service participants can be a useful resource and sometimes we want to increase their degree of involvement. Therefore we can make conscious decisions about the degree of involvement of the patient in the journey. Service blueprinting identifies which parts of the process the patient can see and which parts happen without the patient's full knowledge.

Value-adding steps

A tool used by industry is value-stream mapping. This takes the conventional process map and enhances it with a discussion about which steps in a process add value, in this context from a patient's perspective. This highlights where patients are handed over unnecessarily or participate in unnecessary activities. A recent example from Royal Bolton Hospital showed that a surgical admission process took 84 steps. Of these, only 21 added value to the patient's journey. The other 63 should therefore be eliminated. This allowed staff to devise a plan to reduce the journey to 19 steps, with a consequential journey time reduction of 50% and a 25% reduction in the staff time needed to treat the patient. Originally, the patient was handed over from one member of staff to another 23 times during the journey. This could be achieved in just 13.

Understanding variation

Table 26.1 shows the number of people who did not attend a series of out-patient clinics over 5 weeks. The clinics were approximately the same

Table 26.1 Numbers of patients who did not attend clinics over a 5-week period

Clinic	Week 1	Week 2	Week 3	Week 4	Week 5	Total
A	0	0	1	0	1	2
B	1	1	0	2	0	4
C	1	0	0	0	0	1
D	0	0	1	0	0	1
E	2	1	3	0	0	6
F	0	1	0	0	0	1
G	0	0	0	0	0	0
H	1	0	2	1	0	4
Total	5	3	7	3	1	19

size. Can you see any patterns in the data? Are there any clinics that have a significantly better record than others, whose practices for getting patients to attend without fail should be copied as best practice?

You may well see some patterns in the data. Clinic G has a very good record – what is it doing right? Clinic E is responsible for nearly a third of all patients who did not attend – surely a problem? Was week 3 a holiday week when patients found it difficult to attend?

The real answer is that there is no statistical difference between these clinics in the long term. You are actually looking at a page of random numbers (with a skewed binomial distribution). Now consider the implications if managers do not realize that performance statistics suffer from random variation. We may find that all clinics are asked to copy clinic G's practices, even though this may not produce an overall performance improvement. Hopefully, the manager for clinic E will not be disciplined, as there is no substantial evidence of mismanagement.

When we study the behaviour of systems and processes, two distinct types of variation are classified:

1 *Common cause variation.* This is variation that results from a wide variety of constant causes. Common cause variation will always happen, but we would like to minimise it.
2 *Special cause variation.* Some variation can be assigned to external factors that are not likely to happen constantly. These factors should not cause us to adjust out behaviour completely after assuming such an event will happen each time. We just make contingency plans to respond to special causes.

Statistical process control

Some of the following has already been discussed in Chapter 15, but it is included here for ease of following the argument.

The established way of assessing process variation is called statistical process control (SPC). The method has been used by industry for over 50 years. SPC can be used:

- to monitor a process
- to measure the quality of output from a process
- to develop an understanding of the behaviour of a process
- to measure the effect of a process change on performance.

When SPC is compared with clinical audit methods of assessment, it has two key strengths. First, it does not rely on comparisons of behaviour from two samples taken at the same point in time. This avoids the simple errors associated with conventional hypothesis testing. Second, it reveals how a system works over time, showing characteristics such as the sustainability of change. A problem associated with evidence-based assessment of management interventions is that situations are always multivariate. How do we know that a change in behaviour is caused by the change that we introduced? We cannot provide a statistically valid number of control samples – there are not enough hospitals in the country to do so! Instead, we interpret from control charts, produced at a single case site.

The standard SPC chart

In healthcare, the most commonly found SPC chart is one called the XmR chart. This takes single points of data and assesses the likely spread of those data due to variation. A minimum of 20 data points is needed to provide a meaningful starting estimate. The measure of spread is used to compute control limits above and below the mean value. Fig. 26.1 shows a typical example. (Also see Chapter 15.)

The XmR chart is used because it does not need a lot of data before it can be used satisfactorily. In most situations, the volume of work flowing through healthcare processes is too small to justify alternative sampling methods, which need a lot more data. The 'moving range' is used to

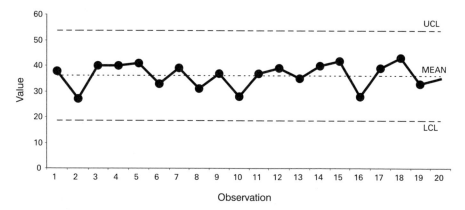

Fig. 26.1 The standard XmR SPC chart.

Table 26.2 Moving range computation from data values

	Observation									
	1	2	3	4	5	6	7	8	9	10
Value	38	27	40	40	41	33	39	31	37	28
Moving range		11	13	0	1	8	6	8	6	9

estimate the magnitude of common cause variation and this figure can be used to derive the 'process control limits'. The control limits are simply the boundaries above and below the mean that indicate 'normal' variation. The moving range is computed by finding the differences between adjacent numbers in the sequence. Table 26.2 illustrates how this can be done. The mean of the moving range figures provides an indication of the spread of the data. Upper and lower control limits are computed by taking the sample mean and adding or subtracting values from the following formulae:

Upper limit = sample mean + 2.66 × average moving range

Lower limit = sample mean − 2.66 × average moving range

These limits usually contain approximately 399 out of every 400 observations. Once in every 400 readings you might see a figure outside of these limits that is not due to a special cause. Once we start to plot new data-points, we can start to interpret the behaviour of the systems we are measuring.

Data examination

There are four circumstances when data need to be checked to see if there is any unusual process behaviour change. Fig. 26.2 shows this. There are four rules to apply.

1 *Data fall outside the control limits.* In such cases, we need to assess whether there has been a special cause event or whether the process performance has drifted without us noticing otherwise.
2 *Seven points above or below the mean or a seven-point trend.* Just like seven consecutive reds on a game of roulette, seven points consecutively above or below the mean is statistically very unlikely. Equally, a seven-point increase or decrease needs investigation.
3 *Trends and patterns.* Sometimes data show patterns such as cyclical behaviour. This indicates some time-based factor that needs to be considered.
4 *Unusual distribution of points.* Where very little data occupy the middle third of the range, this gives us clues that some system behaviour has not been anticipated. Examples would be where we are inadvertently measuring two separate processes with their own different behaviours or the process is affected by two people with different capabilities.

319

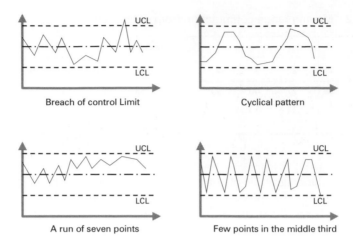

Fig. 26.2 The identification of unusual system behaviour.

For further reading of the application of SPC in healthcare, see the textbooks by Wheeler (2003*a,b*) and Carey (2002). The following examples show how SPC can be used to assess the impact of process changes.

Example 1. The Derby Royal Infirmary 'pitstop'

During work to improve throughput time in the accident and emergency department, staff at the Derby Royal Infirmary decided to develop a multidisciplinary team approach to the receipt of patients by ambulance. The analogy was made between the first point of contact and the fast refuelling seen in a Formula 1 motor racing 'pitstop'. A four-person team was developed to receive, assess, diagnose and dispatch patients rapidly to their next necessary point of contact (e.g. diagnostics). A care plan was immediately devised, so that admission to hospital could be anticipated as soon as possible. Staff wanted to measure the impact of the pitstop.

The SPC chart (Fig. 26.3) showed that the pitstop had an immediate effect on patient throughput time, indicating that the process had been designed effectively. Note that this sample of data does not show the complete data-set, as throughput time was measured continually, from this point on. The median value is used here to counteract the influence of skewed data. Later data showed that the improvement was not easily sustained. The team investigated three possible causes:

1   staff leaving the pitstop at quiet times to do other work
2   staff becoming fatigued by the work at busy times
3   individual performance variation.

The continued use of the charts allowed staff to develop greater consistency of requests for diagnostics. They also rotated staff around the pitstop so that

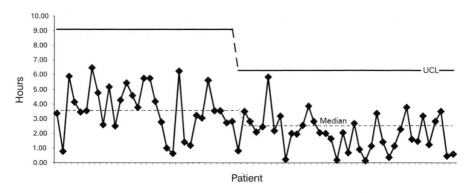

Fig. 26.3 Patient throughput time at Derby Royal Infirmary during the 'pitstop' implementation.

no one was doing the intensive work for longer than 2 hours. This ensured more consistent performance.

Example 2. Use of SPC to evaluate process improvement in mental health

This example relates to an adult in-patient mental health service with 84 beds in four single-sex wards. Service managers had become concerned, as the availability of beds had slowly decreased over the previous 3 years. The hospital was running permanently full, at times using 'client leave' beds to meet excess demand for emergency admissions.

The staff had the impression that the length of stay had been slowly increasing, which was confirmed by an analysis of the run chart for length of stay from 2003 (Fig. 26.4). The average length of stay at the end of each

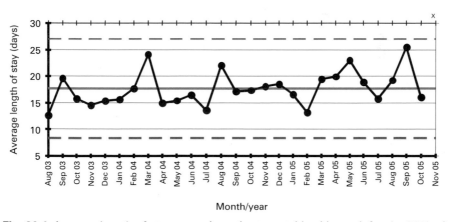

Fig. 26.4 Average length of stay on an in-patient mental health ward, for the 80% of patients comprising the shorter-stay group.

321

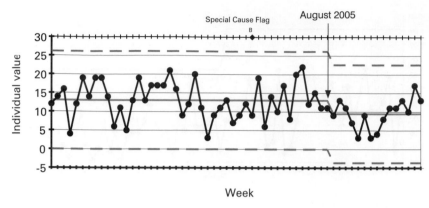

Fig. 26.5 Weekly mental health admissions.

month was calculated and the patients were split into two populations, a larger shorter-stay group, 80% of clients, and a slower stream, 20% of clients. The 80% group showed an increase in average length of stay from 2003, confirming the nursing staff's impression that the transit time through the in-patient system had slowed down.

Two changes were made to the system and measures were used to monitor their effect on the operation of the acute wards. First, the 'inflow' was addressed by the setting up of a crisis team, which worked 24 hours per day and acted as a 'gatekeeper' to all adult admissions, in line with Department of Health policy. The effect of this service development is shown in the weekly admission chart, which shows a drop in admissions per week from August 2005 (Fig. 26 .5).

The second change was to have three dedicated in-patient consultants working just on the admission wards. This increased the availability of expert medical opinion early in an admission ('front-loading') and thereby removed the 'batching' of discharges away from weekly ward rounds towards rapid discharge as soon as the client was well enough to move on.

The effect of this is shown in the daily bed availability run chart, which covers the period from April 2005 to the end of November that year (Fig. 26.6). This chart clearly illustrates the over-occupancy (often above 100%), with the mean occupancy of 83 beds being only 1 bed below the total availability of 84.

Two changes are apparent in this chart:

1   The first drop, from August 2005, is the result of the crisis team reducing admissions by effective gatekeeping, although the rise later in the chart may reflect the effect of the crisis team filling up to capacity and overflowing again into the in-patient unit.

2   The second and bigger drop is the rapid effect of dedicated in-patient consultants speeding up the assessment of admissions and removing the batching in the discharge process.

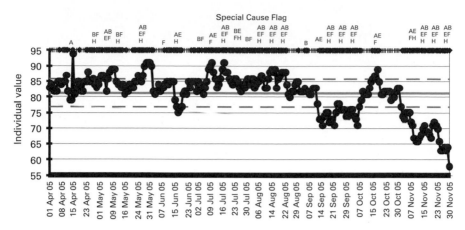

Fig. 26.6 Bed availability.

Conclusion

This chapter has shown how quality management tools used by industry for many years can be used to assist in the improvement of healthcare processes. There is now a growing body of evidence to support such an approach. Although many healthcare practitioners may believe that they have seen this type of work before, it has rarely been sustained, owing to a lack of appreciation of the benefits, a lack of fit with conventional clinical methods of assessment and some unwillingness to use industrial tools.

Healthcare systems comprise a set of interdependent, complex processes. Change to one part of a process has implications for other parts of the system as a whole. This often results in the attempted improvements not happening or the improvement not being sustained. SPC can be used to detect the effect of process change and provides an objective means of assessment, not just of the immediate impact, but also of the sustainability of the change. Once control systems are designed to use SPC, it offers a relatively simple and fast means of providing evidence for the effectiveness of change.

References

Carey, R. G. (2002) *Improving Healthcare with Control Charts*. ASQ Quality Press.

Shostack, G. L. (1987) Service positioning through structural change. *Journal of Marketing*, **51**, 34–43.

Wheeler, D. J. (2003a) *Making Sense of Data*. SPC Press.

Wheeler, D. J. (2003b) *Understanding Variation: The Key to Managing Chaos*. SPC Press.

Womack, J. & Jones, D. (1996) *Lean Thinking: Banish Waste and Create Wealth in Your Organization*. Simon and Schuster.

Part III
Personal development and management

CHAPTER 27

How to manage committees

Charles Marshall

Forming, running and managing committees is all about getting things done: committees should be there to achieve a set of objectives. Far too often, they exist for historical reasons; they meet at set times because that is when they have always met, they rarely revise their membership for fear of offence and their agendas suffer from a lack of focus and direction. Such committees are often an unwelcome intrusion into the working lives of healthcare professionals or impose commitments on people beyond the scope of their everyday jobs. It stands to reason, therefore, that committees and meetings need to be set up for a specific purpose and to have substantial relevance for the people attending. It is not acceptable for people to wander out of meetings wondering why they were there in the first place.

This chapter looks at the responsibilities which need to be embraced by both organisers and participants alike, as well as some ground rules that can be applied to running meetings, be they part of a committee structure or otherwise.

Running effective meetings

Hold only necessary meetings

First, ask whether it is necessary to call a meeting at all. If the meeting involves a large amount of one-way information transfer, it may be more practical to use other means, such as email or letter. Even if there is an element of discussion to be had, then a telephone call should be considered or, where the dialogue involves more than two people, a teleconference, as these can save time and be cost-effective.

Set objectives for the meeting

It is important for all meetings to have a clear purpose. To help formulate this purpose, the following exercise can be useful.

Write down the statement 'By the end of the meeting I want the group to...'. Then note down several phrases and use them as your objectives. Having objectives will help in an evaluation of the meeting afterwards (it is important to assess how successful any meeting has been – see below).

Provide an agenda

Use the objectives which have been decided upon to build the agenda. Also, take advice from the group on issues they want to discuss before the meeting. Rather than have the agenda in the room when people arrive, send it out several days before the meeting and include:

- a brief set of objectives
- a list of topics – who will address each and for how long
- time, date and venue
- any background information.

Once the agenda is in place, *stick to it!*

Assign preparation

For set topics it may be advisable to delegate preparation to individuals. This will save the committee chair a lot of time and has many benefits in terms of providing a wider range of thought processes; it can also act as a developmental process for certain members of the committee or team. For problem-solving tasks, make background information available to the whole group, as solutions may be found only by utilising the strengths of the entire committee. Ensure that everyone attending the meeting understands what is expected of them and that they have the resources to deliver the task.

Control the process

Establish ground rules for the meeting:

- do not allow people to interrupt
- eliminate side conversations
- use a time-keeper
- manage minutes or records.

In order to maintain this kind of process, a wide range of skills need to be utilised (examined below). It is essential to establish a consistent process to save time at each meeting.

Assign action points

All points raised should have a resulting action and, where appropriate, a named person should take responsibility to ensure the action is undertaken.

All objectives should meet the SMART criteria – they should be specific, measurable, achievable, reviewable and time-bound.

Examine the meeting process

Allocate a few minutes at the end of the meeting to review what worked well and what could be improved. All too often, committees and meetings tend to waste time by repeating mistakes. Putting these right quickly can save time and a good deal of frustration. As a result of this analysis, formulate a plan of action for improvements in time for the next meeting

Structure

Meetings of any sort inevitably work better when structured properly. The structure is best designed by allocating specific roles to certain individuals in the meeting; some of these could be undertaken by the same person, but it could be argued that they all warrant a role in their own right.

The chair

This role is expanded upon below; however, as a broad initial overview, the chair is responsible for the set-up, operation and follow-up of the meeting. The chair:

- decides on the why, what, where, when and who in relation to the meeting
- is responsible for publishing the agenda and maintaining adherence to it during meeting
- controls the flow of the meeting, ensures actions are assigned and allocates follow-up to all the action points.
- clarifies decisions and ensures they are published.

The presenter

It could be that people are called upon to present information or a project outline to the committee. There are then certain guidelines which they should be aware of before attendance. They should be told exactly what is expected of them, given an accurate brief for the topic and told how much time has been allocated. On the day, they should provide the required information clearly and concisely, based on a thorough knowledge and understanding of the topic. There may be some unanswered questions and it is important that they are prepared for most eventualities.

A good knowledge of the available audio-visual equipment is important. It can be frustrating for other committee members if they have to waste valuable time waiting for a presenter to set up equipment.

Keeping to time is critical, as there will be other business to discuss. A good understanding between the time-keeper (see below) and the chair will help this process.

The recorder

It is a mistake for the chair to attempt to chair the meeting and take notes. An appointed committee member or dedicated secretary should be available to take minutes. Remaining attentive is clearly important, as is the ability to condense the information into key points. Decisions and actions should be documented and summaries provided as required during the meeting itself. This can help the chair stay on course and get a feel for what has been resolved and what has yet to be tackled. Any minutes from the meeting should be produced and distributed as soon as possible, pending chair approval.

The time-keeper

This could be undertaken by the chair; however, it is useful to have a back-up as the chair can often get side-tracked into process issues and it is all too easy to lose track of time in a particularly intense situation.

The participant

This is a role which should be taken more seriously. Everyone who attends the meeting should feel that their attendance is both necessary and useful. Many committees are populated by individuals who attend because they feel they must or are coerced into doing so by others. Taking a more proactive attitude to attending is the duty of all participants and the responsibility rests squarely with them.

They have a duty to arrive on time and to be well prepared. They should be able to remain attentive and alert throughout meeting, to contribute where appropriate and to be supportive of other team members – maintaining respect, keeping focused and avoiding interruptions.

The environment

It is sometimes difficult to obtain a room which is ideal for the meeting, but the layout and size of the room can have dramatic effects on whether everyone can hear what is being said, the energy levels of participants and general comfort levels (it is hard to concentrate when uncomfortable).

Some opportunity for participants to move around should be built into the meeting and the layout should be suitable for the nature of what is being discussed. Boardroom style is the traditional approach, but for larger groups cabaret style, with tables seating four or five people, works very well, particularly if there is an opportunity for smaller group work.

Process

Chairing the meeting

Leading and chairing meetings is a skill which can drastically affect the power and influence of a committee. In that context, the selection of the chair is critical. The role requires an individual with demonstrable skills in the following areas.

Involvement

While there is an individual responsibility for participants to involve themselves proactively in the meeting, there will always be differences in how comfortable people feel about this. This will give rise to disproportionate contributions from certain individuals and create an imbalance and potentially lead to animosity. It is essential from the outset, therefore, that the chair has the skill to encourage involvement from everyone.

Some kind of warm-up procedure may be advisable for unfamiliar groups, while more established groups may feel comfortable to engage from the outset.

Impartiality

Chairpersons are likely to be tempted to try to steer the proceedings of the meeting or to give their own point of view but, strictly speaking, they should resist this and focus on the process rather than the content (although this is easier said than done).

The main requirement is to ensure that all participants can express their points of view and that all delegates get the opportunity to contribute. There will be times when the chair needs to intervene to move things along, but this is very different from steering the meeting by using the position of chair to champion a particular cause.

Assertiveness

Assertive behaviour in chairing is one of the key skills required to ensure effectiveness. The line between firmness and overbearing aggression may be fine but does exist. Having sufficient respect for one's own point of view needs to be balanced by an equal respect for that of others and their right to express it.

There will be numerous occasions when the chair needs to intervene, move matters along or clarify a point of understanding; the chair needs to have enough confidence to do this without fearing the reaction of those in full flow. It may be necessary to prevent others from dominating and it is often those characters who resent it the most, but it is essential that the chair can bring in all participants and 'protect' their contributions.

Applying the ground rules established at the start is paramount to effective control of a meeting.

Staying on course

It is important to allot time to each topic and to stick to it. It is quite acceptable to call further meetings if issues cannot be resolved; people's busy schedules can jeopardise this, but if the issue is important enough it is worth reconvening. The group will often need to be pushed to reach a decision and it is important that this happens, otherwise discussions become protracted and circular. As part of the planning, enough time needs to be allocated for all topics to be concluded.

Summarising

Summarising is a useful technique as it establishes the end of the discussion, promotes clarity and understanding, and provides an impartial description of the discussion, with a clear next step. It also has the advantage of preventing the revisiting of decisions already made.

Facilitating the meeting

Facilitation is a unique process in itself and is fundamental to running meetings and committees successfully. In order to facilitate effectively, there are some core skills which should be recognised and practised.

Developing empathy and trust

Some key guidelines on the building of empathy and trust relate to the employment of certain behaviours:

- knowing everyone in the group by name
- providing encouragement and acknowledging progress within the group
- intervening only when necessary
- being honest with the group (if the chair has suggested a method and it is not working, then a degree of flexibility and understanding is likely to gain far more respect than rigidly sticking to a course of action)
- involving the whole group
- checking to see whether the group is giving agreement and support
- retaining a sense of humour (which is not to say that flippancy is appropriate, but a realistic sense of humour is important).

Questioning

Questions are the crown jewels of a good chair: they support the development of empathy and also encourage participation. They provide opportunities for clarification and will encourage people to be specific and precise.

Good questions tend to be clear, appropriate, non-judgemental, open rather than closed, and non-threatening. It is advisable to give the group some clear time to respond to questions and it is essential to listen to the answers.

Neutrality

Neutrality means suspending judgement. The chair must respect the right of everyone to their own opinion, no matter who they are and what their opinion happens to be.

- Be assertive not aggressive.
- Reflect questions and comments back to the group.
- Ask other people's opinions.
- Treat everyone equally.

Observation

Looking out for signals within the group is a key skill for good facilitation. What is said is often the tip of the iceberg. Signals provide insight into certain key factors at play within the group.

Energy and activity levels
The group's effectiveness can be seriously reduced if the group have become tired, bored or simply frustrated. A good facilitator should recognise these signs and introduce breaks or variations in activity to maintain good energy levels.

Emotional and comfort levels
A committee's role is to get things done and make things happen. It can fail to achieve its objectives if there are clear signs that members are unhappy or uncomfortable with decisions. These should be recognised and preferably resolved before the group can move forward.

It is not possible to please all the people all the time, but it is essential to be able to recognise when this is happening and to take action to minimise the impact.

Focus
Groups are renowned for straying off the point, not sticking to agendas, running over time and so on. The chair needs to be aware of the group moving outside its remit and must make a decision as to whether the diversion is appropriate or distracting. Assertion is required to move the group back on course.

Seating
The job of chair is made easier when the rest of the group can be clearly seen. Control is difficult if eye contact is not achieved. Seating can also affect group dynamics (who sits near whom, the presence of sub-groups

within the main group). Limiting 'unofficial' conversations is important to the smooth running of the meeting.

Body language
Expressions and gestures can give the chair insight into what is going on. Picking up non-verbal cues is important and may enable the chair to ask clarifying questions when there is a suspicion that something is being felt but not necessarily expressed to the rest of the group.

Intervention
Intervention is an inevitable requirement of a good chair. Timing and appropriateness are key attributes to good interventions. There are some specific points at which intervention is appropriate:

- setting the scene
- encouraging participation
- keeping on track
- time management
- clarifying issues
- helping the group reach consensus
- acknowledging feelings within the group
- monitoring energy levels
- challenging what is not being said
- dealing with individual behaviour
- feedback and review.

Dealing with problems

It would be ideal if every meeting ran smoothly, all participants played their role to perfection and the chair had merely to administer the process and keep everyone on track. The real world, however, is different. Personal agendas, organisational politics and vested interests tend to get in the way. Anyone leading a committee or a meeting therefore needs to be prepared to cope with problems.

Having looked at the various principles concerned with structure and process, we now have to turn to the principles involved with managing people. This is an involved process over and above the usual management issues, as most of the people on the committee will not be directly responsible to the chair in their day-to-day jobs. Any authority must therefore be generated by the personality of the chair rather than purely the role played in the committee.

It is a matter of gaining respect from other members. Use of the skills described above will form a good foundation for this, but there will always be a need to handle individuals, both those who are and those who are not supportive. To highlight the difference, they are described here as heroes and villains. Heroes are supportive of the chair and are driven by basically good intent. Villains play games to undermine the process and disrupt progress. Both come in a variety of types, which are described below.

Heroes

While heroes may be supportive on the whole, they also need to be 'managed' in order to get the most out of them and the rest of the group.

The creative inventor

Creative inventors have a creative genius and large ego. They are vocal and have a tendency to try to dominate. It is sometimes difficult for the group to understand where they are coming from.

They need involvement, recognition and to be delegated to, as they have huge amounts of energy and enthusiasm. They will also need to be focused and controlled in order to stop them running away with ideas and initiatives.

The realist

Realists display focus, objectivity and attention to detail. They are keen to apply and stick to a procedure or process. They can work against the creative inventor as they like concepts to be at least proven and realistic. They are pragmatists who need to have concepts expressed in a tangible setting.

They need opportunity to give input and have their views aired. They will also need time to apply more intangible concepts. They should be encouraged to be more flexible and less judgemental.

The facilitator

Facilitators display the ability to clarify, interpret and summarise. They are good at questioning and may have a tendency to try to 'out-chair' the chair.

They need to achieve some kind of team balance and thrive on support and encouragement. They can be indispensable when deadlock sets in, as they are good at cementing the group and working towards outcomes. Occasionally, their need for consensus can disrupt decision-making.

The mediator

Mediators display wisdom, experience and balance. Their behaviour is driven by a need for team spirit, harmony and non-confrontation with their peers.

While their intent is clearly supportive, it may be necessary to suppress their tendency to trivialise issues, which they may do to avoid confrontation or embarrassment.

The supporter

Supporters display encouraging behaviour, are positive, enthusiastic and have a good deal of energy.

They need harmony, team balance and involvement in order to thrive.

The shy one

These individuals are on the border between heroes and villains, depending upon their motive. If they are genuinely shy, they feel discomfort when pushed into a situation where they have to contribute. They prefer a lack of involvement and a quiet life.

To bring them out of their shell they need space, eye contact, direct questions and support. It is important that they realise, however, the fact that a degree of responsibility rests with their position on the committee and that a significant contribution will be expected of them as befits their role.

The villains

The monopoliser

Monopolisers have a tendency to interrupt, ramble, repeat themselves and generally take over the commentary. Such behaviour is best dealt with by waiting for a suitable space in the proceedings, acknowledging the point they are making and then perhaps bringing another participant into the dialogue. It is important that the chair gives everyone on the committee a chance to express their opinion.

The distracter

These people tend not to be involved in the process of the meeting. They are attention-seeking and tend continually to make irrelevant and verbose side-comments. This may be a consequence of their attention span, the relevance of the topic or a deliberate attempt to undermine the chair. As a result, a fairly direct intervention is required: halt them firmly, restate the objective or topic and ask them a specific question in relation to the topic.

The sniper

Snipers are characterised by their use of side-comments, again, trying to undermine the chair and to put the chair on the spot. There are several ways to deal with this. It may be helpful to ask them to share their comments, rebound their question if it is deliberately misleading or ask the rest of the group for their thoughts and comments.

The sceptic

It is sometimes difficult to separate the sceptic from the realist. It is mainly to do with their motives. Sceptics tend to be critical, negative, unhelpful and resistant to change, whereas realists need things putting into perspective. Sceptics can be turned into realists by gaining their support; ask for solutions, not problems, and apply objectivity to their cynicism.

Judgement

Chairing meetings, managing committees and running groups are all bound by the same basic set of rules and processes. What tends to characterise an effective chair is the ability to make the interventions and apply the principles at the right time and with the correct emphasis. This needs experience and it is important to be prepared to make mistakes.

Trial and error are bound to be the key to developing judgement, but the confidence this brings can make the whole process an enjoyable and stimulating experience.

Postscript

Here are some scenarios which can typically occur in a meeting or committee. Have a look through them and, using the information from this chapter and your personal judgement, make some decisions about what you would do. There are no right or wrong answers, but some actions may produce better outcomes than others!

- Your meetings normally involve about 20 professional people and the seating is horseshoe or boardroom style. The outputs from the meeting are often poor, in terms of both keeping to the agenda and follow-up.
- The meeting has been broken into subgroups for part of the agenda; attendees have been given their discussion assignments and asked to report back at a specific time. After the meeting, one attendee approaches you and says that he cannot stay in the group to which he was assigned because of a personality conflict with one of the other members.
- As you begin your meeting, you sense a great deal of hostility in the room. The attendees' arms are folded in a defensive style and they respond only when called on. This continues even after you have outlined the agenda and asked for comments.
- You are a third of the way through your meeting and are summarising the previous discussion. An attendee blurts out 'I disagree. You are totally out of touch with the real world. That's great in theory but it won't work here.'
- During your meeting, several attendees engage in side conversations. This is not the first time they have done so. You have so far ignored the situation, hoping they would stop on their own, but the situation seems to be getting worse.
- The entire group begins talking among themselves, sidetracking the discussion you are trying to lead. In fact, they seem to be attempting to take control away from you.

CHAPTER 28

Presentation skills

Kalyani Katz and Pramod Prabhakaran

'The whole art of teaching is only the art of awakening the natural curiosity of young minds for the purpose of satisfying it afterwards.' (Anatole France, *The Crime of Sylvestre Bonnard*, 1881)

Presentation is a performance. A successful performance depends on good communication between a presenter and an audience. Most professionals are required to give a presentation at one time or another. Some, for example teachers and doctors, are expected to do so more often than others. Doctors, through their essential duties of training future generations, giving and explaining information to their patients and educating the general public about health issues, need to exercise skills in presenting information in an easily understandable and digestible form. Some doctors are born teachers; others have to learn, develop and master these skills. Once acquired, at a more senior level these can be of use in negotiating and planning the development of new services and in procuring funding in order to implement change.

The basic guidelines set out below should not only help trainee doctors, who are expected to take part in weekly academic programmes involving case presentations and journal clubs: they should also be of use to newly appointed consultants, whose responsibilities include teaching a range of professional groups, such as nurses, occupational therapists, general practitioners and social workers.

The precise style, mode and content of a presentation will depend on the type of meeting, the needs of the audience and the number attending. In all cases, the presentation must be educational, thought-provoking and entertaining. The audience must be made to feel further curiosity about the subject by the end of the presentation; this is a task for the presenter. It will be no great challenge to one who has both a passion for the subject and good communication skills, but, even with these, delivering the same talk over and over again will make the task more difficult. It is essential to revise and update the material each time; there is always scope for improvement, as well as opportunities to incorporate new information. Remember also that communication is a two-way process; we often gain new ideas during the question and answer and discussion time, and we can ourselves learn through teaching others.

The kind of presentation we are dealing with here is quite different from a written article prepared for publication, although this, too, is a form of presentation. Reading aloud at a meeting a published article, or one that is prepared for publication, rarely makes a successful presentation. Changes will always need to be made to such material if it is to be easy for listeners to absorb and assimilate.

There is another basic rule that is often not adhered to. The presenter should never exceed the allocated time. We have all attended lectures where even the most passionate speaker has managed to put off an audience by being overenthusiastic and by speaking for too long. In our view, it is advisable to finish the talk even a few minutes early.

Let us now examine the different components of a successful presentation:

- preparation
- planning
- delivery.

Preparation

The first step in preparation is to collect all the relevant information about the nature and the theme of the meeting and about the topics being covered by other speakers. This is essential before any planning starts. Take for example a talk on depression in the elderly, delivered as part of a conference on healthcare for the elderly. If the talk is aimed at a wide range of medical and paramedical professionals, it will be different from a lecture given as part of an MRCPsych Part II course attended by trainee psychiatrists. It will be different again from a session aimed at helping general practitioners to identify early depression.

Proper knowledge of the particular context will help you to decide on the aims of your own presentation. Be sure to discuss and clarify your aims in advance with the organiser of the meeting. This will ease the process of planning. You may find a list of fairly common aims useful when thinking of the aims for your presentation:

- helping to spread new information (e.g. concerning the withdrawal of a product)
- improving awareness (e.g. of high rates of depression in the elderly)
- introducing change (e.g. the implementation of guidelines from the National Institute for Health and Clinical Excellence)
- inspiring action (e.g. incorporating the use of the 'single assessment process' to reduce the delay in the process of consultation for the elderly).

The second stage of preparation involves finding out more about your audience and how they intend to use your information. It may sometimes help to ask yourself the question: 'What would I wish to learn from this lecture if I were in the audience?' When analysing your audience, consider:

- the size of the audience
- their educational level
- their expectations and needs.

The presentation will not succeed unless your aims match the expectations and the needs of the audience. For example, community psychiatric nurses attending a lecture on suicide in psychiatric patients will want to learn how to assess the risk of suicide in patients. They will not be content to listen to your research findings on neurochemical abnormalities in patients who express suicidal ideas.

Knowing your audience will also help you to illustrate your ideas with relevant examples, ones which relate to their experience. In the long term, people tend to remember stories, rather than theory alone.

Some knowledge of the educational background of those in the audience will allow you to decide on the pitch of your talk; you must always avoid being condescending to those who come to hear you, but equally you must avoid speaking over their heads (if you do so, they will be unable to concentrate on your lecture and will 'switch off').

These days, through increasing media coverage and access to websites, the public has become more knowledgeable and more aware of health issues. It is not uncommon to find that a member of the audience has gleaned some new information from the media which you yourself have yet to hear through professional medical channels.

Planning

After the preliminary work of preparation, you can start thinking about exactly what you are going to say and how you will say it.

What are you going to say?

Start jotting down your ideas as soon as you have accepted an invitation to talk. You may find it useful to discuss your ideas with colleagues; constructive advice is often forthcoming, including suggestions of new reference material you may not have seen.

The next step in planning is to collect relevant material to support and illustrate your ideas. The Cochrane Library is the most comprehensive single source of information on the effects of healthcare interventions. It comprises a collection of databases. You can register for the 'Athens' password for the Cochrane Library at your local library or on the website of the National

Library for Health (NLH) (http://www.library.nhs.uk). Registration allows access to various databases:

- Medline
- Embase
- PsycINFO
- Cochrane Library
- AMED.

These can all be accessed via the website for Health Information for London Online (HILO) (http://www.hilo.nhs.uk) or the NLH website. The internet is of course also a valuable source of evidence and information to draw upon for a presentation. The following are particularly recommended:

- http://www.hilo.nhs.uk
- http://www.library.nhs.uk
- http://www.rcpsych.ac.uk
- http://www.doctors.net.uk
- http://www.nice.org.uk

You may also consult a local librarian; in our experience librarians are always keen to help. Be sure to keep details of references.

Of course, you must decide when to stop collecting material and to start evaluating what you have collected. Resist the temptation to collect too much material; this can cause problems in both extracting and simplifying information. You need reliable evidence to support your ideas. To achieve this, evaluate and exclude information that will not stand up to scientific scrutiny. Allow plenty of time to arrange material in a coherent and logical scheme; this can be time-consuming.

The precise title of the presentation should become obvious at this stage. A bland title can be made more interesting through only a slight change. For example, 'Suicide prevention in the mentally ill' could be made to sound more engaging, and could make a more lasting impression on the audience, if the phrase 'An unachievable goal?' were added. But you must avoid using a glamorous title simply to impress; satisfy yourself that the title really does reflect the content of your presentation.

Be aware of 'political correctness' in expressing your ideas but do not be its slave.

How will you say it?

The mode of the presentation is dictated generally by the size of the audience. The smaller the group size, the easier it is to make the learning more interactive. The interactive model, which is generally thought to be more conducive to learning, cannot easily be used in a larger gathering. An ability to control the group is essential if you are to choose this method.

Despite the derogatory comments we often hear about the workshop model – for example, that it is a way of getting others to do your own work – it can bring advantages, such as spontaneity and audience participation. But there are risks. A presenter may feel exposed by difficult questions, or by encountering members of the audience with their own agendas.

The didactic model, best suited for larger gatherings, has not been popular of late. In a study comparing the interactive and the didactic methods of learning, the assessment of knowledge in postgraduate trainees did not reveal significant benefit in one system compared with the other (Haidet *et al*, 2004).

Whatever the mode of presentation, the use of visual aids is now the norm. There are several advantages in this. For example, visual aids help people to concentrate and they break the monotony of the speaker's voice. It has been said that people generally remember 20% of what they hear but 50% of what they see and hear (Treichler, 1967). Well-prepared visual aids, such as slides or PowerPoint presentations, summarise the text in a concise form and will help the audience to focus on and retain the information. Recently, PowerPoint presentation seems to have become the most favoured option. Previously, slides, acetates and flip-charts were in common use. It may help to have one back-up method in case of technical problems. The choice will depend upon the availability of technical equipment at the venue.

However, visual aids are no more than aids. Do not make them too fancy or gimmicky, or an end in themselves – they can also be distracting. Use key words or phrases for emphasis. If you download images from websites, check the copyright.

The clarity and visibility of projections is very important. Choose an appropriate font size and style, and avoid using block capitals. Each projection should contain a minimum of two and a maximum of five points. It is not a substitute for a detailed text. Avoid very 'busy' slides and avoid projecting those you intend to skip (unnecessary slides give an impression of inadequate preparation and lead to boredom in the audience). Exposure to too many stimuli – the phenomenon referred to as 'stimulus overload' – can raise stress levels and diminish learning ability (Mendl, 1999).

Allow roughly 2 minutes' talking time for each slide. This is a good way of getting the length of your talk right. A printed version of your slides will be useful as a handout, and will save the time you might have spent in preparing separate ones.

The final step in the planning is to arrive early at the venue, in order to familiarise yourself with the surroundings and organise your visual material. Late arrival in a state of panic can seriously affect the delivery of even a very well-prepared talk.

Delivery

It is through the delivery itself that a presentation will make a lasting impact; the delivery is therefore the most important element of the presentation.

The first few minutes of non-verbal communication are crucial in making a positive impression on your audience, and can also help to establish a good rapport. Once you have taken this opportunity, it will be easy to hold the audience's attention and interest; if you lose their attention it will be hard to regain it. It is, of course, advantageous to dress appropriately for the occasion and to walk confidently on to the stage.

Some famous speakers cultivate an image of untidiness and a chaotic personal style. We do not recommend this. Distracting dress may be able to seize the audience's attention, but will not be sufficient to sustain it. Excessive movements of hands, or pacing about on the stage or podium, can betray anxiety, and anxiety is infectious. The same may be said of excessively rapid speech, failing to look at the audience and rushing through the presentation. Smile and adopt a confident posture, for confidence is infectious too.

Make sure that you can be heard clearly by those furthest away from you and that they can see your slides or projections. Aim your delivery at the back row for at least a good part of the time, and certainly avoid speaking to your visual aids rather than to the audience. Learn to use appropriate pauses to emphasise certain points. If English is not your first language, do remember to speak slowly and to be conscious that your accent may be difficult to understand for those unused to it. This is one of the most common reasons why audiences lose attention. Practise speaking clearly and slowly, and ask a friend (a real friend, not just one who will flatter you) to comment honestly, or practise in front of a closed-circuit television to analyse your own performance.

A good introduction, followed by a statement of your plans for your allotted time slot, will help to gain the attention of your audience and keep them interested. It can be very effective to start with a controversial statement, or an event currently in the news, or perhaps an interesting real-life anecdote. It has been said that a good anecdote is worth a thousand pages of statistics. Better still is a good anecdote backed up by statistics.

Most people are averse to arrogance and appreciate some humility in the speaker. Occasional humour can lighten the atmosphere, and a relaxed atmosphere is more conducive to learning. Be cautious with jokes, however – they should be in appropriate taste and should actually be funny. A joke that fails to amuse can alienate an audience.

Dealing with anxiety

Knowing a few simple facts about anxiety should help you to overcome it. Any performance is likely to create anxiety or emotional arousal in the presenter. Performing at an optimal level in fact depends on some degree of nervousness. Fig. 28.1, which depicts the well-established Yerkes–Dodson law, shows how performance improves up to a point, beyond which anxiety becomes an impediment (Yerkes & Dodson, 1908).

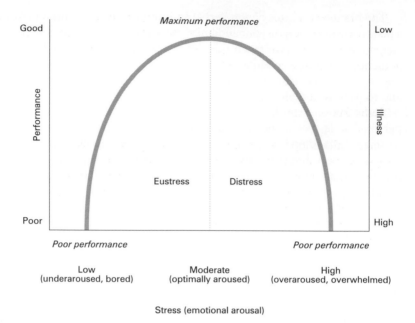

Fig. 28.1 The optimal stress curve. (Yerkes & Dodson, 1908.)

There are certain effective methods of controlling the more severe levels of fear. Use of alcohol, benzodiazepines, beta-blockers or excessive caffeine could be disastrous. Instead, try eating one or two bananas. It is not merely an old wives' tale that a banana has a calming effect. Good preparation and rehearsal are even more effective methods of reducing any apprehension that your performance will fail.

Just before you start, use some breathing techniques of the kind that are now widely familiar. The level of anxiety goes down once you begin. During the lecture, you should treat the audience as friends and try to create a relaxed and informal atmosphere in the room. Making eye contact with individuals certainly helps to reduce anxiety. Slow down and pause between sentences from time to time, in order to focus your thoughts. Use prompt cards or essential notes as a memory aid; under anxiety, it is easy to forget and lose your train of thought.

A common fear is that of not being able to answer questions after the lecture. Prepare yourself by anticipating the obvious questions and practise answering them. You need to remain in charge of the question and answer session. This session also gives you the opportunity to gauge whether the audience has understood your message and it enables you to clarify and emphasise your 'take-home' message. Before attempting to answer a question, it is very often necessary to rephrase it for the benefit of those in the audience who may not have heard or understood it. Entering into a dialogue with just one member of the audience is a common pitfall. To avoid this, direct your answers to the entire audience. If you do not know the answer to a question, do not hesitate to say so, but rather offer to research it and answer it at a later date.

Conclusion

Although all of this might seem like stating the obvious, we feel it is necessary to do so, having frequently sat through some very painful lectures. Richard Smith's article in the *BMJ* summarises the common mistakes that lead to a bad presentation (Smith, 2003). But to achieve success, prepare well, practise adequately, arrive on time, make contact with your audience and do not overrun your time. And try to avoid accepting the time-slot after lunch!

References

Haidet, P., Morgan, R. O., O'Malley, K., *et al* (2004) A controlled trial of active versus passive learning strategies in a large group setting. *Advances in Health Sciences Education: Theory and Practice*, **9**, 15–27.

Mendl, M. (1999) Performing under pressure: stress and cognitive function. *Applied Animal Behaviour Science*, **65**, 221–244.

Smith, R. (2003) How not to give a presentation. *BMJ*, **321**, 1570–1571.

Treichler, D. G. (1967) Are you missing the boat in training? *Film and A-V Communication*, **1**, 14–16.

Yerkes, R. M. & Dodson, J. D. (1908) The relation of strength of stimulus to rapidity of habit-formation. *Journal of Comparative Neurology and Psychology*, **18**, 459–482.

CHAPTER 29

Time management

Jill Sandford

'Time goes, you say? Ah no!
Alas, times stays, we go.'
(Austin Dobson, *Proverbs in Porcelain*, 1877)

Time, and the management of it, have become a familiar component of management books such as this one, and a feature of the self-improvement movement as a whole. The sense of powerlessness we have at the march of time (reflected in the quote above) and the increasing pace of life mean that people often feel that they are managing their time 'badly'. One of the most common issues people have when they come to me for coaching is the management of their time.

Personality styles and time management

Attitudes to time vary from culture to culture and person to person. In the West we tend to have a linear, 'time is money' attitude. We are a product of our cultural upbringing. Your own attitude to time will also be affected by your personality preferences. You may be familiar with the work of Jung and the personality types that can be explored and defined by the use of the Myers–Briggs type indictor. The very notion of time management appeals to certain of these type classifications. It can be a useful starting point for you to consider how you manage your time and why this may, or may not, be important to you.

The Myers–Briggs type indicator identifies whether you take in information with a sensing or an intuitive preference, make decisions with a thinking or a feeling preference and organise your life by judging or perceiving. It also identifies levels of extraversion and introversion – but this is less relevant in time management. Judgers tend to respond to ideas of structure and planning and perceivers want more of an open-ended free flow of events, with less structure. For the purpose of time management I summarise the styles below:

- *Sensing judgers* are often good at time management. They are very grounded in reality but can be rigid when plans have been fixed. They find it hard to relax and the judging preference can make them stressed and 'time anxious'. They will push for a decision to be made and for plans to be clearly established. They like things to be planned in advance.

- *Sensing perceivers* can meet immediate needs well and are less anxious to push for a decision or closure. Their efforts can be scattered. They may get caught up in the moment. They are flexible and can handle schedule change. They are more 'last minute' and will procrastinate about planning for the longer-term future, as they are more grounded in the here and now.

- *Intuitive feelers* are sensitive to needs of others. They may find it hard to say 'no' and neglect their own needs. They believe time is useful to find one's life purpose and are generous with their time.

- *Intuitive thinkers* see time merely as a concept. Once they have thought something through they may not think it necessary to take action. Time is a tool but they may ignore people's needs. They sometimes need to ground their goals in practical plans with deadlines.

Understanding your own time management style in this way can assist you in developing approaches to overcome your shortcomings and in identifying strengths upon which to build. This chapter offers you the opportunity to do this.

The process of time management

What is effective time management? It must be 'getting the desired results in the time available'. Focusing on the bigger picture – the outcome of your role – is one way of managing your time more effectively. The nature of managerial work, in particular, is that it is frequently unbounded and does not lend itself to a clearly defined set of tasks. The demands, particularly when there is an enhanced level of responsibility for people and services, can be great. Managers can therefore easily feel that they have too much to do. Interestingly enough, having too little to do can cause as much stress as being overwhelmed. Time is to some a concept, to others a precious gift, or a horse galloping ahead that we can never catch – always getting away from us.

How we think about time and the attitudes we have about it are complex and deep rooted. This chapter, however, is essentially a practical and pragmatic set of activities and ideas for you to consider. It offers a framework (with some activities) to help you. The stages it outlines are as follows:

1   Identify your own use of time and your strengths and weaknesses (your style).

2   Identify your purpose and main goals in life, and how to plan to achieve these. What is really important to you? What do you want to do more of and less of?

3   Develop strategies for more effective and satisfying use of your time – ones that assist you in achieving your goals.

Identifying your use of time

This is the diagnostic stage. Its purpose is to indicate how you use your time at the moment. This sounds relatively easy but we often delude ourselves that things are better or worse than they actually are. I usually recommend keeping a time log for a few days to monitor how you are actually spending your time. This may seem tedious but it is worthwhile. An example of a time log is presented in Fig. 29.1.

How to use a time log

Make a note of each activity and how long you were engaged on it, by entering a start and finish time. If you were interrupted, then enter each stage as a separate activity and note that you were interrupted. If you get a lot of interruptions, it is important to be aware of this. Which activities were planned? These might be meetings, training, a ward round or a clinic. 'Imposed' means an interruption or an unexpected task given to you by someone else – or yourself! Travel, eating and walking from one place to another all need to be noted as an activity. Do not forget thinking time – even if it is in the car. The extent to which you distinguish between work and home, I leave up to you. If you find work spills over into home and leisure time, then you may wish to log this.

Date:				
Activity	Start time	Finish time	Planned	Imposed

Fig 29.1 Example format of a time log.

It is worth keeping this log for several days. It is not always necessary to wait for a typical day – but it is obviously not a good idea to complete the log when you are on holiday.

When reviewing the log, ask yourself the following questions:

1   Is there a pattern emerging in any of the columns? For example, are many of the activities imposed?
2   Are you able to complete a task without being interrupted?
3   Are you giving adequate time to current activities and to planning for future activities?
4   Which people are you spending most time with? Are these the people you ought to be spending time with?
5   If you have someone to delegate to, are you doing this sufficiently often?
6   How do you deal with interruptions and emergencies? Do you defer these until tomorrow so that you can execute today's plans? Is this always possible?
7   Are you spending a lot of time on your aspects of your job? Is this the right balance?

This should result in an analysis of how you utilised this precious resource over a few days. The purpose of the log is to provide a baseline to come back to in stage 3 (developing strategies). It all depends on what you think you should be doing with your time in the first place. Unless you are clear about this, then you will not be sufficiently motivated to change anything about your personal time management style. Keep the log and your conclusions to one side for the moment and let us move to stage 2.

Identifying purposes, setting goals and establishing priorities

Your role defines your purpose at work. It establishes what you are there to achieve, with whom, for whom and in what timescales. You will work within frameworks and guidelines in order to do much of your work. You may have a greater degree of autonomy and control over *how* you execute the tasks.

If you were to define your role or your purpose as a medic or a manager in one or two sentences, how would you write this? Try it out as an activity for the purposes of this chapter:

• My role/purpose at work is …

It often helps to start this by listing the verbs that best express what your role is fundamentally about. You might 'advise', 'provide' psychiatric diagnosis and treatment for a specific patient group, 'deliver' education and training for junior staff, or 'research and develop' new approaches. You

	Urgent	Non-urgent
Important	1. Crises and deadlines	2. Prevention, relationship-building, recognising new opportunities, strategic thinking, planning, prioritising, long-term processes, recreation
Not important	3. Interruptions, some emails, some meetings	4. Trivia, time-wasters, some emails and calls

Fig. 29.2 Covey's categorisation of the expenditure of time and energy.

might want to have some words like 'prevention' in your statement, too. These are just suggestions to help you get started. Once you have some key words you are happy with, frame them into a sentence. Once you start listing tasks, then you usually find you have gone too far down into the 'how'. A role or purpose statement is about the 'why'.

The key to effective time management is to focus on the important tasks that directly contribute to the successful implementation of your role. I would like to introduce you here to the work of Stephen Covey, *The 7 Habits of Highly Successful People* (Covey, 1999). Covey focuses on being 'on purpose' and the successful fulfilment of things that are important to you. His time management strategies build on the identification of the important tasks, quality time with people, and looking after yourself and your health and development as a professional. The latter is what he calls 'sharpening the saw'. Essentially, he says there is no such thing as time management – only self-management. His categorisation of how we spend our time and energy can be presented as a four-cell matrix, as shown in Fig. 29.2.

Prioritising and planning

The ideal is to get out of the other cells and into cell 2 – important non-urgent tasks. The more time spent doing these key tasks, the more everything else will take care of itself. So a starting point is to plan your time in weeks, not days. To do this, you have to keep an overarching perspective, thinking first of your purpose in life and work. Time spent planning and scheduling is never wasted. Allocate slots of time to do the 'cell 2' things. Ensure you have sufficient time to react to situations that need your attention, but develop an approach that says 'I will spend only so much time on this activity'. Take control of your time and decide what you are going to spend it on.

By now you should have some insights into your own time management, in particular its strengths and weaknesses. Let us now move on to stage 3.

Developing strategies for more effective and satisfying use of your time

Better time management falls into two main areas: organisational skills and interpersonal skills.

Organisational skills

The following areas are all worth considering:

- *Planning and organising work activities* – being clear about what needs to be done and when. Establish lists and use a diary or time management system if this works well for you. Break down the big jobs into smaller tasks and put a timescale against each one.
- *Gathering and using information* – being able to find out the right information and apply it appropriately. Ensure you have the information you need in order to complete tasks.
- *Keeping records simple, accessible, up to date.* If you forget things (as I do!), then write lists and keep notebooks (paper or electronic).
- *Evaluating demands* – creating short- and long-term plans for work and being flexible in the short term but focused in the long term. Stephen Covey calls this 'keeping the end in mind'. Do not lose sight of your goals.
- *Managing and allocating resources* – making the best use of materials and operating within financial constraints.
- *Assessing the effects of change* – adapting and revising plans in response to change, in terms of both the changing needs of individual patients and developing local policies.
- *Managing your environment.* Consider what is the best time of day for you to do tasks that demand all of your attention, the location that is best for you to work in, and so on.

Managing paperwork

There are three ways to deal with paperwork:

1 Read it and deal with it.
2 Read it and pass it on.
3 Put it in the bin.

Sounds too simple?

Read it and deal with it
How many times have you picked up a piece of paper and thought 'I must deal with that'? A novel approach is to put a dot on the sheet each time you move it around – just to see how many dots it gets. If it ends up looking

like a bad case of the measles, you will have wasted a lot of your time. A brave approach is to cut the top 2 cm off the paper each time you pick it up or move it!

More seriously, I am trying to encourage you not to put off dealing with the perhaps boring and unpleasant tasks. It may be the sheer volume of paperwork that makes it daunting. I find an initial sort into the three piles I have indicated above really does help. I deal with the first category straight away by replying or actioning.

A useful technique is to have a 'Bring forward' folder, divided into days of the month. I simply place letters, documents, maps, presentations and so on into the appropriate date slot of the folder. I can then find what I need before the meeting. I can remind myself to reply to a communication on a certain date, too. In conjunction with a diary, I can keep a busy life organised and ensure I do not let people down. You need to remember to look in the 'Bring forward' folder each day. If I want to read something in advance, I simply pop it in the section for the day before.

If you are lucky enough to have a personal assistant, then encourage him or her to use this system on your behalf. You can utilise the Outlook Express diary system, for example, to run a 'Bring forward' folder electronically if you prefer.

Read it and pass it on

Is the paperwork just for information? If so, read it quickly and pass it on to whoever needs it. Copy and keep in files if necessary. I find my reading file tends to get quite big sometimes and often it is ideal train reading!

Put it in the bin

This pile is often easy to deal with. If you are not brave enough for the bin, then put in the bottom draw of a desk or filing cabinet. Clear out every 3 months. I wager you will not have to go into that drawer to retrieve anything.

Email

This probably causes more angst than anything other form of communication apart from other people's mobile phones on the train. It can be a great time waster and is also a boon to communication. I would recommend the following strategies:

- Do not check your email more than twice a day unless an urgent matter is at hand.
- Do not have 'you have mail' signals – you will be tempted to stop what you are doing and review them.
- Approach email communication like a proper letter. Write fully, with proper greetings, constructed sentences, punctuation and courtesy.

Nothing is more irritating that curt communication. Nothing is more confusing than ambiguous emails.

- Read and check emails before sending them.
- Ask yourself whether you would say to this person's face what you have written.

Interpersonal skills

Working effectively with other people

Establish working relationships that are effective and where you can share solutions and good practice with colleagues. This can include the following:

- *Communication (verbal and written, listening and talking).* Be clear at all times. This includes being assertive and saying 'no' in an appropriate way when you need to, especially if you find yourself being distracted out of those important quadrant 2 activities.
- *Valuing colleagues and other professionals.* Show appreciation and respect for others and their time.
- *Being flexible and responsive.* Be open to change, for example adapt and change plans when you need to.

Organising other people

The key here is to delegate effectively. Note, however, that you can delegate only tasks and authority – you cannot delegate accountability. Learning to delegate well can make you more effective, as it will leave you doing the right things.

There are two barriers to delegating:

- giving up some of the jobs you like doing
- the fear of losing control.

Delegating comes down to two issues:

- Which task?
- Who does it?

To delegate appropriately, it is necessary to identify the right person to do a task, and then to brief and support that person. It is therefore necessary to ask two further questions:

- Is the person capable of handling it?
- How long will it take that person to learn?

It may be necessary to make a training plan.

Box 29.1 gives some tips in relation to delegating.

> **Box 29.1** Delegation
>
> - Take your hands off
> - But keep your eyes open
> - Be available for advice
> - Check up on key points
> - Monitor progress
> - Inform others

Conclusion

I hope this chapter has presented you with some practical ways to manage your time more effectively. Remember you will not get it right all the time!

Reference

Covey, S. (1999) *The 7 Habits of Highly Successful People* (revised edn). Simon & Schuster.

CHAPTER 30

Managing people

Manoj Kumar

Employees are the biggest assets of any organisation that provides services. The largest part of the expenditure of the National Health Service (NHS) is devoted to salaries of employees and the NHS is the biggest employer in the UK. Healthcare by its very nature can be delivered only through people and requires a great deal of teamwork. Effective management of the employees, therefore, is the most important aspect of managing healthcare. Because employees represent both the major cost and are the major driver of value creation, changes to 'people management' that lead to even small changes in operational performance can and do have a major impact on outcomes. Management, as an important driving force for the delivery of healthcare, has gained momentum over past two decades.

In today's constantly evolving healthcare and management practice, the role of psychiatrists is continuously changing. By virtue of the nature of their clinical work, psychiatrists are already skilled and experienced in managing human interaction, whether it be with patients or mental health teams, provided that they make an effort to translate their knowledge and skills for such interactions. Teamwork and relatively flat management structures have replaced hierarchical practices. Since people are the most important assets of any organisation, managing them effectively is crucial to the overall performance of a team or organisation. The collaborative nature of multi-agency work also emphasises the importance of interaction with people outside the organisation.

An efficient manager manages people effectively through a reasonably good understanding of human behaviour and by utilising individuals' as well as teams' potential maximally. This is necessary in order to motivate people and to communicate effectively with them. Despite a plethora of literature and theories on various styles of management, there is no single style applicable to all situations and every person. Management involves a complex, dynamic interaction of personalities, motives and situations, especially in the workplace. Great leaders tap into the needs and fears we all share. Great managers, by contrast, perform their magic by discovering, developing and celebrating what is different about each person who works

355

for them and how they can be activated and supported. How do managers carry out their jobs? This 'softer' aspect of management contrasts with a 'harder' facet, concerned with more formal structures and systems. It is helpful to understand why managers, faced with situations which appear similar, behave in different ways.

Management styles

Rowe & Mason (1987) describe four different management decision styles among managers and leaders:

- *Directive* – practical, authoritarian, impersonal, power-centred. This is sometimes also described as 'theory X' management. It assumes that people are lazy and can be made to work only under coercion and clear-cut direction. The traditional 'order and obey' approach may be used to get the workforce to accomplish tasks. This style is particularly useful in crises but can be quite counterproductive if used excessively and continually, as it can suffocate creativity and block communication and feedback, thereby resulting in an unmotivated and uninvolved workforce. In contrast, 'theory Y' management relies on the self-discipline of a skilled and self-driven workforce. Modern literature on management suggests that most people have both 'X' and 'Y' in them in varying proportions and therefore need to be managed accordingly, in the hope of moving them into a predominantly 'Y' configuration.

- *Behavioural* – sociable, friendly, supportive. This style is useful in opening people up and especially in helping new or under-performing staff. It encourages initiative, motivation and loyalty. It is considered a softer style but can often lead to overdependence.

- *Conceptual* – insightful, enthusiastic, personal, adaptive, flexible. This is a relatively more mature and refined management style; it is often observed among senior management. It is particularly useful in managing complex organisations, where collaboration is essential, as well as where long-term planning, innovation and competitive advantage are needed.

- *Analytical* – intellectual, impersonal, control-oriented. With this style of management the manager is constantly analysing and seeking to control the actions of the workforce.

In addition to these, two further management styles can be noted:

- *Coaching*. The emphasis here is on training and acquiring skills, either through coaching by the manager personally or by the manager putting suitable arrangements in place. As with the behavioural style, it is useful for the new or under-performing employee or where a new role is envisaged. However, there are costs involved and an excess of coaching-style management is inappropriate, especially where staff are already skilled and competent.

- *Delegation.* Appropriate delegation is an art. It does not mean simply passing on work. Effective delegation requires adequate preparation and planning, matching the task to personal capabilities and regular feedback. The capability of the workforce will determine the levels of delegation. An insecure and overly controlling manager may find it difficult to delegate, resulting in high levels of stress and reduced productivity.

None of the above management styles is complete on its own. Good management requires a combination of styles, and the precise combination at any particular time will depend upon the situation. In order to identify their own styles and to use them effectively, managers must have good understanding of themselves as well as the team members. Before managing others, managers have to manage themselves effectively, and to be aware of their own strengths and weaknesses. For the purpose of simplicity, however, the task of managing people can be looked at under four broad headings:

- analysing and understanding people
- maximising their potential
- managing difficult situations and relationships
- appraisals and rewards.

Analysing and understanding people

Natural, instinctive behaviour is not always appropriate in the workplace. Therefore it is important to make an effort to facilitate behavioural patterns that lead to productive and effective teamwork. It is natural for people to adopt instinctive and self-protective behaviour, which explains why emotion is a strong force in the workplace, often reflected in strong reactions to criticism and competition. This usually creates a stressful and unpleasant working atmosphere, resulting in reduced productivity, absenteeism and high turnover. Detecting and minimising such behaviour in the workplace, and promoting a more positive interaction are hence necessary. Table 30.1 suggests ways in which some specific types of natural behaviour can be translated into more appropriate workplace behaviour.

Identifying needs

Human motivation and behaviour are driven largely by both conscious and unconscious needs. Apart from basic needs, such as security, salary and good working conditions, employees have higher, self-affirming needs, such as job satisfaction, a sense of achievement, recognition, challenge and a sense of purpose and belonging. The latter are as important as the former

Table 30.1 Replacing 'natural' (negative) behaviour with behaviour appropriate to the workplace

Natural behaviour	Appropriate behaviour
Reacting emotionally when information is received	Establishing the facts using a pragmatic approach
Avoiding risks through fear or insecurity	Taking risk in an entrepreneurial fashion
Fighting fiercely and defensively when under threat	Forming collegiate, collaborative, non-combative relationships
Making snap judgements about people and events	Insisting on detailed analysis before judgement
Spreading gossip throughout the organisation	Practising totally open communication
Competing for status and its symbols	Recognising achievement, not status
Dwelling on past successes	Learning from mistakes
Feeling more comfortable in small factions	Choosing to work in cooperative groups
Always seeking hierarchical superiority	Operating within flat non-hierarchical structures

From Heller (1999), with permission.

and need to be met. Managers need to identify and exploit these needs for optimal productivity.

Managing diversity

Great managers know and value the unique abilities and even the eccentricities of their employees, and they learn how best to integrate them into a coordinated plan of action. Managers will succeed only when they can identify and deploy the differences among people, challenging each employee to excel in his or her own way. A manager's approach to capitalising on differences can vary tremendously from place to place. For example, one manager may use reward schemes to motivate staff, while others may use matching specific strengths to the task.

Identifying and capitalising on each person's uniqueness saves time. No employee, however talented, is perfectly well rounded. Capitalising on uniqueness also makes each person more accountable. The team member should not simply be challenged for his or her ability to execute specific assignments, but should be challenged to make this ability the cornerstone of his or her contribution to the team, to take ownership for this ability, to practise it and to refine it. In addition, capitalising on what is unique about each person builds a stronger sense of team working, because it creates interdependency. It helps people appreciate one another's particular skills and learn that their co-workers can fill in where they are lacking. In short, it makes people need one another.

Fine shadings of personality, although they may be invisible to some and frustrating to others, are crystal clear to and highly valued by great managers. They could no more ignore these subtleties than ignore their own needs and desires. Figuring out what makes people tick is simply in their nature. In order to utilise an employee's potential, there are three things to know about how to manage them well: their strengths, the triggers that activate those strengths, and how they learn.

Effective communication

A good communicator is first and foremost a good listener. To understand people's motivations and attitudes managers need to be open and acutely perceptive to the way in which people communicate. Listening plays a key role in managing meetings, dealing with complaints, appraisals and so on. Asking open questions and providing the opportunity for people to express their feelings will make members of the team feel listened to and valued. Correct interpretation of what is being communicated is extremely important: asking the right questions, clarifications, regular feedback and avoiding selective listening help accurate interpretation. Awareness of and attention to non-verbal communication are vital. Box 30.1 summarises key points to remember for clear and effective communication.

Box 30.1 Key points to remember for clear and effective communication

- Listen carefully and sincerely
- Ask open questions that encourage total honesty
- Always clarify and feed back until you fully understand what the person means
- Be perceptive to non-verbal communication
- Give people enough opportunity to express their feelings
- Keep appointments with all members of staff, regardless of their status
- Use technology for efficiency, not as a total substitute for personal interaction
- Arrange to meet up with staff as regularly as possible, not only in a crisis
- Talk to everybody during away-days and outside visits
- If you need to speak with someone, meet him or her in person if possible
- Take the opportunity to speak to staff on an informal basis
- Ensure to record minutes of formal meetings
- Always make an effort to brief staff about any new changes or policies

---

Nurturing commitment

Working with a highly committed team can be a very satisfying experience. Inner drive, purpose and ambition are key personal attributes for commitment to a job. However, the level of personal commitment is influenced by what the workplace has to offer. Meeting employees' key needs, paying attention, respecting individuality, fostering self-efficacy and personal empowerment, nurturing mutual trust, creating a blame-free culture and appropriate recognition are some of the important organisational attributes which enhance commitment. A manager who has little understanding of such a conducive environment or who lacks the skills to create it is likely to be faced with poor motivation and performance in the team, often manifesting itself in stress and burnout, absenteeism and high turnover. Traditionally, there has been little emphasis on fulfilling the personal and emotional needs of staff. In order to realise maximum commitment from employees, however, you need to address both intellectual and emotional needs. It is also important to keep staff committed over the long term, for example by expanding levels of interest, the variety of tasks to perform (e.g. involvement in management), providing resources and training to learn new skills, appropriate rewards and career progression.

Maximising potential

Conventional wisdom holds that self-awareness is a good thing and that it is the job of the manager to identify weaknesses in staff and create a plan for overcoming them. However, self-assurance (labelled 'self-efficacy' by cognitive psychologists), not self-awareness, is the strongest predictor of a person's ability to set high goals, to persist in the face of obstacles, to bounce back when reversals occur and, ultimately, to achieve the goals set. Effective managers therefore focus on the strengths of their workforce. When people succeed, the great manager does *not* praise their hard work. Rather, even if there is some exaggeration in the statement, the staff would be told that they succeeded because they have become so good at deploying their specific strengths. This, the manager knows, will increase their self-assurance and make them more optimistic and more resilient in the face of challenges to come.

Failures

Repeated failure, of course, may indicate weakness where a role requires strength. In such cases, there are four approaches for overcoming weaknesses. If the problem amounts to a lack of skill or knowledge, that is easy to solve, by offering relevant training, incorporating new skills and looking for signs of improvement.

Another strategy for overcoming employees' weaknesses is to find them support from someone whose talents are strong and complementary in precisely the areas where they are required.

If training produces no improvement, if complementary partnering proves impractical – or perhaps even if no suitable discipline technique can be found – the fourth and final strategy is to rearrange the employee's working world, to render the weakness irrelevant. This strategy will require, first, the creativity to envision a more effective arrangement and, second, the courage to make that arrangement work. The payoff that may come in the form of increased employee productivity and engagement is well worth it.

A person's strengths are not always on display. Sometimes they require precise triggering to turn them on. If the right trigger is squeezed, individuals will push themselves harder and persevere in the face of resistance. If the wrong one is, the person may well shut down. This can be tricky because triggers come in myriad and mysterious forms. One employee's trigger might be the boss, another's independence.

The most powerful trigger by far is recognition, not money, more so in the NHS, although this may be beginning to change. Most managers are aware that employees respond well to recognition. Great managers refine and extend this insight. They realise that each employee plays to a slightly different audience. One employee's audience might be their peers; the best way to praise them would be to celebrate their achievement publicly. Another's favourite audience might be the manager; the most powerful recognition then would be a one-on-one conversation in which the individual is told quietly but vividly why he or she is such a valuable member of the team. For other employees, who might be defined by their expertise, the most prized form of recognition would be some type of professional or technical award. Yet others might value feedback only from clients. Given how much personal attention it requires, tailoring praise to fit the person is mostly a manager's responsibility. But organisations can take a cue from this, too.

Learning organisations

In the 21st century, any organisation, big or small, would neglect staff training and development at its peril. Developing the abilities of staff at all levels is so important that many organisations have their own training and development departments and use both in-house and outside trainers. However, it is important to be clear about the purpose of training (see Table 30.2).

The more multi-skilled staff members are, the more valuable they will be. Having multi-skilled staff also cuts down on costs and time, provides greater flexibility and encourages team spirit and collaboration. Certain skills are vital for every employee in the NHS, such as communication (knowledge skills framework, Department of Health, 2004). In addition, 'soft' skills,

Table 30.2 Purpose-linked training

Type of training	Purpose
Specific	To improve current performance (e.g. risk assessment, audit)
General	To provide wider skills (e.g. computer skills)
Advanced	To prepare for promotion and change (e.g. management)

such as thinking holistically and analytically, should be encouraged, as they can be particularly useful in improving overall performance.

Coaching and mentorship

A manager is a coach and is responsible for feedback on people's performance. Coaching involves giving clear instructions about what is expected and helping to identify strengths and weaknesses, as well as to form ambitions. Sometimes, an employee may need counselling regarding personal problems. Mentorship may be one solution; it is about helping junior colleagues to steer successfully through an appropriate career path.

Leading by example

Team members depend on their leaders and look up to them as role models. It is expected that a manager will set examples of behaviour and performance for the staff to follow. Managers must therefore consistently maintain high standards themselves, but to be willing to help others who fall short of them.

Inspirational managers share several common attributes including competence, supportiveness, directness, fair-mindedness and an intelligent vision. They always encourage more experienced employees to teach others through practice. This ensures that skill resources in teams are shared, which in turn leads to improved understanding and efficiency.

Motivating people

Contrary to popular belief, motivating people is not just about persuasion or giving inspiring speeches. It is a rather complex process which involves identifying the needs and personality styles of the staff and matching them to the task, including them in planning and decision-making, encouraging power-sharing and ownership, and facilitating autonomy and recognition of achievement. Apart from these, there are various other factors which may influence the motivation of an individual, such as relationships at work or outside, personal circumstances and self-esteem.

Managing difficult situations and relationships

Good interpersonal skills are essential for creating a comfortable and productive environment. Creating an atmosphere in which people feel appreciated and valued is a challenge for every manager. It is worth investing time and effort in creating such a work environment. This saves an organisation's resources, by minimising the possibility of future problems.

Managing change

Health services in the UK have undergone rapid evolution, driven by scientific as well as political developments. Increasing emphasis on accountability and evidence-based practice, a move towards community psychiatry, ever-changing management structures and the development of specialist teams have ensured that effective change management is the key task for modern healthcare managers. Recent examples include the development of early intervention, of crisis teams and of home treatment teams. This has led to a cultural shift in the *modus operandi* of mental health teams. In addition, mergers of mental health trusts and the implementation of the European Working Time Directive have led to further changes, testing employees' capacity to adapt constantly.

The behaviour of individual healthcare professionals is influenced by a wide range of factors. The 'social influences' model of behaviour change suggests that individual beliefs, knowledge, attitudes and psychological factors interact with peer-group influences, the culture and attitude of the employing organisation and wider social forces, to shape behaviour in a particular clinical situation. Altering individual behaviour is therefore a complex task and should be approached as part of a wider strategy that takes this fully into account.

Advance planning before any major changes in working practice are implemented should include educating, informing and involving the employees in the change process. To minimise resistance, confusion and resentment in relation to change, it is important to be open while at the same time highlighting the potential benefits and disadvantages of the change and acknowledging the effect on individual employees. It is important to tackle resistance as early as possible. Organising seminars and workshops, conducting audits and giving feedback while providing support to affected employees is helpful. It is advisable always to try to identify 'change agents' in the organisation and to encourage them to come together.

Conflict management

The quest for harmony and common goals can actually obstruct teamwork. Managers get truly effective collaboration only when they realise that conflict is natural and necessary.

Psychiatrists involved in management are uniquely placed to handle conflict within the organisation because of their dual role of holding power through management office at the same time as having credibility as a clinician. Furthermore, their understanding of clinical priorities can help the 'us against them' areas of conflict between managers and clinicians, which as an issue quite often dogs the functioning of the NHS. However, their position alone does not guarantee successful conflict resolution. Conflicts can arise at personal as well as at organisational level and is unavoidable when people interact in any given social structure.

A positive and rational approach to defuse heightened emotions is required to reach a pragmatic resolution. The problem, its nature, stakeholders and solutions – and their implementation and potential complications – all need to be clearly identified.

Disputes often arise because of disagreement about facts; if possible, these should be triangulated from independent sources. Avoiding a win/lose situation helps in the reaching of a constructive resolution and reiterates the impartial position of the manager.

Difficult colleagues

Managing difficult colleagues can be a tricky business and requires patience as well as tact. Fortunately, these occurrences are relatively rare. However, for medical managers, they can consume a great deal of time and resources. The problem could be due to the inflexibility of those colleagues, their obstructive and irrationally challenging behaviour or frequent conflict with other team members. Sometimes they end up being marginalised themselves. Firm but skilful and open-minded communication is vital. Difficult members of staff are often preoccupied with specific personal and narrow-minded issues. There is no fixed way of dealing with such people – they have to be dealt with on an individual basis.

Poor performance

A poorly performing team member can take up a great deal of the team's time and energy. Some circumstances may need stronger action beyond effective day-to-day management or particular attention in individual supervision.

As a team leader responsible for practice standards it is important to involve your team in standard setting. It may be really useful to ask yourself four key questions:

1   Am I clear about my own, the organisation's and the profession's expectations of acceptable behaviour at work, performance standards and ways of negotiating differences of professional opinion?

2   Am I confident that these expectations are explicit and shared within the team I manage?

3   Do my team members tell me about problems and concerns regarding behaviour and standards?

4   Does the whole team have a stated, shared responsibility for ensuring appropriate standards of behaviour and professional practice?

Employers usually have policies and written procedures for dealing with poor performance. These will set out how the organisation distinguishes between various levels of performance, ranging from the good, through the improvable to the unacceptable. Familiarity with the range of options will help you to decide which, if any, of these responses is the appropriate one in the circumstances.

Issues of poor performance and behaviour are particularly difficult to think about on your own and in isolation. Therefore it is always useful to consult colleagues, senior managers or the human resources department at early stages of concern. It is also important to distinguish between poor performance related to professional behaviour (e.g. clinical work of a junior doctor) and to employee behaviour (e.g. lateness, discourtesy).

In the first instance, concerns should be raised informally with the employee, if possible in the supervision session. You need to be polite, clear about your concerns and expectations, and helpful. If you are not the line manager, an informal discussion with the line manager of the person concerned may be preferable. In many cases improvement will not be instant and, depending on the nature of the job and on the effect of substandard performance on the department, the informal process should continue for a reasonable period, which ideally should be agreed with the employee. Depending on the reasons for poor performance, adequate support, which may include training, should be offered. Performance should subsequently be monitored at regular intervals.

If informal management fails, a more formal process may need to be initiated in accordance with the organisation's policies, which may range from a written warning to dismissal. Where the required standard is still not reached, consider other options before dismissal, for example transfer to alternative work, premature retirement either in the interests of the efficiency of the service or on the grounds of ill-health.

Many performance issues can be picked up early through regular formal appraisal.

Appraisal and rewards

Appraisal for trainers will become increasingly important in their portfolios and as part of the signing off of competencies in the new era of training and assessment. Both trainees and trainers must attend appraisal training courses to learn how to maximise the usage of the appraisal process. An effective appraisal process should be able to identify areas of strength and weakness, which turn should direct the personal development plan and training issues.

Good performance should be rewarded with at least an immediate feedback and, wherever possible, openly. Every worker needs to feel valued for their contribution. Rewards could range from simple praise to material incentives and felicitations.

Conclusion

Given the high financial, social and political stakes, people management is a core operational process for any modern organisation and not solely a support function run by the human resources department. Clinicians have a vital role to play in improving productivity, in terms of both business (e.g. clinical) issues and management issues (e.g. how to create an organisational and working environment that fosters productive output). If success in a capital-intensive business comes primarily from making the right investment decisions, success in a people-intensive business comes from hiring the right people and putting in place processes and an organisation that makes them productive.

Managers also need to ensure that employees' interests are aligned with the organisation's objectives and their execution. Organisations often use surveys and other tools to assess how well they are meeting employees' personal goals. Too often, however, these tools focus only on traditional human resources issues, such as work/life balance, benefits and training. But staff satisfaction and engagement are more likely to be destroyed by conflicts at work than by conflicts between work and 'life'. The right survey can help spot such conflicts between employee interests and company objectives. Diagnosing and addressing them – however uncomfortable for the senior line managers who may be the source of the problem – is crucial to keeping employees engaged and productive. People cannot be effectively managed in the absence of relevant performance information – information that can and will be acted upon.

As mentioned above, every employee has a unique combination of thinking, motivation, needs and abilities, which manifests as a personal style of working. Good managers do not try to change a person's style. They never try to push a knight to move in the same way as a bishop. They know that their employees will differ in how they think, how they build relationships, how altruistic they are, how patient they can be, how much of an expert they need to be, how prepared they need to be, what drives them, what challenges them and what their goals are. These differences of trait and talent are like blood types: they cut across the superficial variations of race, sex and age and capture the essential uniqueness of each individual. Like blood types, the majority of these differences are enduring and resistant to change.

A manager's most precious resource is time, and great managers know that the most effective way to invest their time is to identify exactly how each employee is different and then to figure out how best to incorporate those enduring idiosyncrasies into the overall plan. Great managing is about release, not transformation. It is about constantly tweaking the environment so that the unique contribution, the unique needs and the unique style of each employee can be given free rein.

References and further reading

Barber, F. & Stack, R. (2005) The surprising economics of a 'people' business. *Harvard Business Review*, June.

Buckingham, M. (2005) What great managers do? *Harvard Business Review*, March.

Department of Health (2004) *The NHS Knowledge and Skills Framework (NHS KSF) and the Development Review Process*. Department of Health.

General Medical Council (1999) *Management in Health Care – The Role of Doctors*. General Medical Council.

Heller, R. (1999) *Managing People*. Dorling Kindersley.

Naylor, J. (2004) *Management* (2nd edn). Pearson Education.

Rowe, A. J. & Mason, R. O. (1987) *Managing with Style*. Jossey-Bass.

Rowlands, P. (2004) The NICE schizophrenia guidelines: the challenge of implementation. *Advances in Psychiatric Treatment*, **10**, 403–412.

CHAPTER 31

Mental health informatics

Martin Baggaley

Health informatics can be defined as:

'The knowledge, skills and tools which enable information to be collected, managed, used and shared to support the delivery of healthcare and to promote health.'

Mental health informatics applies to mental health services. Computers and the electronic transfer of information are part of normal day-to-day life and are increasingly important in health service delivery, including psychiatry. Psychiatrists need to understand the key principles of mental health informatics both to be able to work effectively now and also to appreciate the opportunities for more effective ways of working in the future which modern information technology (IT) affords.

Personal skills and services

To use IT successfully requires a certain level of personal competency, although it is not necessary to understand the technology or how computer software is written.

European computer driving licence

All staff working within the National Health Service (NHS) require a basic level of competence in health informatics. Basic IT skills are essential to support many healthcare practices. The European computer driving licence (ECDL) has been adopted as the referenced standard for NHS staff; it covers the basic use of IT. It is widely used, in over 140 countries, and is vendor neutral, that is, it aims to cover skills independent of the software supplier. Most trusts offer training to allow clinicians to study for and obtain the ECDL for free. Alternatively, courses are available in adult education centres. The syllabus includes:

- concepts of IT
- using a computer and managing files
- word processing
- spreadsheets
- database
- presentation
- information and communication.

Effective use of email

Email is gradually replacing letters and written memos as the standard way of communicating. To get the most out of email, it is important to understand how to use the software effectively and to be aware of the basic rules of etiquette (see below), which unfortunately are rarely taught.

Microsoft Outlook

Most NHS PCs have Microsoft Office as a standard suite of programs, which includes Outlook as the standard email application. Outlook is like a postbox but it needs a mail system to operate. Many trusts will use an application such as Microsoft Exchange to distribute email around the system.

NHS Contact

Contact is a fully integrated email, calendar and directory service for use by all NHS employees throughout their careers in the NHS. It allows for transmission of patient-sensitive data to another NHS user on Contact using secure encrypted messages. It has a huge flexible database of contact details, which, provided trusts and other NHS organisations keep it up to date, will prove to be a very useful way to contact other people in the NHS. Contact can be used from any PC which is connected to the internet (outside NHSnet) and it is compatible with the use of Microsoft Outlook. Individual NHS clinicians can register to use Contact and over the next few years it is anticipated that all NHS organisations will migrate across to use Contact instead of their own email server. The advantage of Contact is that it offers one address wherever anyone moves in the NHS and allows transmission of patient-sensitive information (within the system). One disadvantage is that email addresses cannot be as easily guessed; for example, most trusts use the format firstname.secondname@trustname.nhs.uk, whereas Contact uses numbers to distinguish same names, for instance john.smith99.

Etiquette

Email is a very powerful tool but can easily be misused. It can be all too simple to send angry emails copied to everyone up to chief executive, which is soon regretted. It is sometimes possible to retrieve emails but do not rely on this to salvage potential disasters. It is a good rule never to send an email

369

when feeling angry – better to calm down and review the matter the next day. It is also easy to appear rude when this was not the intention at all. There are many circumstances when a quick telephone call is better than an email. Typing in capitals to indicate irritation is rude and should not be done. Avoid sending copies to everybody in the trust.

Email psychotherapy

There are some psychotherapists who provide psychotherapy by email. The regulation and ethical framework of such services is difficult to determine, especially when the therapist lives in a different country to the patient. Also, the efficacy of such treatment has not been clearly demonstrated. Nevertheless, some service users appear to appreciate such contact and the impersonal nature of the interaction. Service providers charge per email or time taken over a case. Most internet psychotherapists are based in the USA, although it can be difficult to know exactly where they are based at times.

In the UK, there are few services which offer internet therapy. However, there are therapists and psychiatrists who use emails as a follow-up and as a way of monitoring the progress of patients they also see face to face.

Email is much less intrusive than telephone calls and therapists and patients can read the message at their convenience. There are some web-based cognitive–behavioural psychotherapy treatment programmes which have been shown to be effective in the treatment of depression and anxiety disorders.

Trust intranets

An intranet is effectively an internal internet; thus, people use a browser, such as Microsoft Explorer, to look at web pages, but these are not accessible to those outside the firewall (a firewall is software which prevents unauthorised access to computers connected via a network). A trust can use an intranet to share information which might otherwise clog up the email system. For example, instead of sending an email to everyone, notices of interest can be posted on the intranet.

Internet and NHSnet

The internet, then known as ARPANET, was brought online in 1969 under a contract let by the renamed Advanced Research Projects Agency (ARPA), which initially connected four major computers at universities in the south-western US (UCLA, Stanford Research Institute, UCSB and the University of Utah). The internet was designed in part to provide a communications network that would work even if some of the sites were destroyed by nuclear attack. If the most direct route were not available, *routers* would direct traffic around the network via alternative routes. Since then, the internet has expanded globally to become a key communication tool, especially now that broadband connections have become common in the UK.

Theoretically, every clinician in the NHS has access to the internet through NHSnet. NHSnet is a virtual private network that operates throughout the NHS and is inaccessible to non-NHS organisations. It provides access to both NHS-specific websites (prefixed nww.) and the worldwide web (www.). Clinicians now have an enormous amount of clinically relevant material available at their desk, if they are able to access that material effectively. In addition, patients and carers have access to much of the same information through the internet, which means that the patient and carer may know as much or more about a particular topic as the attending clinician. One un-resolved difficulty is communication to key stakeholders outside NHSnet, such as private providers and social services. It would be useful to exchange patient-sensitive data with such agencies but at present this raises difficult security issues.

Knowledge management

Clinicians are faced with an exponential growth of new knowledge, including new research and new guidelines and policy directives. This knowledge is available electronically, which allows clinicians to access it at their desktop, as required, even when seeing service users. Many services can be configured to send alerts when relevant research is published. Online searches can be performed and the relevant abstracts retrieved and saved or printed out. Librarians are changing function from managing books to becoming experts on electronic information management. It is possible simply to use an intranet search engine to try to look up suitable material. However, it is usually more effective to access a site which can act as a gateway to relevant resources via hyperlinks. Such sites for psychiatrists might include the Royal College of Psychiatrists' website and the NeLH mental health site (see below).

The National electronic Library for Health (NeLH)

The National electronic Library for Health programme is working with NHS libraries to develop a digital library for NHS staff, patients and the public. This includes access to other NHS agencies, such as the National Institute for Health and Clinical Excellence (NICE), the National Patient Safety Agency (NPSA) and information resources such as Prodigy (which gives advice on managing primary care problems) and Bandolier (on evidence-based medicine). There are also subject-specific specialist libraries, including one on mental health contained within the new National Library for Health (NLH).

Athens account

All NHS employees can apply for an 'Athens' password, which allows access via the internet to a large range of electronic resources, including Medline, the Cochrane database and a specialist library for mental health (see above). This includes many full-text articles of original papers.

Map of Medicine

This product should be available via the local Care Records Service in England (see below). Currently, it includes over 250 patient journeys, with 1300 flow charts detailing clinical pathways, the equivalent of more than 5000 text pages. These journeys appear in a unique graphical representation that enables the user to follow a pathway more easily. These journeys also provide access to clinical thinking and process in digestible chunks, with the ability to retrieve more detailed information as required (http://www.mapofmedicine.com).

Confidentiality and security

All medical data are potentially sensitive and information regarding mental health especially so. The principles of confidentiality and security with regard to medical records are not fundamentally different for electronic notes as for paper systems. The former cause greater concern because of the potential ease of browsing vast numbers of records, but in fact most electronic systems can be more secure than the paper equivalent, for example by having an audit trail of who has accessed what page. The National Programme for IT (see below) uses the principle of role-based access (i.e. the access to data is dependent on nationally determined roles, such as doctor, administrator etc.) and having a legitimate relationship to the patient. Access is controlled by a smart card and password, and is checked via the Spine (see below) once the individual logs onto the system. Other systems typically use password and user-name access only.

There is always a tension between making information available so that it is useful to service users and clinicians and making it absolutely confidential. The greater the control, in general the slower the system is to log on to and the greater is the chance of the information not being available because the clinician has insufficient access rights. In order to reassure both clinicians and members of the public, in 2006 the Secretary of State for Health Lord Warner issued what is known as the Care Records Guarantee (Government News Network, 2006), which provides that:

- individuals will be allowed access to their own records
- NHS staff's access to records will be strictly limited to those with a 'need to know' (i.e. in order to provide effective treatment to a patient)

- information will not be shared outwith the NHS unless individuals grant permission, the NHS is obliged to do so by law or failure to share would put someone else at risk, and any sharing without permission will be carried out following best-practice guidelines
- if individuals are unable to make a decision about sharing health information on their own behalf, a senior healthcare professional may make a decision to do so, taking into account the views of relatives, carers and any recorded views of the individual
- where healthcare is provided by a care team that includes people from other services, the NHS and patient can agree to share health information with the other services, bearing in mind the effect failure to share might have on the quality of care received
- individuals can choose not to share information in their electronic care records, although this may have an effect on the quality of care received
- there will be a complaints procedure
- individuals are entitled to check and correct mistakes in their record
- the NHS must enforce a duty of confidentiality on its staff and organisations under contract to the NHS
- the NHS must keep the records secure and confidential
- the NHS must keep a record of everyone who looks at the information held in the service (individuals will be entitled to ask for a list of people accessing their records and details of when they looked at the records)
- the NHS must take enforcement action if someone looks at records without permission or good reason.

There is some discussion as to whether patients should opt in or opt out of having their data included in the Care Records Service. There is the concept of the so-called 'sealed envelope', where some information is not shared, for example with the Spine or other service providers. This is somewhat problematic. For example, if information about a depressive episode is kept from the Spine yet the service user is on antidepressant medication and this information is on the Spine, the information would nevertheless indicate depression. It is considered unsafe to give only partial medication information and therefore it is the current position that all medication information would be omitted in such a case.

Data protection

The current UK legislation is the Data Protection Act 1998 (a complex piece of legislation). It contains eight principles regarding the handling of personal data. These state that all data must be:

1   processed fairly and lawfully
2   obtained and used only for specified and lawful purposes

3   adequate, relevant and not excessive
4   accurate and, where necessary, kept up to date
5   kept for no longer than necessary
6   processed in accordance with the individual's rights (as defined)
7   kept secure
8   transferred only to countries that offer adequate data protection.

Freedom of Information Act 2000

The Freedom of Information Act 2000 gives a general right of access to all types of recorded information held by public authorities, with full access granted in January 2005. The Act sets out exemptions to that right and places certain obligations on public authorities. It requires all organisations in the NHS to set up and maintain publication schemes that tell the public what information is held.

Caldicott guardians

'The Caldicott principles and processes provide a framework of quality standards for the management of confidentiality and access to personal information under the Leadership of a Caldicott Guardian.' (Department of Health, 2002)

The name arises from the work of Dr Fiona Caldicott, a past President of the Royal College of Psychiatrists. Chief executives were required to appoint a Caldicott guardian by 31 March 1999 and in 2002 this responsibility was extended to councils with social service responsibility (CSSRs). There are approximately 1000 Caldicott guardians throughout the NHS and in CSSRs. The Caldicott report (NHS Executive, 1997) established a clear set of principles, reflecting best practice in the handling of confidential information:

- *Justify the purpose.* Every proposed use or transfer of information within or from an organisation should be clearly defined and scrutinised, with continuing uses regularly reviewed by an appropriate guardian.
- *Do not use patient-identifiable information unless it is absolutely necessary.* Patient-identifiable information should not be used unless there is no alternative
- *Use the minimum necessary patient-identifiable information.* Where the use of patient-identifiable information is considered to be essential, each individual item of information should be justifiable, with the aim of reducing identifiability.
- *Access to patient-identifiable information should be on a strict need-to-know basis.* Only those individuals who need access to patient-identifiable information should have access it.

- *Everyone should be aware of their responsibilities.* Action should be taken to ensure that those handling patient-identifiable information, both clinical and non-clinical staff, are aware of their responsibilities and obligations to respect patient confidentiality.
- *Understand and comply with the law.* Every use of patient-identifiable information must be lawful. Someone in each organisation (the Caldicott guardian) should be responsible for ensuring that the organisation complies with the legal requirement.

Electronic patient records

It is intended that, in due course, all healthcare records, including those for mental health, will become electronic. Some general practices have become paperless, but few mental health trusts are even close to such a position. Mental health stands to gain particular benefit from such systems, especially if they are widely networked, given that mental healthcare is usually community based. This means that patients are liable to present at various sites, such as a community team base or an accident and emergency department or a hostel. An electronic patient record (EPR) provides the right information at the right time at the right place. There are important safety gains in implementing a full EPR, particularly with electronic prescribing, which has been shown to reduce drug errors by 85%.

An EPR also should improve the availability of information for both service users and carers, as it is possible to print off or even email copies of care plans, drug information leaflets and so on for them.

Most trusts, as they move towards a paperless system, will still keep paper records for a transitional period. This requires careful management and may in itself represent a risk, as vital information may remain in the paper records while the community mental health team (CMHT) uses more up-to-date electronic information, unaware of the existence of relevant past material. A recent serious incident occurred at a trust with a well-used electronic information system when a patient was admitted to the in-patient unit. There were extensive electronic records going back 3 years which were used during the admission but the paper records were not examined. The patient carried out a serious assault which mimicked almost exactly one 4 years previously, which had resulted in a forensic assessment which was in the paper but not electronic record. Had the existence of the assessment been known, the incident might have been avoided.

EPRs will inevitably change the way psychiatrists practise. The practice of an old-fashioned clerking will probably go, to be replaced by an electronic multidisciplinary assessment, which will be updated and edited from already existing information.

National Programme for IT

The National Programme for IT in the NHS, delivery of which is the primary work of NHS Connecting for Health, will bring modern computer systems into the NHS in England to improve patient care and service. It will connect over 30000 GPs to almost 300 hospitals and give patients access to their personal health and care information, transforming the way the NHS works (Connecting for Health, 2005). Currently, the National Programme for IT (NpfIT) covers England only, but there are some similar initiatives beginning in Wales and Scotland. NpfIT is a vast ambitious programme which includes various subprogrammes, including: the Spine; the Care Records Service; electronic transfer of prescriptions; N3; and 'choose and book'.

The Spine

The Spine is a national database with demographic information on the entire population of England. This is known as the PDS (patient demographic service). All EPR systems will be able to use the PDS as their patient master index, rather than using a local patient master index. The Spine will also contain key summary data, such as active problems or diagnoses, allergies, current medication prescribed, medical history and the details of other clinicians involved in the patient's care. This potentially will be very useful in psychiatry, where patients commonly present to services other than their own. However, having a national database raises concerns about confidentiality. These are covered in what is known as the Care Records Service Guarantee.

Care Records Service

This is the provision of an EPR. England has been divided into five clusters (South, London, North East, North West and West Midlands, and Eastern). Each cluster has a local service provider (LSP), a large commercial company that is contracted to supply the service, and a software supplier that is contracted by the LSP to build the system. The plan is for the Care Records Service to provide an EPR which allows clinicians with a legitimate relationship to access patient-centred information across all care settings. It should allow care pathways to be developed and support the government initiative to move care from hospital to the community.

Electronic transfer of prescriptions

This programme is not for electronic prescribing but for the transfer of prescriptions electronically. Patients would be given a prescription, which, provided they had nominated a chemist where they want to collect the prescription, would be sent electronically to that chemist, who would dispense the medication. The process of the chemist invoicing for the prescription would be dealt with electronically.

N3

This is the programme to upgrade the network for the NHS to provide broadband access throughout England.

Choose and book

The relevance of choose and book (C&B) for psychiatry has yet to be determined, as, in England, most services are related to general practice and require social service involvement, and it is not possible to choose to receive services from one local authority in preference to another. It would be difficult therefore to choose to refer a patient with schizophrenia, say, to one of four community mental health teams.

UK government policy

Mental Health Information Strategy

The Mental of Health Information Strategy was published in March 2001 by the Department of Health. It was therefore written before the roll-out of the National Programme for IT, but the principles which it covers have not changed. For more information see http://www.icservices.nhs.uk/mentalhealth/mh-is/pages/documentation.asp.

Mental Mental Health Minimum Data Set

'The Mental Health Minimum Data Set has been developed to improve information on mental health services usage and need. The data set describes the care received by service users during an overall SPELL OF CARE. It is person-centred so that all the care received by individuals can be studied, and includes details of clinical problems, treatments given, outline aspects of social care and outcomes. Geographic markers allow analysis by any type of health, GP or local authority administrative categories. The prime purpose of the data set is to provide local clinicians and managers with better quality information for clinical audit, and service planning and management. From 1 April 2003, when the data set became mandatory for MH service providers, central collection will provide improved national information, facilitating feedback to trusts and the setting of benchmarks.'

The Mental Health Minimum Data Set (MHMDS) is an aggregated data-set which should provide useful comparative information for service managers to compare how one service performs compared with another. It should be extractable from routinely collected clinical data, although in many cases the appropriate information system from which such data can be collected is not available. Further information is available at http://www.icservices. nhs.uk/mentalhealth/dataset/pages/default.asp.

Royal College of Psychiatrists

Mental Health Informatics Working Group

This is a College committee that works closely with the Mental Health Informatics Special Interest Group and reports to the Public Policy Committee of the College. It meets on a bi-monthly basis and is able to advise the College on matters of relevance and to raise issues of concern from College members. The minutes of its meetings are available on the 'Members' section of the College website (http://www.rcpsych.ac.uk). College members are required to register to be able to use parts of the site.

Mental Health Informatics Special Interest Group

This Group holds meetings, produces a newsletter and runs training workshops at College meetings for College members. Details are available via the College website.

The future

Mental health informatics is a rapidly developing topic, driven by continuing technological advance, which is certain to change the way mental health services operate and psychiatrists practise. Hand-held devices, perhaps 3G mobile phones, will allow EPRs to be accessible in service users' homes. Service users may be able to download their medical records to flashcards or access information via a website. There will always be differing levels of enthusiasm for such systems and progress will always seem slower than it might be. However, if psychiatrists can understand the basic principles, they will be in a better position to obtain real benefit from developments in informatics, rather than feeling that the technology is being imposed on them.

References

Connecting for Health (2005) 'NHS Connecting for Health: better information for health, where and when it's needed.' http://www.connectingforhealth.nhs.uk/resources/ comms_tkjune05/nhscfhsummary.pdf

Department of Health (2002) *Implementing the Caldicott Standard into Social Care. Appointment of 'Caldicott Guardians'* (HSC 2002/003:LAC (2002)2). Department of Health.

Government News Network (2006) Health Minister sets out electronic patient record details. http://www.gnn.gov.uk/environment/fullDetail.asp?ReleaseID=237651&NewsAreaID=2

NHS Executive (1997) *Report on the Review of Patient-Identifiable Information (Caldicott Report)*. Department of Health.

CHAPTER 32

Stress management and avoiding burnout

Frank Holloway and Jerome Carson

We live in an era of moral panic about stress in the workplace. Declining morale among the medical profession appears to be a worldwide if poorly understood phenomenon that probably relates more to changes in the 'psychological compact' between the medical profession, employers, patients and society than to issues of pay and workload (Edwards *et al*, 2002). In the past, experienced doctors could expect, after considerable early sacrifices in their working lives, a high degree of autonomy in their work and to be treated with deference and respect, in return for good-quality clinical care (as defined by the doctor). Contemporary medical practice is characterised by an ever-increasing level of accountability, team-working, a 'patient-centred' approach, openness to evaluation by non-professionals and exposure to an increasingly litigious, risk-averse culture. This shift in expectations on doctors may be particularly difficult because of the personality traits that traditionally characterise the medical profession. Consultants characteristically enjoy autonomy and innovation, want their decision-making to be based on logical analysis and need to be able to control their working life (Houghton, 2005). These traits are at apparent odds with the demands of the consumer-oriented, protocol-driven, team-based and rather chaotic culture of contemporary health services.

Mental health workers face increasing demands to provide treatment for people who experience workplace stress. It is therefore more than a little ironic for psychiatrists as a professional group to be described as being particularly prone to stress, burnout and suicide (Fothergill *et al*, 2004).

There is a perceived crisis in the recruitment and retention of psychiatrists, with large numbers of experienced consultants opting for early retirement (Kendell & Pearce, 1997). The reasons people give for leaving the profession early are both poignant and provide insight into the (potentially remediable) sources of distress that the profession as a whole has experienced (see Box 32.1). These include: the effects of serious adverse events, such as patient suicide, serious violence or homicide; a pervasive feeling of accountability without power to influence the actions of others; and alienation from the edicts of a 'management' that is perceived as remote, critical and unaware of day-to-day clinical reality.

Box 32.1 Selected reasons for early retirement given by consultant psychiatrists who retired prematurely in 1995 and 1996

- A consultant colleague committed suicide in 1994. I did not want to be next.
- A recurring feeling that I was failing despite working long hours.
- I had no wish to be 'crucified' in a future hospital inquiry into a suicide/homicide.
- Persistent awareness of a disaster about to happen at any time.... I realised it was only a matter of time before I was in the dock [i.e. a homicide enquiry] despite all my best efforts.
- Stress, stress, stress.
- I feel I let a patient down ... with serious consequences.
- I was tired. I had nothing left to give.
- I was unable to give enough time to many needy people because of imposed changes in practice.
- Increasing fears for personal safety.
- The level of violence against staff ... and the level of violence committed by my patients.
- The night work got too demanding.
- A total disregard for the views of the clinical team in planning services.
- An impossible medical director.
- Unable to meet the conflicting demands of NHS work and university work.
- Appointment of a colleague as clinical director for whom I had no respect.
- I was always in the cross-fire between medical colleagues and non-medical managers.
- I was deeply disenchanted by the fact that I didn't have any influence over long-term or day-to-day plans, though ultimately I carried the can.
- Only negative feedback from managers.
- The main reason was a feeling of being unappreciated/unsupported by management – an atmosphere of alienation – 'us and them'.
- Appalling attitude (hostility and grossly inadequate funding) to psychiatry of the purchasers.

Source: Kendell & Pearce (1997).

In this chapter, we provide a brief review of the concepts of stress and burnout and present what is known about the factors that lead to and protect from stress for mental health professionals. Then, drawing on what empirical evidence exists and our own experiences as a clinical psychologist with a particular interest in staff stress and a medical manager, we give some practical suggestions as to how psychiatrists can manage the stresses they inevitably experience.

These suggestions are largely targeted at the individual practitioner. However, it is important to emphasise that medical and service managers must take the issue of staff stress seriously, since a distressed workforce will be an ineffective workforce (Firth-Cozens, 2003). It is also sobering to note that how we experience our job in terms of its demands and the latitude we have over decisions has a very significant effect, independent of other risk factors, on the occurrence of fatal coronary heart disease (Kuper & Marmot, 2003). High demand and a restricted latitude in decision-making are potentially dangerous – and increasingly characterise the lot of the mental health professional. If taken seriously, this finding has profound implications for the responsibilities of the employer and specifically for job design.

The concepts of stress, burnout and stress management

Stress in the workplace

'Occupational stress' is a fashionable and rather generic term. It may be more helpful to talk in terms of the stress process (Carson & Kuipers, 1998). A model of this process comprises three levels: external stressors, potential moderating factors and stress outcomes (see Fig. 32.1).

External stressors include specific occupational stressors, hassles and uplifts, and major life events. Psychiatrists face a number of job-specific

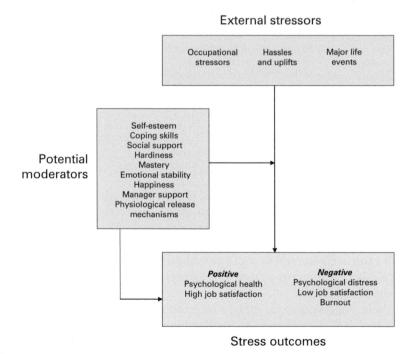

Fig. 32.1 The stress process model.

work stressors, which are not shared to the same degree by other mental health professionals. These include, for example, responsibilities under the Mental Health Act, the prescribing of psychotropic medications, decisions surrounding hospital admission and discharge, and the ever-present fear of criticism following a serious adverse incident. Hassles are the sort of minor irritations that can have a cumulative effect on our sense of feeling stressed. They can range from commuting difficulties to arguments with others. Uplifts reflect the positive aspects of personal and professional life. None of us is immune from the effects of major life events such as bereavement, marital breakdown, financial pressures and family problems and, cumulatively, they all take their toll.

Whether stressors cause positive or negative *stress outcomes* depends on the range of *moderating factors* available to us as individuals. These can be *internal factors*, such as self-esteem, coping skills and hardiness, or *external factors*, such as having the support of a line manager and colleagues. Hence a member of staff with a robust sense of self-esteem may be better able to deal with external stressors than a more fragile colleague.

Stress outcomes can be positive or negative. The former include psychological health and high job satisfaction. The latter involve psychological distress, low job satisfaction and the occupational burnout syndrome (see below).

While this stress process model provides a way of conceptualising the complex issue of staff stress, it is not comprehensive. For instance, while the issue of life events is highlighted, significant stress can also be generated by 'non-events,' such as failure to get a job or win a promotion. There are also significant difficulties with the attendant stress literature, which is heavily reliant on cross-sectional rather than prospective studies.

Burnout

The concept of burnout originated in the USA. The best definition has been provided by Schaufeli & Enzmann (1998, p. 36):

'Burnout is a persistent, negative, work-related state of mind in normal individuals that is primarily characterised by exhaustion, which is accompanied by distress, a sense of reduced effectiveness, decreased motivation and the development of dysfunctional attitudes and behaviours at work. This psychological condition develops gradually but may remain unnoticed by the individual involved. It results from a misfit between intentions and reality in the job. Often burnout is self-perpetuating because of inadequate coping strategies that are associated with the syndrome.'

The main psychometric measure used to assess burnout is the Maslach Burnout Inventory (Maslach & Jackson, 1986). This has 22 items which assess: the degree to which individuals are *emotionally exhausted* by their jobs; their level of *depersonalisation*, or their ability to feel for their patients; and their level of *personal accomplishment*, or the degree to which they feel they are effective or are rewarded by their jobs.

383

Psychiatrists and the stress process

There is a small and very diverse body of literature investigating aspects of the stress process as experienced by psychiatrists. There is evidence that consultant psychiatrists experience higher levels of stress than consultants working in other specialties, despite their lower objective workloads (Deary *et al*, 1996*a*). Perhaps surprisingly, psychiatric trainees report higher levels of stress than consultants (Guthrie *et al*, 1999). It is also now recognised that the transition from trainee to consultant is often experienced as particularly difficult.

A wide range of stressors for psychiatrists have been identified. These include changes within the health service, changes in community care, personal stresses, management and resource issues, and lack of time (Benbow & Jolley, 1997). Some studies have identified patient characteristics, particularly the management of the violent or potentially violent patient, as major stressors (Guthrie *et al*, 1999). Patient suicide is experienced as a highly stressful event by psychiatrists. Relationships with work colleagues, both psychiatrists and doctors in other disciplines, can be problematical, although, interestingly, this was not identified as a problem by old age psychiatrists (Benbow & Jolley, 1997).

The moderating factors most explored in the stress outcome literature for psychiatrists relate to what might loosely be termed 'personality factors'. Low self-esteem, neuroticism and negative coping strategies (such as worrying, self-blaming, anger, irritability and losing sleep) are, rather predictably, associated with poor stress outcomes (Deary *et al*, 1996*b*; Thomsen *et al*, 1998; Rathod *et al*, 2000). Work climate and workload also affect stress outcomes. Perceived support, being able to participate in the organisation and good leadership have a positive effect (Thomsen *et al*, 1998). There is some evidence that different styles of working are associated with different stress outcomes (Mears *et al*, 2004). These issues are discussed in more detail below.

Stress management

Given that stress can be conceptualised as a process with three different levels, it is hardly surprising that stress management can also be viewed at different levels. Cooper (1996) sees workplace stress interventions as fitting into a primary, secondary or tertiary prevention model.

1   In the *primary* prevention of workplace stress, the aim is to reduce or eliminate stressors and positively promote a supportive and healthy work environment.

2   *Secondary* prevention is concerned with the prompt detection and management of depression and anxiety, by increasing self-awareness and improving stress management skills. The aim here is to help

workers evaluate the psychological effects of stress and to develop their own personal stress control plans. The majority of work stress management programmes focus on the secondary level.

3   *Tertiary* prevention is concerned with the rehabilitation and recovery process of those individuals who have suffered or are suffering from stress-related disorders. The main forms of help at the tertiary level are workplace counselling and employee assistance programmes.

Stress management interventions often include the following elements (Dollard & Winefield, 1996):

*   changing, increasing or enhancing coping responses and resources
*   teaching arousal reduction techniques, such as relaxation or medita-tion;
*   changing perceptions or appraisals of work stress via cognitive re-structuring.

While there have been over 100 empirical studies of the stress process in mental health professionals, there have been very few intervention studies. Nurses form the focus of most studies and there are no published studies of stress management interventions solely for psychiatrists. A conventional stress management programme proved difficult to recruit to (Kunkler & Whittick, 1991). In one of the few randomised trials, Ewers *et al* (2002) showed that training in psychosocial interventions led to significant improvements in knowledge of and attitudes to psychosis, as well as reduced burnout in ten forensic nurses. Other interventions have included risk management (Sharkey & Sharples, 2003), clinical supervision (Berg & Hallberg, 1999), educational programmes (Milne *et al*, 1986), primary nursing (Melchior *et al*, 1996), assertion training (Gordon & Goble, 1986) and relaxation training (Watson, 1986). Carson *et al* (1999), in a randomised controlled trial, found no benefits from a social support programme for nursing staff in comparison with feedback only. In a review of the stress management literature, Reynolds & Briner (1994, p. 75) stated that:

'Occupational stress reduction is … one of the many fads initiated by academics, commercialised by consultants and embraced by managers but that ultimately fail to deliver the panacea-like solutions which they promise.'

The disappointing results to date from stress management interventions underline the need for further research in the area and the likely value of primary prevention as opposed to therapeutic strategies.

Reducing stress: what can be done?

The generic occupational literature identifies a range of interventions that (potentially) decrease stress in the workplace (see Box 32.2). Five issues are discussed in some detail: working styles (i.e. the characteristics of the job);

Box 32.2 Potential areas for intervention in the workplace to decrease stress

- Role characteristics – issues of clarity of role and workload
- Job characteristics – attending to the design of the job
- Interpersonal relationships – improving communication in the workplace
- Organisational climate and structure – encouraging decentralisation and participation by the workforce in decision-making
- Human resource management – recruitment and selection policies that select staff for the task in hand, and the establishment of effective mechanisms for supervision, appraisal and performance management
- Physical aspects of the work environment – quality of the physical environment, safety issues, adequate personal space

---

effective working within teams; achieving a work/life balance; relationships with medical colleagues; and training.

Working styles

The practice of psychiatrists, like that of all doctors, is changing rapidly. A National Steering Group (2004) has reviewed the role of the psychiatrist in the context of the 'modernisation' of mental health services. Traditional models of working within adult psychiatry, which involve both high individual case-loads within out-patient settings and responsibility for all patients on the case-load of the team, are associated with higher levels of stress than models with a more 'progressive' role (Mears *et al*, 2004). This 'progressive' working style is characterised by smaller personal case-loads, protected time for professional development, ability to react to unforeseen situations and much scope for delegation within the team. Clarity over the consultant role and perceived levels of support from the multidisciplinary team and service managers were also associated with lower levels of stress and burnout. It does appear to be clear that having some form of boundary on workload is important. This has obvious implications for the future design of consultant jobs. However, a job that was so well designed that it offered little or no direct patient and carer contact, made no intellectual demands or did not require the post-holder to feel responsible for the service would be unlikely to attract high-quality applicants (or much in the way of remuneration).

Teamwork issues

For mental health staff in general, colleagues within the multidisciplinary team are the main perceived source of support (Reid *et al*, 1999). Mutual support and respect from colleagues can buffer the adversities that inevitably occur within the life of a mental health professional. Effective teams can offer a valuable sounding board for discussing problematic cases and have subtle ways of supporting a colleague who is temporarily finding things difficult. Good teams do not, however, tolerate established poor performance. This partly reflects team culture, but also follows from the fact that good teams tend to have good managers.

A core skill of the contemporary consultant is the ability to work effectively within the multidisciplinary team. Some consultant behaviours will encourage good team-working, but others will consistently erode the support potentially available from the team (see Chapter 8). Although an adequate degree of technical competence, effective decision-making and specialist expertise are important to mental health teams, it is the 'softer', interpersonal competencies that dominate the relationship between the psychiatrist and the team. Putting the issue another way, it is the experience of most medical managers that their consultant colleagues rarely cause problems because of lack of technical competence: problems much more commonly arise because of issues of personality or personal style and consequent emerging conflicts with their teams or consultant colleagues.

Much more difficult than working well within an effective team is to support the transformation of a failing team. The failing team will increase the burden on the consultant in a number of ways, for example by colleagues refusing to share responsibility for the case-load, engaging in poor decision-making and not carrying out agreed tasks. The medical manager needs to support consultant colleagues where teams are failing, although the remedies tend to lie with the team leader and service manager. One particularly important but much neglected aspect of team functioning is the administrative support to the team.

Work/life balance

In the past, a male-dominated consultant workforce generally relied on a support system comprising a wife and family. Women entering higher levels of the profession were required to make choices between their role as a parent and as a professional, either by forgoing parenthood altogether or by depending on full-time domestic support.

One core demand of contemporary doctors is to achieve an appropriate balance between work and other aspects of life (Dumelow *et al*, 2000) and there is some evidence that women physicians who work their preferred hours have the best family and work outcomes (Carr *et al*, 2003). Doctors are seeking jobs that can offer a reasonable work/life balance, with part-time posts becoming increasingly popular among both women and men. There is also a requirement for career pathways that allow for less demanding jobs to be available towards the end of one's working life (which, for demographic reasons, is set to become significantly longer than in the past).

Job planning offers an opportunity to introduce flexibility into the consultant job description. Medical managers also need to consider developing more part-time posts that will be attractive to those seeking to improve their work/life balance. Part-time posts do, of course, have implications for the organisation of the service, raise the issue of providing continuity of care and are, because of the negotiated structure of the job plan, more expensive than full-time posts.

Working with medical colleagues

In contemporary, community-based practice, consultant psychiatrists tend to have much more regular and frequent contact with their multidisciplinary teams than with their consultant colleagues. This may be the explanation for the surprising finding that consultants frequently report their contacts with their colleagues as being a source of stress (Guthrie *et al*, 1999). There are a number of drivers to improving the links between consultant colleagues working within a service. Appraisal is based on an implicit model of the 'good doctor', who will be in regular communication with peers to discuss and review standards of practice and clinical outcomes. Accreditation for continuing professional development requires the doctor to participate in a peer group, which should be both supportive of and challenging to its members (see Chapter 20). Simple measures can improve working relationships, such as grouping consultant offices together and meeting colleagues regularly in both a work and a social context. Traditionally, case conferences and academic meetings have offered opportunities for consultant medical staff to meet. We have found particular value in regular informal meetings that discuss clinical issues which consultants are finding problematical (a 'risk forum').

Medical managers need to be aware of interpersonal difficulties occurring within a consultant group, although effective interventions are extremely difficult. There are particular sensitivities where consultants share medical responsibility for a team or service, which is likely to become increasingly common as part-time working increases. Working within a job share or with a co-consultant can be experienced on a spectrum from enjoyable and supportive to the deeply dysphoric.

Training issues

The literature on stress provides no clear guidance on how training for the consultant role and continuing professional development could help improve stress outcomes. The stresses that trainees experience are quite different from those that consultants identify (Guthrie *et al*, 1999), although patient suicide, hostility from patients and carers, complaints and serious untoward incidents are significant stressors for all psychiatrists. Training should provide all staff with the technical competence for the roles they undertake, and the ability to identify when they must seek additional expertise. All staff should have a thorough grounding in the ethical aspects of clinical practice: many of the most stressful situations psychiatrists experience are the product of the ethical dilemmas, which are an inevitable part of working within mental health services.

Our experience suggests that a thorough grounding in the theory and practice of the assessment and management of risk is helpful in reducing stress, but in a much more thoughtful way than mere familiarity with the local risk assessment documentation (Holloway, 2004). Specific training for appearing in the coroner's court, often a peculiarly distressing experience, may be useful. All psychiatrists should develop an understanding of how teams work and how they can work effectively within a team. These 'soft' competencies are not formally taught, but deficiencies are often picked up by trainers. Difficulties with management are frequently identified as sources of stress for consultants. This book, which seeks to provide an insight into the management process, should help psychiatrists learn to use their managerial colleagues more effectively. Health services are undergoing continual change: specific training in leading processes of service redesign and change management can allow psychiatrists to feel empowered rather than disoriented and distressed.

Conclusion

The stressors that psychiatrists experience are largely external to any particular mental health service and the propensity to experience stress (and to attract stressful experiences) seems to relate significantly to personality. However, it is possible to produce some suggestions to the psychiatrist for long-term professional survival. Individual clinicians need to identify whether they prefer the stimulation of the varied professional life of the generalist to the usually more boundaried role of the specialist, and to recognise when they need to change from one to the other. In psychiatry, the pace of service change is such that one can expect to undertake a number of roles within a professional lifetime, adapting generic skills to each new role and learning additional skills as necessary.

In an era obsessed with risk assessment and risk management, consultants need to adopt effective strategies that do not leave them paralysed by fear or vulnerable to criticism should disaster strike: the simplest strategy is, if in doubt, 'phone a friend'. Discussion with colleagues is an under-used resource and a degree of humility in the face of complex situations is a valuable trait. Humility also helps one embrace the processes now in place to review serious untoward incidents and complaints, by looking honestly for lessons that can be learned. It is also valuable for the consultant to have particular areas of interest for which there is protected time and which boost the individual's self-esteem and sense of autonomy – what might be described as 'hobbies'. These may, for example, be clinics that require specific expertise, medical management roles, teaching, research or even private practice. In choosing jobs, consultants need to think carefully about their working environment, and to pay at least as much attention to the quality of medical and multidisciplinary colleagues and service management as to simple workload parameters.

The literature clearly shows that medical managers can contribute to psychiatrists' stress (Kendell & Pearce, 1997). Service modernisation, which implies job redesign, offers the opportunity to reduce work pressures. Setting up mentorship schemes can be helpful for the younger consultant, who will benefit from the opportunity to discuss frustrations and difficulties with a more experienced colleague (Roberts *et al*, 2002). Above all, medical managers need to promote an open, respectful and positive organisational culture that offers all staff the opportunities to experience a sense of autonomy in their working lives and ensures that staff have the skills to undertake their tasks and roles.

References

Benbow, S. & Jolley, D. (1997) Old age psychiatrists: what do they find stressful? *International Journal of Geriatric Psychiatry*, **12**, 879–882.

Berg, A. & Hallberg, I. (1999) Effects of systematic clinical supervision on psychiatric nurses' sense of coherence, creativity, work related strain, job satisfaction and view of the effects from clinical supervision: pre–post design. *Journal of Psychiatric and Mental Health Nursing*, **6**, 371–381.

Carr, P. L., Gareis, K. C. & Barnett, R. C. (2003) Characteristics and outcomes for women physicians who work reduced hours. *Journal of Women's Mental Health*, **12**, 399–405.

Carson, J. & Kuipers, E. (1998) Stress management interventions. In *Occupational Stress: Personal and Professional Approaches* (eds S. Hardy, J. Carson & B. Thomas), pp. 157–174. Stanley Thornes.

Carson, J., Cavagin, J., Bunclark, J., *et al* (1999) Effective communication in mental health nurses: did social support save the psychiatric nurse? *NT Research*, **4**, 31–42.

Cooper, C. (1996) Stress in the workplace. *British Journal of Hospital Medicine*, **55**, 569–573.

Deary, I., Blenkin, H., Agius, R., *et al* (1996a) Models of job related stress and personal achievement amongst consultant doctors. *British Journal of Psychology*, **87**, 3–29.

Deary, I., Agius, R. & Sadler, A. (1996b) Personality and stress in consultant psychiatrists. *International Journal of Social Psychiatry*, **42**, 112–123.

Dollard, M. & Winefield, A. (1996) Managing occupational stress: a national and international perspective. *International Journal of Stress Management*, **3**, 69–83.

Dumelow, C., Littlejohns, P. & Griffiths, S. (2000) Relation between a career and family life for English hospital consultants: qualitative, semistructured interview study. *BMJ*, **320**, 1437–1440.

Edwards, N., Kornacki, M. J. & Silversin, J. (2002) Unhappy doctors: what are the causes and what can be done? *BMJ*, **324**, 835–838.

Ewers, P., Bradshaw, T., McGovern, J., *et al* (2002) Does training in psychosocial interventions reduce burnout rates in forensic nurses? *Journal of Advanced Nursing*, **37**, 470–476.

Firth-Cozens, J. (2003) Doctors, their well-being, and their stress. *BMJ*, **326**, 670–671.

Fothergill, A., Edwards, D. & Burnard, P. (2004) Stress, burnout, coping and stress management in psychiatrists: findings from a systematic review. *International Journal of Social Psychiatry*, **50**, 54–65.

Gordon, V. & Goble, L. (1986) Creative accommodation: role satisfaction for psychiatric staff nurses. *Issues in Mental Health Nursing*, **8**, 25–35.

Guthrie, E., Tattan, T., Wiliams, E., *et al* (1999) Sources of stress, psychological distress and burnout in psychiatrists. *Psychiatric Bulletin*, **23**, 207–212.

Holloway, F. (2004) Risk: more questions than answers. *Advances in Psychiatric Treatment*, **10**, 273–274.

Houghton, A. (2005) The importance of having all types in a workforce. *BMJ Careers*, 5 February, 56–57.

Kendell, R. E. & Pearce, A. (1997) Consultant psychiatrists who retired prematurely in 1995 and 1996. *Psychiatric Bulletin*, **21**, 741–745.

Kunkler, J. & Whittick, J. (1991) Stress management groups for nurses: practical problems and possible solutions. *Journal of Advanced Nursing*, **16**, 172–176.

Kuper, H. & Marmot, M. (2003) Job strain, job demands, decision latitude and risk of coronary heart disease within the Whitehall II study. *Journal of Epidemiology and Community Health*, **57**, 147–153.

Maslach, C. & Jackson, S. (1986) *Maslach Burnout Inventory*. Consulting Psychologists Press.

Mears, A., Pajak, S., Kendall, T., *et al* (2004) Consultant psychiatrists' working pattern: is a progressive approach the key to staff retention? *Psychiatric Bulletin*, **28**, 251–253.

Melchior, M., Philipsen, H., Abu-Saad, H., *et al* (1996) The effectiveness of primary nursing on burnout among psychiatric nurses in long stay settings. *Journal of Advanced Nursing*, **24**, 694–702.

Milne, D., Burdett, C. & Beckett, J. (1986) Assessing and reducing the strain of psychiatric nursing. *Nursing Times*, **82**(7), 59–62.

National Steering Group (2004) *Guidance on New Ways of Working for Psychiatrists in a Multidisciplinary and Multi-agency Context*. Department of Health.

Rathod, S., Roy, L., Ramsay, M., *et al* (2000) A survey of stress in psychiatrists working in the Wessex Region. *Psychiatric Bulletin*, **24**, 133–136.

Reid, Y., Johnson, S., Morant, N., *et al* (1999) Improving support for mental health staff: a qualitative study. *Social Psychiatry and Psychiatric Epidemiology*, **34**, 309–315.

Reynolds, S. & Briner, R. (1994) Stress management at work: with whom, for whom and to what ends? *British Journal of Guidance and Counselling*, **22**, 75–89.

Roberts, G., Moore, B. & Coles, C. (2002) Mentoring for newly appointed consultant psychiatrists. *Psychiatric Bulletin*, **26**, 106–109.

Schaufeli, W. & Enzmann, D. (1998) *The Burnout Companion to Study and Practice: A Critical Analysis*. Taylor and Francis.

Sharkey, S. & Sharples, A. (2003) The impact on work related stress of mental health teams following team based learning on clinical risk management. *Journal of Psychiatric and Mental Health Nursing*, **10**, 73–81.

Thomsen, S., Dallender, J., Soares, J., *et al* (1998) Predictors of a healthy workforce for Swedish and English psychiatrists. *British Journal of Psychiatry*, **173**, 80–84.

Watson, J. (1986) A step in the right direction. *Senior Nurse*, **5**(4), 12–13.

CHAPTER 33

How to get the job you *really* want

Dinesh Bhugra

In order to get any job that you really want, a number of factors have to be considered. To become a consultant is a culmination of training in the right specialty and the right type of experience in training, teaching and research. In view of the number of vacancies that are currently in the system at the consultant level, to get a consultancy job is not impossible, provided you have the right aptitude, knowledge and skills. To get the job you *really* want requires technique and background work. This chapter aims to help the trainee look at a job and apply the right skills to obtain it.

There is little doubt that for those in hospital practice, becoming a consultant is important: if not a pinnacle of achievement, at least a stopover to bigger achievements. The task of assessing a job and going after the one you really want must be seen as a professional task. The art of getting such a job is not a battle that has to be won but a courtship, in which potential employers and colleagues have to be wooed. When planning to go out on a date, you decide whether there is any long-term potential in the relationship and will prepare accordingly (where to go to, what to wear, what food to order, what wine to drink). Similarly, applying for a consultant job requires careful thought, preparatory work and rehearsal, all of which should make the actual performance of the task easier. This should enable you to show yourself in a strong light in the pre-interview visits and reflect your glory in the actual interview.

Failure to get a job is often due to inadequate preparation, not being clear about why you would like that particular job and your own career plans, and poor performance at the interview. Appearing for an interview and becoming a consultant requires long-term and short-term planning.

In relation to long-term planning, most candidates for consultant jobs in the UK will have done exactly the same period of training in similar rotations, although their administrative, teaching and research experiences will be more varied. For this reason, in addition to having the MRCPsych examination or equivalent (for the latest guidelines consult the Royal College of Psychiatrists), having other research diplomas or degrees, such as an MD or PhD, will make you a more attractive candidate. You have to make sure that you have a CCT (Certificate of Completion of Training) or are eligible for it.

The focus of this chapter is on short-term planning. Once you know your date of completion of training and the date on which you will obtain the CCT, you should start to look around for jobs. You may find it helpful to break down the process of gaining a consultant job into the following steps:

- opening a job file
- preparing an up-to-date curriculum vitae (CV)
- preparatory visits and homework
- the interview.

In addition, if you are offered the job, there will be negotiations over the contract, but these are beyond the remit of the present chapter.

Opening a job file

The job file should contain every bit of information that you need to prepare for the particular job. If you cut out the advertisement and paste it on to a blank sheet you can also write a time line for that application on the same sheet: when the advertisement appeared, closing date, pre-interview visit, the date of the interview and so on. You can then decide on what other specific information may be helpful. Within such a folder or ring binder you could include specific questions and proposed answers, and relevant documents and papers such as summaries of the NHS Plan or of the National Service Framework (on which, see Chapter 5).

The job file should also be the place where you list why you want the job, what problems you envisage in the job, what the responses of various people (whom you have been to see) are, what your plans will be and what your CV's strengths and weaknesses are. You may wish to include recent medico-political documents as well as the responses to those from the Royal College of Psychiatrists and the British Medical Association (BMA), for example.

Thus, the file will give you comprehensive information even when you need it in a hurry. During this phase, talk to others who may have participated in recent interviews either as an interviewer or a candidate. This will give you an idea of the questions likely to be asked and also how to deal with pressures and different styles of interviewing. It is not always likely that you will be asked the same questions but at least this may give you some hints.

Preparing a CV

You cannot be interviewed unless you are shortlisted and your shortlisting depends on your CV and how you have presented yourself. The shortlisting is on the basis of the CV and makes a distinction between definite candidates and probable candidates. Even when job application forms are used, a CV provides useful background.

Different people have different ideas about the layout and the contents of the CV. The aim is to impress your potential colleagues sufficiently to make it on to the shortlist. Therefore the CV should be neatly laid out and well ordered. It is important to read the instructions for application very carefully and to submit the right number of copies if required, with adequate time to spare. Intra-hospital handling of the post may add another day or two to the delivery time, so take that into account. If the employers have asked for 26 copies of the CV, then 26 it will have to be.

A suggestion for the ordering and content of the CV is presented in Box 33.1.

All institutions have equal opportunity policies and no discrimination on the basis of race, age, gender, marital status or sexual orientation is allowed. Thus you do not need to give these details unless specifically asked.

Undergraduate training and education should be mentioned briefly, as should basic schooling. Dates of entry, graduation and any awards, distinctions and prizes should be mentioned. A complete list of qualifications with the years in which they were obtained should be given, followed by details of posts. Giving a list of all the posts in a tabular form with details of overall experience gained in the text below the table is often helpful.

Box 33.1 Suggested contents and ordering of a CV

- Name
- Address
- Contact details (including mobile phone number and email address)
- Sex
- Qualifications (year/school/degree)
- Distinctions
- General education
- Current post (also note experience – clinical, administrative, research and teaching)
- Previous posts
- Administrative experience
- Teaching experience (medical – undergraduate and postgraduate – and also non-medical)
- Research (current experience)
- Publications (peer reviewed, invited, commentaries, editorials, chapters, abstracts)
- Membership of learned societies
- Career plans
- Other interests
- Referees

Previous posts should be in chronological order. The most common format is to give the most recent job first and then to work backwards to pre-registration house officer (PRHO) jobs. Try to highlight your relevant experience in each job, as this allows you to draw the reader's attention to your suitability for the job on offer.

The sections on administration, teaching and research should give a succinct summary of your relevant experience. Depending on the type of job applied for, you may need to detail the relevant experience accordingly. For example, if applying for an academic job, academic components (i.e. research and teaching) will take precedence over clinical experience. Administrative experience may well be more useful for jobs that contain clinical lead roles.

The list of publications should be up to date and accurate. Either the Vancouver or the Harvard style may be used, but consistency of style is important. In multi-authorship papers, your name should be underlined or in bold letters. A long list of publications can be divided into those in peer-reviewed journals, reviews, editorials, book chapters; or it could be divided according to subject. Details of membership of learned societies may be given if these reflect appropriate experience. Scientific communications or presentations may be added if required. For administrative experience, it is not sufficient simply to state that you were a member of however many committees: your roles and responsibilities must be stated. Similarly, teaching experience can be divided into undergraduate, postgraduate, non-medical and so on, rather than simply listing lectures.

You will be required to provide names and contact details of two or more referees. It is important to have the right referees for each application. If you are applying for an academic job or a job in a teaching hospital, you should give the professor's or academic head's name if you have worked with him or her directly; otherwise, you may need to give the names of other academics in the department with whom you have worked. All jobs will require a referee from your current placement and unless there are exceptional circumstances you should provide those details. A third referee could be another person you have worked for. Thus, one clinical and one academic referee are helpful and if the job is clinical the third referee could be a clinician, or an academic if the job is academic. It is advisable to name referees you have worked with in the past 5 years. You must obtain your referees' permission before giving their names and keep them informed by sending them an up-to-date copy of your CV and the job description of the post you have applied for, so that they can tailor the reference accordingly.

Before submitting your CV, show it to the scheme organisers, consultants and colleagues who have had experience of shortlisting. Get their advice and do not leave writing and updating of your CV to the last minute. A slovenly written, misspelt, shoddy CV will certainly lose you the shortlisting, no matter how brilliant you are. Having your CV on a PC with regular updates and spellchecks is helpful. When updating, you may need to change the tone of the CV rather than simply add on bits of experience. You should also be aware that if you are sending the CV for different jobs, you should amend it accordingly and the CV must flow well. Within the CV you should have no more than a paragraph stating what your career plans are and how this particular job fits in with those.

A covering letter should accompany your application. Some trusts use standard application forms which will be used for recruiting other members of staff as well, and therefore will not be adequate for your purpose. Under these circumstances, fill in all the sections as appropriate and if there are gaps that cannot be filled you can draw the employer's attention to the relevant sections in your CV. Some employers may ask that the accompanying letter be handwritten, in which case do so on plain paper and not on hospital headed notepaper.

Homework and preparation

After you have read the job description, get others – colleagues, consultant or scheme organiser – to cast an eye over it to identify areas of potential problems, such as office space, secretarial support and potential changes in service development.

You need to be clear as to why you want this particular job in this particular area and why the appointments committee should take you seriously. You have to be certain that you meet all the essential and most of the desirable criteria and person specifications. You should try to get hold of trust annual reports and 5-year plans. You should explore your fixed-session commitments and resources. The actual contract will be issued only after you have been offered the job, which you should discuss with BMA representatives.

Use both formal and informal channels to gather information about the job. Informal visits before the interview are encouraged, although some hospitals prefer that this occurs only after shortlisting. You may, of course, need to make more than one or two visits. Have a list of questions with you, some of which will be suitable only for medical colleagues, others for managers and some for both. When you arrange a visit by contacting the relevant clinical director or human resources people, you should arrange to see as many people as possible or, if it is impossible to do so, at least talk to them by telephone or correspond via email.

You need to find out if it is a new job or a replacement. If the latter, find out how long the post has been vacant and whether there have been problems in recruitment, and if so, what the reasons are. You may get some of the information from the regional advisor of the Royal College of Psychiatrists, who can also tell you whether it is approved for purposes of training. You must explore the number of sites that you will be expected to work at and the distances involved. You need to know about staffing levels and whether there are trainees in post and any impending changes. You may wish to find out about further education, study leave, details of removal and travelling expenses, research facilities and support. You should have your own list of priorities and arrange to see all those who may give you an overview. You should attempt to visit the site and talk to members of the multidisciplinary team. You may find it helpful to talk with some trainees, who may be able to tell you things which are pertinent to your application. You must arrange to see the chair of the trust, the chief executive and managers who are responsible for the specialty or sector. These managers will be able to give you details of potential changes which may affect the job in the long run. You should review the retention/attrition rate in the trust, which will give you a clear idea of what the trust's priorities and attitudes are.

The visit is for mutual appraisal, in that you need to find out about the job and the people, and the employers need to ascertain your strengths and weaknesses. The visits also serve another purpose, in that you may feel less anxious during them and may benefit if your performance in the interview is below par. Take extra copies of your CV and the job description with you and arrive in plenty of time for your appointment.

Also make sure that the secretary and the individuals concerned are aware of your arrival. It is acceptable to take notes but this may be distracting. If you do not, try to do so as soon as possible after the visit, as you are likely to forget vital information. After finishing your visit, you may wish to drive around to get a feel for the area if you are not familiar with it. You may also wish to take your family around and may choose to discuss the visit with your referees. You must make an effort to meet with other key people, such as the head of social services. Always ask the people you are seeing whether there is anyone else they think you should be seeing.

The interview

The interview is a vital process, which, although meant to select the best candidates, does not always do so: it selects those candidates who are good at being interviewed.

View the interview as another stage in the courtship ritual: you have to show yourself as confident, enthusiastic, honest and charming.

The consultant appointment procedures are enshrined in law and you can find out the most up-to-date information on the structure of the panel by checking relevant websites. For consultant advisor appointments, committees include a lay member (often the chair of the trust or another non-executive director), a College representative, the chief executive (or a board-level executive or associate director), the medical director (clinical director), a consultant from the trust and a university representative (especially if teaching and/or research commitments are part of the job description). These are core members and the committee may not proceed if any core member (or an appointed deputy) is not present. Trusts are free to add additional members but the balance of the committee must have a medical majority. Further details of the actual procedure can be obtained from the Department of Health (2005) document *The NHS (Appointment of Consultants) Regulations*. For academic appointments, the head of the department, one or two external assessors and at least one other member of the department should be on the committee. A representative of the human resources department is also in attendance.

The committee is looking for a competent, dedicated and sensible individual and it has been known for committees to appoint a more suitable candidate over a 'preferred' or favoured candidate.

You should appear neat and well dressed, relaxed and assertive. Even if you feel anxious (which you should and are entitled to be), try to hide it. As a consultant, you will be expected to contain other people's anxieties and to try to deal with them in non-pharmacological way. Ensure that you are properly dressed – old school ties may prove disadvantageous. For women, jewellery should be unobtrusive and make-up minimal. Before you are called in, ensure that your mobile phone is switched off and set your watch so that it does not beep.

When you are called in, greet the chair politely; the chair will then introduce the panel and set the rules for the interview. Try to relax and control your nervousness. Do not flop in the chair; sit erect and maintain eye contact with members of the panel.

Mock interviews and use of video may make you aware of your good and bad points. A good interview combines preparedness with spontaneity and naturalness. You may be asked to do a 10-minute presentation before the interview or at a separate time. Prepare your subject carefully, avoid jargon and do mock presentations. You may be asked to do a presentation to users' groups, where you may be asked questions about your attitudes to different types of treatment such as electroconvulsive therapy.

In the interview, the questions will be quite sophisticated and divided broadly into general, factual, philosophical/political and academic categories. If there is more than one candidate, each panel member is expected to ask the same questions. The first few questions are designed to set you at ease. A list of questions you may be asked is given in Box 33.2. There is no fixed length of the interview, but it is rare for it to exceed 40 minutes.

The chances are that the output of a specialist registrar research day will be assessed either formally in the interview or informally. The perceived output must include peer reviewed publications, either in press or published. The role and utilisation of special-interest sessions will also be explored, especially in the context of the job for which the individual has applied or is being interviewed.

The signing off of a record of in-training assessment (RITA) (grade C) is necessary for promotion to consultant grade. Yearly educational objectives should be part of the process of RITA. Increasingly, 360° appraisals and assessments will start to become part of the assessment.

Box 33.2 Questions likely to arise in interview

General

- Why this job? (To say it is a challenge is a cliché)
- Why are you suited for this job?
- Why this hospital/academic department?
- Why this area?
- What do you see as deficiencies in this service?
- How would you improve efficiency?
- What are your plans over next 5–10 years? (Talk about both professional and personal aims)
- What special skills do you bring?
- What are your special interests?
- How would you fit in?

Factual

- Largely to do with your CV
- Gaps in CV
- Why did you do this and not that?
- Why did you do/not do an MD?
- Why did you decide to become a psychiatrist?

Political/philosophical

- Views on NHS reforms? (Avoid party line – use your BMA/College views)
- Views on ... patients with intellectual disability
  - changes to the Mental Health Act
  - capacity for consent
  - mental health capacity
  - the Postgraduate Medical Education and Training Board
  - the European Working Time Directive
  - *Modernising Medical Careers*
  - clinical audit
  - the role of clinicians in management
  - revalidation/appraisal
- How would you reduce your budget by $x\%$?

Academic/research

- How would you organise teaching for undergraduates, postgraduates?
- How would you organise journal clubs?
- What journals do you read?
- How would you organise and supervise research?
- How would you organise rotation?

Additional

- Your strengths and weaknesses
- Your views of the area
- Hobbies, relaxation and so on

When the panel has finished asking questions, the chair will ask you if you have anything to add or any questions for any member of the panel. This is your opportunity to clarify major points, but no more than one or two. This is not the time to ask for designated car parking space or to ask banal or facetious questions. It may be worthwhile stating that you have already been to the place and seen relevant people, who have been very helpful in answering all the questions you had. Indeed, if you have done your homework, you should have had all your questions answered by the time of the interview.

At the end of the interview, thank the chair and the panel and leave. You may be asked to wait for the decision or the chair may ask you to provide contact details so that the committee can let you know their decision. The committee is advisory and they will make a recommendation to the trust board.

The procedure of interviewing has problems of its own. The important factor to bear in mind is selling your uniqueness. For women and doctors trained overseas, there may be additional factors that come into play. Questions about personal circumstances and private lives have to follow guidelines for equal opportunity legislation and conform with the code of good practice. It is unacceptable to ask a woman any questions which are not asked of men. In the event of a complaint regarding racial or gender discrimination, members of the panel may be required to give evidence.

It is important to be clear about the job you are applying for, the reasons for your choice and the commitment required.

Be yourself and you cannot go far wrong. Good luck!

References and further reading

Asbury, A. (1985) Assess a job. In *How to Do It* (Vol. I) (2nd edn) (ed. S. Lock), pp. 81–85. BMA Publications.

Department of Health (2005) *The NHS (Appointment of Consultants) Regulations*. Department of Health.

Drife, J. (1985) Be interviewed. In *How to Do It* (Vol. I) (2nd edn) (ed. S. Lock), pp. 92–95. BMA Publications.

Gray, C. (2005) Fair interviewing is harder than it looks. *BMJ Careers*, **331**, 68–69.

Hobbs, R. (1985) The interview. *British Journal of Hospital Medicine*, **33**, 220–222.

Naeem, A., Rutherford, J. & Kenn, C. (2005) From specialist registrar to consultant. Permission to land. *Psychiatric Bulletin*, **29**, 348–351.

Poole, A. (2005) What not to do at an interview. *BMJ Careers*, **331**, 65–66.

Rhodes, P. (1983) Applying for jobs. *BMJ*, **286**, 618–620.

Rhodes, P. (1983) Interviews: sell yourself. *BMJ*, **286**, 706–707.

Rhodes, P. (1983) Interviews: what happens. *BMJ*, **286**, 784–785.

Rhodes, P. (1983) Women doctors. *BMJ*, **286**, 863–864.

Rhodes, P. (1983) Overseas doctors. *BMJ*, **286**, 1047–1049.

CHAPTER 34

Surviving as a junior consultant: hit the ground walking

Mark Salter

Whatever the quality of your specialist registrar training, or the resource-fulness and resilience of your personality, the early years of your first substantive post as consultant psychiatrist will be a time of challenge and more than a little stress. Nothing can fully prepare you for this. Upon start-ing work, you will encounter a sudden hike in the range and complexity of your responsibilities, and the demands made of you by others, senior and junior, in terms of decisions, actions and calls for leadership and support. You will need to balance your responses to these demands against the seemingly ever-changing motives and agendas of countless other individuals, from many backgrounds, clinical and managerial. Many of these people will be total strangers and will bring with them all the unpredictable quirks and foibles that human nature is heir to.

In the early months, you will also need to assimilate a large amount of critical, need-to-know information – names, places, telephone numbers, faces and so on – while at the same time handling a vast increase in seemingly less crucial information that reaches you, via meetings, telephones, pigeonholes, pagers, faxes and emails. Much of this will prove useless; some of it will be invaluable. Few people will tell you which is which. Against this blooming, buzzing backdrop, you will also need to continue to practise the clinical psychiatry for which you have trained, and grapple with the ever-present problems of work in an under-resourced and stigmatised service. Occasionally, you will need to make quick decisions about high-risk situations, possibly involving suicide or even homicide, with incomplete information. If you have any energy left, you might even try to maintain a life outside work.

None of this need be half as forbidding as it sounds, provided that you think about these matters before and during the first months of the job. All of the key issues have been well described elsewhere in this book. It is useful to reiterate them here in a simple maxim: surviving as a junior consultant can be made easier – fun even – by looking after six things: objects, time, systems, information, people and yourself. (See how these themes define the opening paragraphs of this chapter.)

Box 34.1 Essentials from the start of the job

- Dedicated office
- Dedicated secretary
- Telephone
- Fax
- Computer, with full internet and intranet access
- Dictating machine
- Mobile phone
- Signed contract
- Pension agreement
- Clear understanding of annual leave, study leave, sabbatical allowance

Get the hardware to work the way that you want

Never start work without at least the essential tools of the job. Think about this well before the start date. Research into the availability of a personal office, dedicated secretarial support and access to the rest of the world, by telephone, fax and email, should form an essential part of your pre-interview reconnaissance. It is also a handy filler for that 'Is there anything that you want to ask?' part of the job interview. The reply will say much about the department. Mental health services are usually cash-strapped and many consultant posts, especially new ones, are created with scant thought for administrative support, in spite of the massive expansion in paperwork and communications in recent decades. Your own private space is an absolute must. Never agree to share an office with a colleague: if they really want you, they can hire a Portakabin. Box 34.1 gives a full list of the essential items that you should demand on, or before, the first day of the job.

Having secured these tools, learn to use them properly. Of all the skills that can transform your consultant life, confident use of a dictating machine and ten-finger typing are by far the most valuable. If you are not already literate in Word, Outlook and PowerPoint, arrange for your trust to send you on a course (see also Chapter 30). The computer and mobile phone are essential tools for controlling the flow of information through to you, but make sure you control these devices and not vice versa. Technology allows you to manage a crucial aspect of consultant life: availability. Be available, but not too available.

The only piece of kit more essential than the computer is the humble diary. Never keep more than one, but make sure your secretary keeps a regular back-up. It is debatable whether this should be of the paper or electronic variety, but only one will survive a drop down a flight of stairs on a council estate. Cultivate the art of diary husbandry from day one: a well-kept diary is the secret to mastery over time and systems.

Know your network: the teams they are a-changin'

A disconcerting aspect of life as a new consultant is the impression that everyone else seems to have a much better idea of how things work. This is largely an illusion. Instead, they are just a little more familiar with the chaos and unpredictability inherent in any large system. The National Health Service (NHS), with its burgeoning management and ever-shifting arrangement of teams, is no exception. The truth is that no one, anywhere, really knows how best to make it work. A useful lesson that derives from this inherent chaos is to ask not *how* various teams, clinics, managers and meetings function, but *why*. Although people tend to do things better with familiarity, it also blinds them to alternatives. It may seem hard to believe on day one, but your lack of familiarity with the way things work is an asset. Try to keep the 'why' question alive in your head throughout the early months of the job, and never accept 'That's just the way it is' as a reasonable answer.

Your timetable is a case in point. If everything can change, then so can your timetable. Never commit yourself to a fixed timetable in the early months, whatever it said in the job description. No matter what you are told about the immovable nature of this clinic or that ward round, ignore it. Devising your own timetable – which usually means changing someone else's – is essential for your survival. It is hard to overstate the importance of customising your timetable early in the job. Every clinical session generates about two-thirds as much work again in telephone calls, dictation, proofing and countless other tasks. Build these into your timetable from week one and make sure that you allow at least two weekly sessions for personal time. This means time dedicated to whatever activity you wish: study, read, talk, lecture, visit, anything. If you find yourself doing routine work in this time, stop and ask yourself how you intend to move it to a more appropriate place in your working month. A useful rule of thumb is a ratio of 3:3:2 for clinical: administrative:personal time. Defend those last two sessions as though your life depended upon them. In a year or two, it possibly will.

At the outset, your clinical work will not have reached full pressure, and so these carefully carved spaces may have an uncomfortably cavernous feel to them. Do not fall into the trap of filling them with other people's problems. All of us, in our first consultant job, arrive with a blend of energy, insecurity and ingenuousness that is both the pity and the envy of our more experienced colleagues. This makes it easy for us to rush in and offer too much in attempt to make a favourable impression. Resist this urge at all costs – do as little fixed work as possible in the first month of the job.

Instead, spend this precious time and clarity of vision learning about the local terrain. No clinical service functions in isolation. Rather, we all work

403

Box 34.2 Sensible things to do – or not do – early on in the job

- Check your contract is signed and agreed
- Check that you exist in the eyes of payroll, pension and human resources
- Go on an induction course
- Get yourself a mentor or enrol with a peer group
- Pay a visit to the chief executive of your trust
- Check out the local non-statutory services
- Do not commit yourself to a fixed timetable in the first 2 months
- Watch more experienced colleagues in action
- Do as little clinical work as possible

---

in a rich lattice of teams, roles and organisations. The ubiquity of mental illness means that there is much overlap between the work of many services, both inside and outside your trust. These overlaps are important: they are a common source of border conflict, as well an opportunity to pass work on to others. Pay special attention to the work done by local non-statutory organisations in your area. A sensible investment of early energy is to pay a visit to your local day centres, hostels, homeless units, Samaritans, MIND, local counselling services and anyone else you think may be useful to meet. If there are leaders of important minority groups living on your patch, go to say hello. A list of sensible things to do and to avoid in the early weeks is given in Box 34.2.

Within your trust, you can afford to familiarise yourself with systems and faces a little more slowly. You should have visited the human resources offices within days of starting, but also attend early on to those facets of the department that are usually invisible: the security office, the front desk, the switchboard, the cleaners and every other organ of that vast creature that is a mental health trust. It always repays itself in time.

Information overload: hello real world, goodbye perfection

We are drawn to psychiatry because it reflects the richness of human nature itself; psychiatry is the one branch of medicine that touches upon politics, biography and philosophy as much as biology. Non-psychiatric colleagues tease us for the detail of our letters and summaries; what they are really doing is acknowledging the bewildering complexity of mental illness. Psychiatry is a data-rich specialty. We all work within a lattice of teams and organisations. It is useful, therefore, to view your work in terms of information flowing between points in a complex, abstract system. Learning how to control this vast flow is a major challenge to the new consultant. There are two key aspects to all this information: its quantity and its objective quality.

The way we gather, consider and act upon clinical information varies greatly with experience. Medical training teaches us to abandon data quantity in favour of quality. Medical courses start 'bottom up', encouraging students to accumulate large amounts of information – most of it redundant – through which we then sift for significance. By the time we reach specialist registrar level, most of us have this sifting down to a fine art, but the habit of wanting to know everything dies hard.

The catch comes with the move to consultant level, because a massive hike in the things that we think we need to know inevitably accompanies this move. Much of this is non-clinical. It is difficult at first to apply our well-honed sifting skills to such strange new material and so we fall back on the habits of our training. Probably the greatest challenge of surviving as a junior consultant lies in learning how to stop thinking and acting like a specialist registrar. Or, put another way, the secret of survival as a junior consultant lies in learning that *you don't need to know everything*. There are many ways to do this, some more drastic than others. First, get technology working for you. Your computer can be set up, for example, so that your secretary – or even the machine itself – sends you only filtered data. Second, surround yourself with reliable people and make sure that you share a clear understanding of exactly what you want and expect from each other. Third, ration your availability to less-experienced staff. You have been appointed as a consultant because you can do the job better than most of the people around you, but this does not mean you should do it. Instead, start delegating from day one and make a habit of it. This skill is not easy to acquire, for good reason: one of the hardest things in the world is to give an important job to someone else, knowing that they will screw it up.

Having learnt to handle the torrent of information that reaches you, next turn your attention to the issue of quality. What do you really need to know? In clinical terms, this usually relates to matters of risk, capacity and responsibility. Despite 5000 years of human civilisation, mental illness has remained perplexing; if there were simple answers to the questions posed by madness, sadness and consciousness, we would have found them by now. Part of the job of a consultant lies in helping people feel less uncomfortable with the truth that there are no easy answers to the big questions that psychiatry considers as stock in trade. Get used to answering the unanswerable.

Fortunately, deciding what non-clinical information is worth knowing is usually easier, and derives from a combination of common sense and spotting the key players in your network, great and small. Meetings are a good place to gather large amounts of this information in one swoop, but, *caveat salutor* (let the visitor be wary), seven out of every ten meetings are a waste of time, and you cannot tell which is which until afterwards. In the early months, it is sensible to attend as many meetings as possible – as this is also a useful way to start practising non-availability – but attend, listen carefully and no more. Try to say as little as possible, and never, ever volunteer to do anything. Afterwards, ask yourself whether the meeting really changed anything. If it did, return, but never attend a meeting whose sole purpose is to decide whether or not to have a meeting.

Hell is not necessarily other people

Whoever said 'Liking your colleagues is a bonus' was a curmudgeon, but probably right. We choose psychiatry for many reasons, but a decent social life should not be top of our list. Mental health attracts an extremely wide range of professions and personalities, and it is unrealistic to expect to get on with all of them all of the time; however, attention to the way we relate to all of our colleagues is always rewarded. Of course, much of the way we act towards others relates immutably to our own personality, but much besides remains under our control.

Pay careful attention early on to the standards that you demand from junior medical staff. Decades of under-resourcing have overstretched the workload of many senior house officer posts, especially on in-patient units. As a junior consultant, it is tempting to allow for this by lowering your expectations. Instead, work to raise resources rather than lower standards.

Supervising juniors is another source of discomfort for some. Lack of familiarity with a post can create the illusion that we really know little more than an experienced senior house officer and that our senior status is somehow as yet unjustified. The wisdom gap with specialist registrars is, of course, even narrower. Fortunately, the rules do not allow us to train such colleagues until we have worked for a year or two.

Aside from the fact that your own secretary is a form of minor deity, treat all administrative staff like royalty. Although much of what they do may seem so uneventful as to be taken for granted by many, their memories are a precious repository of data that can transform your working life. If you think a piece of administrative work has been well done, or made a particular difference, say so. Wherever you see excellence, it is your responsibility as a consultant to nourish it.

Identify and pay special respect to those who have been around for much longer than you. Take time to identify their likes and dislikes. Machiavellian perhaps, but if you want a permit for that new parking zone outside your office, it helps to be on good terms with the person who fills out the application forms.

Similarly, cultivate relations with your local managers. Try to think of the key issues in your service from their point of view and work out what lines of compromise might be reasonable in the event of conflict. Most importantly, in these litigious, risk-averse times, read and reread your local 'untoward incident' protocols and discuss them with your managers before, rather than after, your first near miss. Try to build storm-proof bridges with management before it starts to rain. Most management work is effectively invisible when it is done well.

Of all the managerial staff worth getting to know, none is as important as the chief executive of your trust. It is a good idea to pay him or her a visit a month or two after you have settled into the job. When you go, do not take along a particular agenda. Have a few points to talk about, certainly, but try to make 'getting to know each other' the primary purpose of the meeting. Surprisingly, few consultants actually do this. Your chief executive will certainly remember you and will usually welcome the meeting as a chance to pick up news from the front line. When the brown stuff hits the fan during a tricky case in the years to come, that visit can prove very useful indeed.

As a junior consultant, you should also consider the way that you relate to your colleagues for reasons beyond duty, common sense and human civility. Your transition from specialist registrar to consultant brings with it an ineluctable progression to a leadership role, for which no amount of training can truly prepare you. People will look to you for certainty and clarity in the face of the inexplicable and will make demands – some of them unreasonable – unaware that you are simultaneously dealing with many similar requests from other quarters. Few jugglers begin their practice with five balls, standing on a log, but this is roughly what it feels like in the early years of your consultancy. Of course, each of us deals with these first anxious moments differently, but by far the commonest way is inadvertently to look to others around us for reassurance.

Be very careful whom you turn to in these moments. Be no less careful about the way you reveal your discomfort. Some, in a rush to obtain positive affirmation, go to lengths to prove that they are still 'just one of the lads'. Others may inadvertently offer to take on work of others. More cynical colleagues – often those closer to burnout – may exploit this. Take on extra work if you must, but only ever do so if there is more in it for you than a shoulder to lean on. Another urge to resist when things get tough is pouring your heart out to junior staff, especially if this involves criticism of others. The urge to let off steam can sometimes be very strong, particularly when your listener seems sympathetic but, ultimately, such reassurance-seeking behaviour will inhibit your growth as a leader. Leaders must display more strength, confidence or skill (or a combination of all three) than those whom they choose to lead.

The stark truth is that you are no longer one of the lads. The sooner you incorporate this into your working style, the easier it is to survive as a consultant. A valuable way to spend time in the early weeks of the job is to sit in on the clinics or rounds of several more experienced colleagues who are doing broadly similar work to your own. Watch someone whom you respect, as well as someone you do not, and think about what it is that makes them different.

407

There has been an interesting shift in the way our culture views authority. Not long ago, leadership brought with it automatic respect. This respect is nowadays qualified, and rightly so. The emphasis on equality in multidisciplinary teams and 'flat management structures' is a laudable response to the arrogant paternalism of the past, but these shifts have raised new problems, which are acutely felt by junior consultants. One is that the zeitgeist of egalitarianism obscures the undying truth that humans will always need leaders in any tough job; working with mental illness in our culture is about as tough as it gets.

Another problem is the modern tendency to view a leader as a victim of the situation. This is reflected in current talk about burnout, early retirement and other gloomy themes. The job *should* be tough and sometimes thankless. But it should also be enjoyable and it should never be lonely. The shift of consultant work away from the time-honoured familiarity of the hospital base to community teamwork can lead to isolation. An important goal of the early months of the job is to establish a vestigial network to counter this. There are many ways to build such a support system: regular academic, clinical or management meetings, mentoring, peer groups, sharing the occasional breakfast or drink after work, or whatever. Clearly, some are more formal than others, but whatever the method, choose it and use it.

Conflict and confrontation

Another interpersonal challenge concerns conflict. Most of us dislike and avoid confrontation, but the status that comes with consultancy usually obliges us, sooner or later, to impose our will on something that needs to stop, start or change. Asserting yourself in the early years of the post, especially with senior colleagues, can be uncomfortable and is easily mishandled. Successful assertion requires confidence and experience, commodities that are often in short supply early on. In this state, it is easy to make two errors. The first is to confuse the personal with the professional. The second is to act prematurely. The first is an error of emotion; the second is an error of rationality. To put it another way: keep your powder dry and do not shoot until you can see the whites of their eyes.

Many of us mistakenly assume that conflict is an emotional process. It is not. Try to confine the basis of your challenge to purely factual matters and make sure well in advance that your information is high in quality and quantity. It is pointless confronting someone simply because you do not like what they are doing, or when you are basing your argument on only a few instances. If you manage to score against someone who annoys you, then fine, but that must never be your primary objective. Try to amass adequate grounds before making a move. Pay careful attention to your language, too. Successful negotiation is always phrased in verbs and nouns rather than adjectives; be especially careful when putting your assertiveness into writing. Pages of passionate complaint may or may not achieve their aim, but they can be stored easily and used to weaken the objectivity of your argument at a later stage. Angry letters can become hostages to fortune, so do not write them. Instead, cultivate a cool, calm and succinct style, especially for the things you feel strongly about. This is how experienced negotiators get results.

Look after yourself: charity begins at home

Of all the things that require your care and attention from day one, none is as important as your own head. Doctors make lousy patients and it is a curious irony that we spend much of our working day asking about the very things that we ignore in ourselves. The medical profession is renowned for its dark humour, its myths of indefatigability and excessive partying. Pay close attention to the predominant emotional themes of your workaday thinking, and keep a low threshold for the auto-diagnosis of tetchiness and gloom. Irritability in the workplace is almost always abnormal. It is best defined as disagreeing with more than one colleague in any one 24-hour period. Watch your sense of humour – assuming you have one, that is – for signs of drift towards the gallows.

Do not watch only what comes out of your mouth: watch also what goes into it. The early years of consultancy can be a taxing time for the hardiest of souls, and more than a few of us bump up our intake of booze and other substances in the early years. Disconsolation born of fatigue or frustration is an insidious thing, like gas in a coalmine. It can creep up on you subtly, in a way that is often hard to notice. Try to be as honest as you can with yourself about your thoughts and feelings about your work and make sure that you share these thoughts, light or dark, with someone. Your peer group, or mentor, or whoever or whatever, should provide a helpful – and private – yardstick for deciding when enough is enough in these matters. Do not listen just to your peers, listen to what your body tells you. Be honest with yourself about your pattern of sleeping and eating, and if it is even a little out of kilter, ask yourself what you would say to a patient in that situation. Most of us have a musculoskeletal weak point in our bodies that twinges whenever we are overdoing it. If that left eyelid does not stop twitching after a weekend off, then it is time for a holiday.

Holidays, from the occasional well-crafted bunk to the fully declared 3 weeks of annual leave, are an essential part of the job. You will have familiarised yourself with your annual and study leave entitlements in the first days of the job. Make sure you use them; only fools fail to take their full quota. Be careful, too, about what you get up to on holiday. Taking work on holiday is absolutely contraindicated. A good holiday should pass Taub's test: it should require an effort to recall the code for the office door on return to work.

Holidays, however, should not become the only way to recover from the accumulated angst of months on the clinical front line. Pay scrupulous attention to your work/life balance. Think very carefully before taking work home. Of course, psychiatry would not be the fascinating job that it is if we did not carry some aspects of it over into the rest of our lives, but just make sure that there is a rest of your life to bring it home to. Work taken home is less mentally toxic if it differs in some way from day-to-day clinical tasks. Some take the view that coming home with work of any kind is a first step on the road to burnout, and many, looking back over their working lives, often date the start of their consultant life as the point at which they gave up those Serbo-Croat evening classes. Whatever you do, make sure work comes through your front door only when you want it to. Make sure you are ex-directory and, having made sure that the hospital switchboard can always contact you in an emergency, switch off your pager if you are not on call.

Having learnt to monitor yourself and your life for the signs of work-related distress, keep an eye out for the same in your colleagues, senior and junior, especially after near misses and serious incidents. Occasionally, you will spot someone who displays some quiet, early sign of buckling under the weight of it all: a hint of excess irritation, bags under the eyes, a sustained loss of sparkle or the faint whiff of booze on a Monday morning. No matter how tired you are, be good to them. Listen to them. Young consultant or old, it is your job to help them if you can.

Conclusion

The entirety of this chapter has tried to emphasise how successful adjustment to a consultant lifestyle lies in setting out the skeleton of a balanced working life early on. Strive to keep this skeleton bare at first. You will definitely put on the flesh as the years go by. A well-kept diary, well-honed connections with the key players around you and a firm grip on the flow of data into and out of your head should allow you to read the road ahead, long term and short. But, above all, do not go in search of work. Let it find you, as it surely will. What truly separates the tyro from the veteran is the knowledge that time and nature are the greatest allies a doctor will ever have. Until you learn this for yourself, make sure you hit the ground walking.

CHAPTER 35

How to work with the media – and survive

David S. Baldwin

Working with the media – a range of opportunities

Misunderstandings about the nature of mental disorder, its origins and consequences, its prevention and treatment are widespread among our patients, their carers, our colleagues and broader society. Reducing ignorance about psychiatric illness and tackling unhelpful attitudes towards those with mental health problems are important parts of the workload of all psychiatrists.

The External Affairs Department of the Royal College of Psychiatrists actively engages with all forms of the national media, and utilises the goodwill of health professionals and patient organisations in its liaisons with the media in efforts designed to improve the plight of those with mental health problems and those who care for them, and to reduce the stigma that is still so damagingly associated with most forms of mental disorder. This is achieved: through the identification of public education officers and media spokespersons with detailed knowledge about particular mental health problems; through the activities of the Public Education Committee, including the publication of books and fact-sheets; and through a series of public education initiatives, such as the 'Partners in Care' campaign.

Of course, many other organisations are also concerned to confront stigma and to provide accurate information to the media about the nature of mental health problems and their treatment. For those interested in improving public understanding of psychiatric illness, the College has the experience and resources needed to optimise the impact of your activity, but many psychiatrists might wish to undertake this role away from the centre, working in collaboration with university or trust press offices and local patient support groups.

A personal statement

My working relationship with the national media started in January 1992 and ended 10 years later. At first, by working with colleagues in the management committee of the 'Defeat Depression' campaign, I strove enthusiastically to engage a multitude of national, regional and local radio and newspaper journalists, hoping to convey its public education messages. With time, some of us became frustrated by the cynical attitudes of many journalists, and disappointed by the often partisan and superficial coverage of the important aims and activities of this 5-year initiative. Putting creeping personal misgivings to one side, I continued to participate in media events organised by the Public Education Committee, and feel proud of most of the activities we undertook, in particular the continuing expansion of the College 'Help is at Hand' booklets and the development of the series of patient fact-sheets about various aspects of psychiatric practice.

After 10 years I thought it preferable to stand down from these College roles. Journalists still occasionally telephone or email with queries relating to anxiety and depression and their treatment, but I stress to them that I do not formally represent any particular institution when providing answers. I also hope that, soon, public education initiatives will be just that: aimed directly at an increasingly sophisticated public – patients, potential patients, carers – through multi-layered web-based information and other resources, without the involvement of interposed media, spinning their way from mental health 'issues' to their next 'story'. This is my background and current viewpoint: the following paragraphs summarise thoughts based on my experience, which is, I hope, neither too idiosyncratic nor too distant to be of at least some use to others.

Why do it?

A simple question. We all want to do our bit to increase public understanding and reduce stigma, but there is a world of difference between undertaking these roles within the setting of clinical practice and attempting to address these matters through liaison with local, regional and national media. Take time to reflect on whether you have the necessary clinical expertise and communication skills, as well as the time and personal resources to undertake an additional role in public education. Consider how other aspects of your workload might be affected, and imagine the sentiments that might be aroused in you through being misquoted or ridiculed in the media, with little opportunity for redress.

The problem, of course, is that if you are talented in liaising with the media your name will become known, resulting in progressively more calls to your office. Speaking with journalists can at first be rather exciting, compared with the often humdrum nature of some aspects of your work, and potentially reinforcing. On the other hand, it might become easier for a journalist to contact you than to seek out the opinion of others with potentially greater knowledge, which is to the detriment of all concerned: you can acquire the reputation of being a 'rent-a-quote' doctor, the scientific accuracy of the story might be compromised and the target audience could be misinformed. This damages the reputation of you and the journalist, and may have unfortunate consequences for patients.

What is your area of expertise?

The next step, therefore, is to define and limit your area of expertise. Desperate journalists sometimes cast around for anyone available to comment on a particular news item, but most want the opinion of someone familiar with the subject area, able to place study findings, policy initiatives or emerging controversies within the context of clinical practice. It is clearly foolish to make yourself available to comment on a story relating to Alzheimer's disease when you work as a child psychiatrist and have not seen a patient with a dementing illness for over 20 years. Defining the boundaries of your expertise can be difficult, however. For example, you may feel tempted to answer a query relating to a particular new pharmacological treatment, but if your clinical practice is predominantly psychotherapeutic, it would be hard to place the relative benefits and drawbacks of this drug in the correct context.

Think about the clinical situations in which your colleagues come to you for advice, as it is in these areas that you are considered an expert. Avoid taking on media activities outside your area of expertise and feel confident in being able to state that probing questions need to be addressed elsewhere, if you begin to feel you that you are straying into unfamiliar territory.

Do you need to undergo media training?

With a reasonable degree of self-awareness, you should know whether you can communicate clearly and effectively. Problems in these areas should have been addressed at medical school and during your training as a psychiatrist. Reflect on whether you have the ability to make simple, accurate and interesting statements, delivered in a way likely to engage an audience. If you have no problems in this area, there is no need for media training. But attendance at a brief course can be most instructive, in revealing any behavioural peculiarities or verbal idiosyncrasies that may interfere with effective communication. Consider whether you are so perfect that media training is unnecessary. Most people find it surprisingly helpful.

How can you prepare for a media interview?

If you are speaking on behalf of an organisation, you will probably have been told who made the initial contact, the nature of the enquiry, the format for the interview and whether others are also involved; you may have already been provided with a press briefing and a summary of relevant facts and figures. Most journalists work to tight deadlines and often hold unrealistic expectations of having almost immediate access to nominated spokespersons, but it is essential to have at least some time to prepare for an interview.

Think about what you would like to say and how you intend to say it, and what might follow. Identify the key message and think about its relevance to the audience. Anticipate potential questions and prepare your answers. Consider whether it might be helpful for the journalist to have some written material to read before the interview, such as the abstract of the scientific paper when describing research findings, or a public education leaflet when discussing a particular medical condition.

Do you have a conflict of interests?

It is commonplace to preface presentations in scientific meetings with a disclosure regarding sources of funding and press releases relating to research findings typically list sources of financial support. These explicit statements acknowledge the often considerable investment from the funding agency and can enhance the appraisal of scientific information. At present, such declarations usually relate to research support from the pharmaceutical industry, but most who work in professional positions will have potential conflicts of interest, through allegiances or hostilities to particular groups or organisations, that may influence judgements or actions excessively.

Think about your position, roles and responsibilities, and how these could affect any comments you might make on emerging stories. Sources of potential conflict may not be immediately apparent. For example, it may be tempting to comment adversely on the effect of certain mental health services on clinical outcomes when you have been arguing forcefully for a different pattern of resource distribution. Remember that you are a clinician, that your first concern should be to improve health, and that unacknowledged conflicts may mislead colleagues or prejudice patient welfare. Consider whether you should preface your comments with a statement of interests. In general, it is sensible to declare anything that might cause embarrassment if currently undeclared but revealed in the future. Write down what you declared, for your records.

How is a press briefing organised?

Busy clinicians do not have the time or expertise to mount what can be a complex and nail-biting media operation: this task is normally undertaken by the parent institution (e.g. the College, a university press office or an interposed public relations or communications company). Typically, the date of a briefing will be chosen to avoid similar news events and the timing selected to ensure the maximum potential for press coverage. Journalists will have been lured to the meeting by the promise of individual discussions with key opinion leaders, so it is important to ensure you are able to remain at the venue for a while after the initial presentations are complete, to avoid disappointing them.

It is often helpful to rehearse the presentations before the meeting, but it is important that the final presentations are delivered in a fairly spontaneous and flexible way. The chair will identify each speaker in turn; will refer the attending journalists to the written material (the press release); and will encourage each speaker to talk for only a few minutes, to allow plenty of time for questions. The chair will ensure that any patient representative is treated courteously and sympathetically, and that questions are not monopolised by a specific journalist.

It is sensible to record the proceedings, to verify what was said should there be inaccurate or misleading coverage in the aftermath of the meeting.

How should you conduct yourself during the interview?

Be certain that the journalist knows your name and affiliation, and whether you are speaking on behalf of an organisation such as the College or whether you are giving only your personal views. Ensure that you will not be interrupted and do not be tempted to undertake another activity (such as reading your emails) during the course of a telephone interview. When speaking, remember that you are the expert, not the journalist, and do not let yourself be interrupted or intimidated. Keep the message simple, verifiable and, wherever possible, relevant to clinical practice. Do not be tempted to digress into areas that were not specified in advance of the interview and be sure to avoid rampant speculation.

While most journalists strive to ensure the coverage of a story is balanced and accurate, newsworthy and a good read, some have an agenda that is completely at odds with yours. Do not take this personally. Correct any stated untruths (it is perfectly acceptable to use phrases such as 'I'm afraid that is quite wrong: the real situation is…') but otherwise restrict the discussion to what you had intended to say and ensure this is reported accurately. No prizes are given for repeated attempts to give a balanced account when a journalist is interested in giving only one side of a story. Accept this: there will be other opportunities to convey the message more sympathetically, elsewhere.

Should you comment on individual cases?

No. The Royal College of Psychiatrists believes it is unethical for a psychiatrist to offer a professional opinion unless he or she has conducted an examination and has been granted proper authorisation for such a statement, and other organisations, such as the American Psychiatric Association, have given similar advice. It may be tempting to speculate on the psychological motivations of celebrities caught in the glare of publicity, but without personal knowledge of the person or his or her permission this is highly inadvisable, and could prove damaging to you and to the profession. The most you might do is to make a general statement about the behaviour being discussed and to stress that it would be unprofessional to comment on other aspects of the case.

Most dealings with the press relate to less-sensational matters. Professional bodies usually maintain a list of former or current patients who are prepared to speak to the media about their experience of illness; and journalists will often accompany an otherwise rather dry account of research findings or health service changes with an illustrative personal interest story. If you feel the effect of a news item might be increased through illustration with a relevant clinical case, keep the account simple and ensure the patient is not identifiable.

What happens if you are misquoted?

You should be expected to be misquoted, occasionally. Adequate preparation before an interview and clarification of any uncertainty during the discussion will reduce this chance, but factual errors can creep into most articles, given the need to keep them brief and punchy. One strategy is to ask journalists to send you a draft version of any material they intend to print for your approval, but looming deadlines and the desire for press freedom make many reluctant to agree to this request. Should you discover that some aspects of a report are incorrect, pause to reflect on whether this inaccuracy is inadvertent, and if so whether it adversely affects the tenor or importance of an otherwise helpful article. Keep a record of what you said, and what appeared, and note the differences. If you feel that you have been deliberately misrepresented, it may be worth contacting the editor of the newspaper to arrange a prompt 'correction', but any delay in expressing your concern substantially reduces the chance of such a piece being printed. Console yourself with the memory of all the other times when liaison with the media went well, and rest assured that the opinions of your colleagues will not be swayed by partisan and antagonistic news reports.

Should you do live interviews?

The audiences for many radio and television programmes far outstrip the circulation of even national newspapers and if the message is important it should be addressed to as many people as possible. But particular care is needed when preparing for live interviews: establish who will be interviewing you, the questions they would like to raise, the duration of the transmission, and who else is being asked to comment on the story. It is rare to be given the chance to speak to the interviewer before 'going live' but editorial staff should provide this information and may even let you know the gist of the first question you are likely to receive. Make yourself familiar with the news events of the day, as an interviewer may well seek to place a topical spin on an otherwise dull press release.

During the interview, do not be disappointed if the questions seem rather elementary, but take the opportunity to make simple statements of broad relevance to the audience. When asked detailed questions on specific problems, reply in kind but try to place your comments in a broader context, as most of the audience will not be interested in endless discussion of minor points. Be certain when the interview has ended: do not make statements 'off the record', as programmers may find it hard to resist the temptation to broadcast contentious comments.

How should you appear on television?

Before a television appearance, most experience some anxiety about what to wear. Communication companies offer much advice about how to dress for television interviews. The most important considerations are: to dress smartly but not too flashily; to avoid checks and stripes, as these 'fuzz' distractingly on the screen; and to remember that you may perspire a lot in the studio environment. Men should shave to avoid the impression famously conveyed by Richard Nixon, and should expect that any shiny foreheads will be powdered; women will be made-up in a fashion considered rather scary in other environments. Do not have a drink before the interview 'to steady the nerves': an inebriated psychiatrist is not a good advertisement for the profession. During the interview, look at the presenter, rather than the camera; sit back in your chair; smile when appropriate; and remain courteous and polite, despite hostile questioning.

This all seems quite alarming – is it worth it?

Working with the media has its irritations and carries some potential hazards. Most of these will be avoided by remembering you are a clinician, not a celebrity. The most tiresome aspect of media liaison is being asked the same question repeatedly, by journalists who have clearly not bothered to read a press briefing, only to find your efforts sidelined in an article driven by another agenda. Excessive cynicism about the media is not conducive to the effective delivery of the message, so if ennui starts to characterise your dealings with journalists, it is time to stop.

Do not undertake public education activity in the hope of raising your personal profile, for that would represent a waste of resources and a perversion of its aims. Think about the bigger picture. The greatest reward for your efforts should be to read a sympathetic account of the plight of those with mental disorder, in which the good efforts of mental health professionals have resulted in substantial and sustained improvements for their patients; and to learn some time later that it was articles such as this which encouraged others with the same condition to seek psychiatric help, having avoided doing so for years.

CHAPTER 36

Consultant mentoring and mentoring consultants

Bryan Stoten

It appears to be unusual that, at a time when the evidence base for clinical practice has never been so eagerly sought within the National Health Service (NHS), a process of continuing professional development has emerged which seems to be not susceptible to measurement and to be subject to a wide variety of definitions.

The concept of 'mentoring' has been interpreted across a continuum from the remedial or therapeutic intervention to 'buddying' and the entirely informal. Specific benefits are hard to identify within the available literature. However, Rodenhauser *et al* (2000) refer as follows to the kind of outcomes that can be obtained from the process:

'guidance with socialisation into the profession, assistance with stresses along the way, help with the choice and fulfilment of a career path and inspiration for meaningful involvement in activities such as research and administration.'

However difficult it is to measure in a quantifiable way the benefits of mentoring, there has emerged, over the past decade, a consensus among the healthcare community that mentoring schemes do add value.

What is mentoring?

The trend in recent years to hold professionals to account for their practice has seen the emergence of a number of management innovations. In the NHS, appraisal schemes, often associated with discretionary awards, have become universal. Similarly, together with appraisal, coaching schemes, mentoring programmes and similar interpersonal development initiatives for hospital doctors have become increasingly common.

A general consensus has emerged around the definition of mentoring produced by the Standing Committee on Postgraduate Medical Education of the British Medical Association (BMA):

'[mentoring is] the process whereby an experienced, highly regarded empathic person (the mentor), guides another individual (the mentee) in the development

419

and re-examination of their own ideas, learning and personal and professional development. The mentor who often, but not necessarily, works in the same organisation or field as the mentee, achieves this by listening and talking in confidence to the mentee' (Oxley, 1998, p. 1).

None the less, and not surprisingly, there are a variety of other definitions, which have more or less congruence with this approach. For example, Roberts *et al* (2002) describe the mentoring phenomenon as:

'the offer of a confidential, professional supportive relationship, by an experienced colleague, able and willing to share his or her knowledge and experience to a protégé or mentee.'

It is interesting that Roberts *et al* introduced the term protégé as equivalent to mentee, having, as it does, a sense 'sponsorship' and even 'preferment'. Although such covert patronage has always played a part in the career development of some successful (and unsuccessful) managers, it may be seen to challenge a fair employment policy. We should be only too aware that mentorship takes a variety of forms and that such forms can range from the specifically remedial and even therapeutic through to the sense of favouritism and privileging of one individual colleague over another as result of acquiring a specific mentor.

Mentoring, then, is clearly susceptible to a number of interpretations and, in consequence, a variety of attitudes have emerged regarding the appropriateness of mentoring in organisations and the kinds of relationships it is appropriate to address through a mentoring scheme.

The Royal College of Obstetricians and Gynaecologists (2005) answer the question 'Who needs a mentor?' with the response 'every obstetrician and gynaecologist throughout training and career'. The variety of situations in which mentoring is seen to be valuable by the College includes: career change, appointment to a consultant post, returning to practice after absence, returning following sickness or maternity leave, during or after suspension or exclusion, and generally at times of personal development and stress. Clearly, each of those situations requires a rather different mentoring relationship and presents the mentor with very different challenges and expectations. None the less, it accords with the BMA's general advice that 'mentoring should be encouraged at all levels throughout one's medical career' (British Medical Association, 2004).

Who should do it?

There is surprisingly little discussion in the literature about the characteristics of mentors and, consequently, little consideration has been given to their training needs. Perhaps the most common approach is that of the Royal College of Obstetricians and Gynaecologists (2005), which specifies the following characteristics of a good mentor:

- a good listener
- respected as a professional
- approachable and accessible
- non-judgemental
- enthusiastic, encouraging
- wise, experienced
- challenges but not destructively
- ethical, honest and trustworthy
- good interpersonal and communication skills.

More specifically, Gupta & Lingam (2000) stress the importance of giving mentors good communications training. Clearly too, they point out, mentors will need a specialist understanding of the law relating to medical practice and all mentors in this field will need to have an understanding of the role of the General Medical Council.

There are indications that the training of mentors significantly improves the satisfaction which both mentors and mentees have from the mentoring encounter and, indeed, some evidence that the training of mentees before they enter a mentoring relationship adds even more satisfaction.

An approach based upon personality type theory

Over a period of 4 years an organisation, Health Partnerships, with the guidance of experienced health service managers, clinical leaders and senior business leaders, has offered a training programme specifically for experienced hospital consultants preparing themselves to offer mentoring for newly appointed consultants within their own hospital organisation, though not necessarily within their own discipline. This approach was informed by the experiences identified by Sir Ian Kennedy in his review of the difficulties experienced in Bristol (1998–2001) (Bristol Royal Infirmary Inquiry, 2001).

The approach developed was also responsive to the demands of both the Royal Colleges and the BMA, for, as Jolyon Oxley (2004) points out, the evidence suggests that more informal mentoring arrangements tend to be more successful. However, if such success is to be generalised there need to be some formal structures in place to increase the likelihood that those wishing to have access to a mentor will be able to find one.

The framework for consultant mentoring

The literature contains many references to the idea of 'co-mentoring' and 'non-hierarchic mentoring' as offering a significant variant on the common definitions with which this discussion started. At the heart of a hospital consultant's practice lies the principle of collegiality and peer

421

relationships. Notwithstanding the reality that some consultants will have more experience than others, and hold positions of greater responsibility than others, such hierarchic factors may often be balanced by the sapiential authority of more recently qualified younger colleagues.

Mentoring between fellow consultants, then, must start with an implicit understanding that the mentor–mentee relationship is based on a voluntary desire, on both sides, to improve practice by tapping into the additional experience the mentor has and, often, the familiarity with research and current practice in the given discipline possessed by the newly qualified consultant. More especially, we were most anxious in this initiative to avoid any suggestion that the mentoring relationship involved teaching, counselling, remedial development or therapy. Rather, the purpose was to accelerate the personal and professional development of newly appointed consultants by:

- allowing them to 'embed' into the organisation
- providing support for moments of stress not encountered in a training grade
- offering a sounding board to help the newly appointed deal with the pressures organisations make on neophytes
- bringing to their notice opportunities and developments of which they might otherwise be unaware.

In developing this approach, we were also aware of the general exhortations in the literature that the role of mentors should not be simply to give instructions in the performance of the role. Rather, both the mentor and the mentee will do better in a relationship based on personality type preferences (see Myers, 1995). For example, Freeman (1997) calls for a:

'mentor ... deep enough and brave enough to support both the professional and the personal self of their mentee, not to make false divisions between the two dimensions in order to keep the mentoring relationship comfortable – making the task easier for the mentor but short changing the mentee.'

While we can observe that for some mentors such behaviours will be both natural and easily accomplished, for others this may go against their own personality type. Furthermore, it will certainly be the case that such an ability to move easily between the personal and the professional, while positively sought by some mentees, may appear alarmingly intrusive to others. In consequence, the mentoring training which has been developed has had a central place in it for the notion of personality type and the likely behaviours which an understanding of personality type theory will encourage the mentor to accommodate.

Establishing the ground rules of a mentoring relationship is fundamental to ensuring that the relationship starts off with a reasonable chance of longer-term success. Any successful mentoring relationship must be voluntary (on both sides) and all our examples of such schemes in NHS trusts have adhered to that principle. Furthermore, within the requirements to place patient safety as paramount, the confidentiality of the exchanges between mentor and mentee must be treated as sacrosanct. When it comes, however, to other issues, these are likely to be determined by the personality of the mentor and the mentee. Such issues include:

- the extent to which the mentor feels able to engage with the personal as against professional aspects of the mentee's concerns
- the availability of the mentor to the mentee
- the context within which the mentoring relationship is conducted
- discussion of the mentor's wider social ambience in the mentoring relationship.

The Myers–Briggs Type Inventory

The success of mentoring relationships which involve extensive extramural socialisation, engagement with the participants' families and the choosing of informal settings within which the mentoring relationship can take place appears self-evident to some commentators and yet is clearly dependent on the personality type preferences of the individuals involved. The Myers–Briggs Type Inventory (MBTI) was chosen as a means of legitimating differences in mentoring styles and relationships and as a tool for exploring the different demands which mentors and mentees can place upon the relationship as it develops.

The MBTI is widely used throughout the NHS and, indeed, some organisations routinely offer it to their clinical staff as part of a wider development programme. The MBTI offers four dimensions:

1 *Introversion/extraversion preference.* This dimension reflects the extent to which one engages with the world 'out there' or the world in one's head. Extraverts may accord with the popular use of the term and introverts appear aloof, but the dimension enables access to more subtle aspects of this dichotomy. An extrovert mentor may feel an introvert mentee is unenthusiastic and reluctant to engage with or even to approach the mentor except when scheduled, while introvert mentors may find extrovert mentees demanding and intrusive.

2 *Sensing/intuiting preference.* This dichotomy identifies the way in which information is obtained about the world through the five senses or through that additional or intuitive sixth sense. Mentees with a sensing preference will seek factual information and precision, and live in the 'here and now'. Those with an intuitive preference will be much more interested in exploring the possibilities of the situation rather than the actuality. Mismatching mentor and mentee may lead either to too much 'blue sky thinking' or to too much unchallenged acceptance of the world as it is rather than an exploration of the developmental possibilities. However, mentors with a sensing preference may have difficulty in relating to the intuitive mentee who is focused on future

possibilities rather than the practicalities of the present, while a mentee with a sensing preference may find an intuitive mentor too non-specific about actual dilemmas and practical information to be worth taking seriously. At least an understanding of such differences may make it easier, especially with some humour, to gain benefit from complementary or differing preferences between mentor and mentee.

3   *Thinking/feeling preference.* This dimension reflects how one makes decisions about the world. Identification of this preference in oneself really does require considerable self-awareness. People with a different preference will make different crucial decisions about their work and professional development. The thinking/feeling dichotomy may be of particular importance in determining whether or not a mentor and mentee can form a productive relationship. The critical, analytical mode of thinking exhibited by those with a thinking preference can seem harsh and unappreciative to mentors with a feeling preference, while mentors with a thinking preference may be uncomfortable with the amount of personal exposure which a mentee with a feeling preference may wish to offer in the mentoring relationship. Particularly where discussion of the relationships developed by the mentee may form a crucial part of the mentee's early induction into the professional role and practice, a mentor with a thinking preference may seem unhelpful and lacking in the kind of insights necessary to the process. Conversely, a mentor with a feeling preference may, if able to establish good rapport with a mentee with a thinking preference, help enormously to develop the interpersonal skills to which the thinking preference will initially give little priority.

4   *Judging/perceiving preference.* Finally, the extent to which one wishes to feel in control of one's world is a function of the judging or perceiving preference. People with a judging preference will seek an ordered, predictable process, lacking in ambiguities and uncertainty, whereas perceiving types are much more prepared to 'go with the flow'. A mentee of the perceiving type may seem to a mentor, especially one with a judging preference, as possibly more lackadaisical and uninvolved in the relationship, failing to observe a clearly scheduled process of meetings with any ordered agenda or specific purpose. Indeed, Grainger (2002) argues that 'the key to choosing a mentor is first deciding what you want to achieve and whether mentoring is the most appropriate way to achieve it'. In reality, for perceiving types, no such clarity is likely to occur when embarking on the mentoring relationship, while for judging types it is key. For those with a perceiving preference, the goals and purpose are likely to emerge over time and be 'retro-fitted' to their circumstances rather than provide the framework for their future professional development. None the less, a mentoring relationship between two consultants with a perceiving preference may well flounder, because it has no particular direction.

It is circumstances like these which encourage us to recommend the use of the GROW framework (see below), which, while being of less immediate attraction to perceiving types, does at least enforce a framework which is purposeful and directed.

Using the MBTI

The MBTI is capable of affording complex and subtle appreciation of individual and group interactions. Mentoring training for hospital consultants, however, is unlikely to allow sophisticated development of these insights. None the less, by making consultants aware of the broad parameters of the taxonomy and the four key dimensions, it becomes possible to offer two key insights:

1   A failure to establish an appropriate 'chemistry' between mentor and mentee becomes easier to handle and removes 'blame' from the decision to withdraw from the mentoring relationship.
2   Understanding something of the characteristics of one or other of the eight preferences gives more experienced mentors a better understanding both of how their own preferences can be used positively and of how the mentee's preferences may need to be accommodated in order to obtain the best from the relationship. We are struck again and again by the enthusiasm with which hospital consultants fall upon the MBTI taxonomy to inform not merely their approach to mentoring but also their interpersonal behaviours more generally.

Active listening

The well-worn aphorism that 'God gave us two ears and one mouth, but they are rarely used in those proportions' is especially relevant when observing the training of mentors. For many potential mentors, active listening is the most difficult skill to acquire. This will be especially true of mentors who are:

- introverts (preoccupied with their own thoughts and priorities)
- intuitives (living in the 'there and then' rather than the 'here and now')
- thinking types (constantly analytical and critical).

For them, the likelihood of suspending their own thought processes until sufficient information has been derived from a mentee is diminished.

Setting off with the best of intentions, the active listener is sidetracked again and again by:

- looking for congruence in what is heard with their own values
- testing the content of what is heard against their own empirical observations

425

- constructing their response and advice
- completing the mentee's thought processes by anticipating what will be said next
- developing an awareness of stimuli from outside the setting
- succumbing to the distraction of a busy agenda and time diary.

Yet having the undivided attention of another is both startlingly motivational and enhances the self-esteem felt by the recipient of such attention. Successful politicians understand this and elicit frequently the response 'he seemed completely focused on what I was saying'. Whether merely a technique or genuine passion, such active listening is enormously empowering for the mentee. None the less, in practical sessions in which such active listening is modelled, we find the greatest difficulty expressed by most participants in not succumbing to the interruptions, distractions and interjections mentors employ to break up their periods of listening. Perhaps for clinicians it is especially difficult to be non-directive, withholding guidance and advice and, rather, encouraging self-expression and exploration. Trained to take a medical history in as time-efficient and ordered a way as possible, it may be that such socialisation hampers a listening mode which is less controlling and directional.

Encouraging practical exercises which look for meaning, not merely in the content of the words but through expression and body language, does appear to increase the ability of mentors in training to encourage mentees to say what they want to say, not what their mentor appears to want to know.

The GROW model

The combination of clinical experience, organisational maturity, some insight into the behavioural differences of different personality types and a restraint on the natural clinical urge to advise and prescribe may all contribute to establishing some rapport and mutual confidence in the coming together of mentor and mentee. However, if mentoring is to be purposeful, a basic framework for development seems to be helpful. Milestones in the mentoring process usually help and the GROW model – goal, reality, options and will – creates a shared process which enables both mentor and mentee to 'keep on track'.

Goal

Establishing what the mentoring session is to focus on – however broadly – gives purpose and direction. Answering the question 'What would you like to get from this session?', particularly if asked a day or two in advance, places the responsibility for the direction which the mentoring relationship takes firmly in the hands of the mentee – where it should be!

Reality

Establishing the 'facts' as they are allows for some ground clearing in the earlier period of the mentoring relationship and establishes the differences between the mentee's perceptions, feelings, goals and aspirations, and the perceived constraints, problems and opportunities, which can be empirically tested.

Options

Options – courses of action – are best when they are the product of the mentee's intelligence rather than the mentor's experience. The mentor's job is to facilitate the sifting of wheat from chaff, the quantification of subjective judgements ('Would that be twice as difficult, three times as difficult, no more difficult?') and the mentor has licence to go on asking the crucial question 'And what else could you do?' beyond the point when the mentee might reasonably cease enquiry.

Will

Finally, no mentoring session should end without testing what it is that the mentee intends to do afterwards. If the mentoring process is to be purposeful and the mentoring relationship is to flourish, then a key part of the process must be testing the preparedness or 'will' of the mentee to take something of the mentoring encounter into his or her professional life. In general, we discourage note-taking during mentoring – at least by the mentor – but when testing the preparedness to act positively following the mentoring session, a single line which records 'the next step' reinforces the importance of the session and provides a starting point for the next one.

Conclusion

Mentoring opportunities abound within the NHS. The accelerated rate at which junior hospital doctors can now expect to pass through their training grades into a consultancy post, together with the increasing managerial complexity which intrudes on clinical practice, means mentoring by the experienced 'grey heads' in the profession is endorsed by all the professional bodies.

It is appropriate to issue warnings: mentoring as a rehabilitative or remedial activity will bring the process into disrepute. Mandatory mentoring schemes not merely fall foul of BMA guidelines but will simply reduce some schemes to a tick-box routine. Schemes which offer maximum choice to mentees and encourage the emergence of informal mentoring arrangements will be more successful than those which simply allocate mentor to mentee.

Schemes in which mentors are first trained and schemes where both mentors *and* mentees are trained before they enter the mentoring relationship will have more success. Peer mentoring and non-hierarchical mentoring – as with consultant mentoring schemes – will have higher satisfaction levels than schemes which encourage the mentoring of trainees by faculty members and senior staff.

Roberts *et al* (2002) observe:

'the progressive dispersal of consultant psychiatrists in multidisciplinary, locality based teams, has simultaneously been accompanied by relative isolation from their peers.… Nearly 70% of consultants attending our study days on mentorship stated that they no longer have time for coffee or lunch with their colleagues owing to work pressures – times when "continuing professional development" occurred naturally.'

Such is the pressure in the NHS generally now, and the target culture so all pervasive, that this description of the situation in psychiatry might be applied across many more disciplines in medicine. Never before has it been so important that newly appointed consultants be offered a supportive framework for their professional development as a matter of course and good management practice throughout the NHS.

References

Bristol Royal Infirmary Inquiry (2001) *Learning from Bristol: The Report of the Public Inquiry (October 1998–July 2001) into Children's Heart Surgery at the Bristol Royal Infirmary 1987–1995* (CM 5207). TSO (The Stationery Office).

British Medical Association (2004) *Exploring Mentoring*. British Medical Association.

Freeman R. (1997) Toward effective mentoring in general practice. *British Journal of General Practice*, **47**, 457–460.

Grainger, C. (2002) Mentoring – supporting doctors at work and play. *BMJ*, **324**, S203.

Gupta, R. C. & Lingam, S. (2000) *Mentoring for Doctors and Dentists*. Blackwell Science.

Myers, I. (1995) *Gifts Differing*. Davies-Black.

Oxley, J. (ed.) (1998) *Supporting Doctors and Dentists at Work: An Enquiry into Mentoring*. Scopme.

Oxley, J. (2004) Mentoring for doctors. *BMJ Career Focus*, **328**, 179.

Roberts, G., Moore, B. & Coles, C. (2002) Mentoring for newly appointed psychiatrists. *Psychiatric Bulletin*, **26**, 106–109.

Rodenhauser, P., Rudishill, J. R. & Devorak, R. (2000) Skills for mentors. *Academic Psychiatry*, **24**, 14–27.

Royal College of Obstetricians and Gynaecologists (2005) *Mentoring for All*. Royal College of Obstetricians and Gynaecologists.

Index

Compiled by Caroline Sheard

personality disorder, policy and guidelines 124
PFI 22–3, 32, 83–4
pharmacists 96
PMETB 24–5, 90, 129, 238
Poor Law 1834 3
poor performance, dealing with 291–302, 364–5
population estimates 69–70
postcode lottery 73
Postgraduate Medical Education and Training Board 24–5, 90, 129, 238
potential, maximisation of 360–2
PPI forums 209, 223
PPPs 23
practice-based commissioning 70, 73–4
prescriptions, electronic transfer 376–7
presentations 338–9
  and anxiety 343–5
  delivery 342–5
  learning models 341–2
  planning 340–2
  preparation 339–40
  visual aids 342
press briefings 414–15
primary care groups 19
primary care trusts (PCTs) 22, 32, 34–5, 36, 74
  National Service Framework for Mental Health 61
  resource allocation by 72–4
  resource allocation to 69–71
PRiSM Psychosis Study 273–4
Private Finance Initiative 22–3, 32, 83–4
probity and revalidation 244
process net 175
processes
  bottlenecks 178–9
  mapping 173–7, 316
  matching demand and capacity 179–83
  pathology of 178–83
  redesign 177–8
  re-engineering 177
productivity in healthcare 79–80
professions 48–9
psychiatrists
  core attributes 284
  international recruitment 94–5
  professional standards 243–4, 284
  recruitment and retention 380–1
  and stress 384
psychotherapy, internet 370
public bodies, disclosure of patient information to 254–7
public education, involvement in 411–18

Public Guardian 169
Public Health Act 1848 4
public–private partnerships 23

quality
  development of concept in the NHS 205–6
  improvement tools 313–23
  NHS Quality Improvement Scotland 136–7, 208
  role of medical director 41
  see also clinical governance
quality cycle 177–8

Raising the Standard 150
RAWP 13
RCA, complaints 234–5
recertification 287
record of in-training assessment 89
references, preparation of 300
Reforming the NHS Complaints Procedure: A Listening Document 223
registration 245
research and development, resource allocation to 71
Research and Development Directorate 71
Resource Allocation Working Party 13
resources 28–30, 68–9
  accounting for 82–4
  allocation by PCTs 72
  changes in allocation by PCTs following 'system reform' 72–9
  distribution 69–72
  and foundation trusts 80–2
  management in the current environment 36–7
  for mental health services 84–5
  and post-1997 NHS development 30–6
Rethink 263
retirement 95
revalidation 42, 238–9, 283
  and appraisal 240–2, 286
  and good medical practice 242–4
  and registration 245
risk
  and disclosure of patient information 254–7
  forums 388
RITA 89
role modelling and leadership 195
root cause analysis, complaints 234–5
Royal College of Physicians 3
Royal College of Psychiatrists
  and continuing professional development 243–4